Laparoscopic Surgery:
The implications of changing practice

Current Surgical Practice Volume 8

Laparoscopic Surgery:
The implications of changing practice

Current Surgical Practice Volume 8

Edited on behalf of the
Royal College of Surgeons of England by

Michael Hobsley, TD DSc PhD MChir FRCS
Emeritus Professor of Surgery, University College
and London Medical School, London, UK

Tom Treasure, MD MS FRCS
Professor of Cardiothoracic Surgery, St George's Hospital,
London, UK

and

John M.A. Northover, MS FRCS
Consultant Surgeon, ICRF Colorectal Cancer Unit, St Mark's Hospital,
Northwick Park, Middlesex, UK

with a Foreword by
Sir Rodney Sweetnam, KCVO CBE PRCS
President of the Royal College of Surgeons of England

A member of the Hodder Headline Group
LONDON • SYDNEY • AUCKLAND
Co-published in the USA by
Oxford University Press, Inc., New York

First published in Great Britain 1998 by
Arnold, a member of the Hodder Headline Group,
338 Euston Road, London NW1 3BH

Co-published in the United States of America by
Oxford University Press, Inc.,
198 Madison Avenue, New York, NY10016
Oxford is a registered trademark of Oxford University Press

British Library Cataloguing in Publication Data
A catalogue record for this book is available from the British Library

Library of Congress Cataloging-in-Publication Data
A catalog record for this book is available from the Library of Congress

ISBN 0 340 60760 2

Publisher: Annalisa Page
Project Manager: Robert Chaundy
Production Editor: James Rabson
Production Controller: Sarah Kett
Cover Designer: Julie Delf

Typeset in 10/11 Century Old Style by
J&L Composition Ltd, Filey, North Yorkshire
Printed and bound in Great Britain by
St Edmundsbury Press, Bury St Edmunds, Suffolk and Bookcraft Ltd, Bath.

Contents

SECTION III: SURGICAL APPLICATIONS OF LAPAROSCOPY

SECTION IV: OTHER CONSIDERATIONS

Foreword

This volume marks a departure from usual practice in this series. This time, instead of up-to-date accounts across the broad field of surgery, Michael Hobsley, Tom Treasure and John Northover have compiled and edited an edition entirely confined to laparoscopic surgery for general surgeons.

Ten years ago, in Volume 4, it was predicted that 'Peritoneoscopic surgery may herald a new era in abdominal surgery in the next few decades'. Wisely, it was added a little later that 'There is a very real danger of carrying the procedure beyond its limitations, thus surely bringing it into disrepute'. The final advice was that clinicians 'should temper wizardry with wisdom, enthusiasm with equilibrium'.

This volume, with contributions by a host of experts, does, I believe, temper enthusiasm with equilibrium. Laparoscopic surgery, just like arthroscopic surgery earlier, has now won its spurs; it is here to stay. The authors present a balanced view of the present position, and stress the importance of controlled trials and audit, measured whenever possible against accepted benchmarks. Training is all important, and I am pleased that the Royal College of Surgeons of England, with the generous support of the Wolfson Foundation and the Department of Health, have, with their sister Surgical Colleges, taken the lead. Once again, we owe a debt of gratitude to the editors and authors. Their wisdom in devoting the whole of this volume to this important and rapidly developing area of surgery is self-evident.

Sir Rodney Sweetnam
President, Royal College of Surgeons of England
August 1997

Preface

Previous volumes in this series have been dedicated to covering growing points across the whole field of surgery and have been based to a considerable extent on lectures that have been given at the Royal College of Surgeons of England. The result has been that each book has helped candidates for the old Final Fellowship examination by drawing to their attention areas of current interest which might well be expected to be in the minds of their examiners and therefore in the subject matter of the examinations.

Changes in graduate surgical training introduced by the Royal Colleges have resulted in a new examination structure. The main examination in the generality of surgery is taken at an earlier stage and is more fundamental in its approach. There is a greater emphasis on the basic principles including the scientific infrastructure of surgery and less on the complicated details of surgical operations. Such details, together with the minutiae of surgical management in specialist fields, are reserved for the new final test. This new assessment is not made until the second or third year of specialist training, and is designed separately for each of the surgical sub-specialities.

We have therefore decided, at least for the present volume, to alter the plan of *Current Surgical Practice* so that the book becomes an exposition in depth of a particular field of surgery in which progress has recently been made. We anticipate that the book will therefore be most relevant to a particular group of aspiring surgeons. Nevertheless, since it represents the acme of knowledge and skill in its area, we expect that many qualified surgeons will find the volume a useful way of keeping abreast of the latest advances.

The definition of a field of interest is not necessarily made in terms of anatomy, physiology or pathology. The present volume is indeed an example of the fact that technique might be a foundation for a volume: in this case, we concentrate on laparoscopic surgery, a subject of wide interest to the surgical profession.

Unfortunately, Professor Alan Johnson has found it necessary to step down from joint editorship of the series. TT and MH greatly regret this but accept Professor Johnson's departure in the light of the increased responsibilities that he has taken on elsewhere. TT and MH have great pleasure in welcoming John Northover to replace him as one of the three general editors.

Michael Hobsley
Tom Treasure
John Northover

Contributors

GH Barsoum MD, FRCSEd
Consultant Surgeon, Solihull Hospital, Birmingham, UK (formerly Research Fellow, Department of Colorectal Surgery, Cleveland Clinic Florida, Fort Lauderdale, Florida, USA)

GS Carr-White BSc, MBBS(Hons)
Formerly House Officer, St George's Hospital, London, UK

AS Chilvers MA, MB, MChir, FRCS
Consultant Surgeon, St Helier Hospital Trust, Carshalton, Surrey, UK; Honorary Senior Lecturer, St George's Hospital, London, UK

A Cuschieri MD, ChM, FRCSEng, FRCSEd, FRCSGlas(Hon), FRCSI(Hon)
Professor and Head of Department of Surgery and Surgical Skills Unit, Ninewells Hospital and Medical School, University of Dundee, UK

A Darzi MD, FRCS, FRCSI
Professor of Surgery, Academic Surgical Unit, Imperial College School of Medicine, St Mary's Hospital, London, UK

A D'Hoore MD
Consultant Surgeon, Department of Abdominal Surgery, University Hospital, Gasthuisberg, Leuven, Belgium

L Demoulin MA
Economist-Researcher, Centre for Health Services and Nursing Research, University of Leuven, Leuven, Belgium

AGTW Fiennes BSc, MS, FRCS
Senior Lecturer, Department of Surgery, St George's Hospital Medical School, Honorary Consultant Surgeon, St George's Hospital, London, UK

CG Fowler BSc, FRCP, FRCS(Urol)
Consultant Urological Surgeon, Department of Urology, The Royal Hospitals NHS Trust, London, UK; formerly Tutor, Minimal Access Therapy Training Unit, The Royal College of Surgeons of England, London, UK

N Gallegos MS, FRCS
Consultant Surgeon, Weston General Hospital, Weston-super-Mare, UK

H Gajraj MS, FRCS
Consultant Surgeon, Yeovil Hospital, Yeovil, Somerset, UK

G Gillett DPhil(Oxon), FRACS, MSc
Professor, Bioethics Research Centre, University of Otago and Department of Neurosurgery, Dunedin Hospital, Dunedin, New Zealand
GB Hanna FRCS
Specialist Registrar, Department of Surgery, Ninewells Hospital and Medical School, Dundee, UK
JE Hartley BSc, FRCS
Senior Surgical Registrar/Lecturer, The University of Hull, Academic Surgical Unit, Castle Hill Hospital, Cottingham, North Humberside, UK
AJN Iroatulam MD
Research Fellow, Department of Colorectal Surgery, Cleveland Clinic Florida, Fort Lauderdale, Florida, USA
K Kesteloot PhD
Professor of Economics, Department of Applied Economics, Centre for Health Services and Nursing Research, University of Leuven, Leuven, Belgium
A Loh MS, FRCS
Consultant Surgeon, Barnet Hospital, Barnet, Hertfordshire, UK
AL Magos BSc, MD, MRCOG
Consultant in Obstetrics and Gynaecology, Minimally Invasive Therapy Unit and Endoscopic Training Centre, University Department of Obstetrics and Gynaecology, The Royal Free Hospital, London, UK
OJ McAnena MCh, FRCSI
Consultant General Surgeon and Lecturer in Surgery, University College Hospital, Galway, Ireland
RF McCloy BSc, MD, FRCS
Senior Lecturer and Consultant Surgeon, Pancreato-Biliary Service, University Department of Surgery, Manchester Royal Infirmary, Manchester, UK
JRT Monson MD, FRCSI, FRCS, FACS
Professor of Surgery, University of Hull, Academic Surgical Unit, Castle Hill Hospital, Cottingham, North Humberside, UK
SS Mudan BSc, MS, FRCS
Senior Registrar in General Surgery, St George's Hospital, London, UK
R Nair MS, FRCS
Visiting Registrar, University Department of Surgery, Manchester Royal Infirmary, Manchester, UK
F Penninckx MD, PhD
Professor of Surgery, Department of Abdominal Surgery, University Hospital, Gasthuisberg, Leuven, Belgium
RKS Phillips MS, FRCS
Consultant Surgeon, St Mark's Hospital, Harrow, UK; Dean, St Mark's Academic Institute, Harrow, UK; Honorary Senior Lecturer, St Mary's Hospital Medical School, London, UK
AV Pollock BSc, MB, ChB, FRCS
Retired Consultant General Surgeon, Scarborough Hospital, Scarborough, North Yorkshire, UK
RE Richardson BSc, MRCOG
Research Fellow, Minimally Invasive Therapy Unit and Endoscopic Training Centre, University Department of Obstetrics and Gynaecology, The Royal Free

Hospital, London, UK; Lecturer in Obstetrics and Gynaecology, Academic Department of Obstetrics and Gynaecology, Chelsea and Westminster Hospital, London, UK

RCG Russell MS, FRCS
Consultant Surgeon, 149 Harley Street, London, UK

S. Sarkar FRCS
Late Basic Surgical Trainee, St George's Hospital, London, UK

JH Scurr FRCS
Consultant Surgeon, The Middlesex Hospital, London, UK; Senior Lecturer, University College, London Medical School, London, UK

RJ Stacey FRCS
Surgical Registrar, Charing Cross Hospital, London, UK

RS Taylor MS, FRCS
Consultant Surgeon, St George's Hospital, London, UK

TV Taylor MD, ChM, FRCSEng, FRCSEd, FACS, FACG
Professor of Surgery, Baylor College of Medicine, Houston, Texas, USA; Chief of General Surgery, VA Medical Center, Houston, Texas, USA

A Vleugels MD, PhD
Professor, Hospital Administrator at the University Hospitals, and Director, Center for Health Services and Nursing Research, University of Leuven, Leuven, Belgium

SD Wexner MD
Chairman and Residency Program Director, Department of Colorectal Surgery, Chairman, Division of Research and Education, Cleveland Clinic Florida, Fort Lauderdale, Florida, USA

EG Weiss MD
Staff Colorectal Surgeon, Department of Colorectal Surgery, Cleveland Clinic Florida, Fort Lauderdale, Florida, USA

SECTION I

Introduction

1

The case for minimally invasive general surgery

A.S. Chilvers

Introduction

Minimally invasive general surgery took the surgical world by surprise. For most of us, it has an active history of around eight years. Prior to that surgery had changed little over many years. The constant referral in nearly all publications to the past and past principles has suggested that general surgery has been a backward, rather than forward looking activity. The basis of training in general surgery has been the apprenticeship system, with the overriding principle being 'do as I do' and follow the accepted, but often unproven line.

During ones training, one moved from boss to boss, seldom questioning basic surgical techniques. I well remember, when still a senior registrar, being told proudly by my then consultant that his first registrar had returned to England from Australia and had watched him perform a partial gastrectomy. At the end of the operation, the ex-registrar said 'It's wonderful Mr . . . you still do your gastrectomies the same way as you did 25 years ago'.

Criticism of the past is, of course, dangerous as most of us rely on the past for our surgical well-being. Suddenly, however, our surgical bedrock has been shaken by the emergence of a technique which has brought about a radical change in surgical thinking. Past surgical technique had bare scientific support – the technique of Minimally Invasive Surgery has almost none.

Inevitably, at this time, a discussion on the merits of minimally invasive surgery must be an emotional one rather than a scientific one. There is not enough scientific data to prove the case one way or the other. This will come in later years. Rather belatedly in its long history the Royal College has introduced the discipline of audit, so, it is hoped, we will have data in a few years which will help us to arrive at a scientific conclusion rather than one based on surgical impression. At this stage then, we have a near uncontrollable bandwagon of new technique and we need to question why we are doing it.

I do not propose to indulge in a prolonged retrospective survey of the history of minimally invasive surgery. This has been done extensively elsewhere, almost as a necessary ritual and I feel serves very little purpose. The fact is that today we have superb electronics producing pictures beyond our dreams, instrumentation that is breathtaking in its ingenuity and a standard of anaesthetic that can cope with all the new requirements. Yet at the end of the day the technique is new, difficult and demanding. Why do we do it?

Clearly I am an enthusiast. This then is a biased chapter and I cannot be ashamed of it. In order, therefore, to understand my arguments in favour of minimally invasive surgery, it is necessary to understand my surgical origins. I qualified in 1963 and have only held surgical jobs. In the 1960s and 1970s ones general surgical training was rough and tough. Not a good thing, but one either sank or swam as an artisan. I later specialized in vascular surgery and it is interesting to note that in the UK more vascular surgeons have become active in minimally invasive surgery than any other speciality. In the early 1970s as well as being a vascular surgeon I became seriously converted to staples and have not hand sutured bowel from 1976 to the present day. I therefore see myself as a surgical engineer rather than one practising the 'art of surgery'. The gadgets of minimally invasive surgery therefore appeal to me greatly. I have always felt that one of God's great errors was to give surgeons hands. I believe that any intrusion into the human body should be by instrumentation rather than by rough probing fingers. The blunt dissection techniques are not for me.

Adopting a new technique ─────────

To consider the adoption of a new technique as radical as minimally invasive surgery raises two basic areas of discussion. The first is what is in it for the surgeon and the second is what is in it for the patient? Some may also ask what is in it for the administration? This last, though important, is not worthy of this chapter.

It may be thought that my first two considerations should be reversed. I believe that unless the surgeon is happy, confident and relaxed in what he is doing, then the patient will not benefit. We have all seen done, and in fact have done, operations we are not happy with and the results are never satisfactory. Therefore the surgeon must be the first consideration.

There are two parts to a minimally invasive operation. There is the laparoscopic technique and there are the operative manoeuvres. It is interesting that gynaecologists have for years used laparoscopy as a diagnostic tool, but have done little that is therapeutic. Laparoscopy is not an easy technique and few general surgeons have years of experience behind them. The tricks of laparoscopy and the interplay between laparoscopist and anaesthetist are important. There is a vast difference between peering through a telescope and viewing a modern television colour monitor. For me the first attraction of minimally invasive surgery using modern techniques, is the superb view of the part of the patient one is

interested in. Although, I, like most others, began with laparoscopic cholecystectomy, it was only when I viewed the thoracic cervical chain during laparoscopic
sympathectomy that the full impact of this technique hit me. Later on when I
began performing laparoscopic appendicectomy and was able to view the pelvic
organs in young women with right iliac fossa pain, but a normal appendix, that
the full value of laparoscopy was apparent. Having established a first class
magnified view of the operative field, the next advantage of minimally invasive
surgery is that the instrumentation can be arranged so that it is moving at an
angle as near as possible to 90° to one's line of vision. The problem with so much
open surgery and particularly those cases performed through small holes is that
often the instruments are moving down one's line of sight. To me this is a most
important criticism of the mini-cholecystectomy, where a very small hole is made,
but then the instrumentation is practically in the same line as the view into the
abdominal cavity. If this instrumentation is arranged as near as possible at a right
angle to the line of vision, the fact that there is no stereoscopic vision is unim-
portant as the movement of the instruments is unobstructed and it is easy to see
what one is doing. Although there are already recommended positions for the
introduction of operative ports, these should not be considered as being the only
positions possible. It is important for each surgeon to develop his own technique
so that he is happy with the position of the operating instruments. It is, of course,
vital with minimally invasive surgery that there should never be any sort of
instrumentation failure. It is extremely unusual for the electronics to go down, but
there is no doubt that using non-disposable instruments leads to greater problems. A grasper that does not grasp or a pair of scissors that are blunt or a
sucker that does not suck properly can cause great problems during the course of
a laparoscopic operation. The maintenance of these very fine instruments is a
great problem, and for this reason, we try and use almost exclusively disposable
instruments.

Disadvantages of minimally invasive surgery

It has been argued that one of the disadvantages of minimally invasive surgery
is that one does not have the opportunity to touch or feel the tissues. The
sensations of feeling different tissues is an extremely subjective one and one
that the surgeon only develops after many years of practice. So it is with
minimally invasive surgery. With practice similar sensations can be achieved
using the instruments in the operating ports. It is possible to do a full laparotomy without opening the abdomen. Usually it can be done more efficiently
than with an open operation as vision is always available whereas in an open
laparotomy often the hand only can be inserted into the abdomen and there is
no view of the tissues felt.

Minimally invasive surgery is often criticized because it takes a great deal
longer and is therefore more frustrating for the surgeon and more dangerous for
the patient. It must not be forgotten that the majority of people performing
minimally invasive surgery in the 1990s came to it with no previous experience

and it is therefore quite natural that these operations should at first have been done very slowly. Now that surgeons are becoming more experienced and, in particular, as younger surgeons in training are learning the techniques it is noticeable that the operative time is being rapidly reduced and is approaching that of the open operation. Indeed, in some cases, such as bilateral laparoscopic inguinal hernia repair, the operation is quicker than in bilateral open operative repair.

One of the main disadvantages of laparoscopic surgery is, however, fatigue. When the technique was first introduced, surgeons were only performing perhaps one laparoscopic operation per operating list, but now that the technique is established and surgeons are becoming quicker, it is not unusual to do three or four laparoscopic cases in one operating list. The ergonomics of laparoscopic surgery have not been fully perfected as far as the surgeon is concerned. The operative position, often with the elbows raised, is extremely tiring and also the repeated use of the scissor type grips on the ends of the instrumentation can be quite tiring on the thumbs. The most fatiguing aspect of the technique, however, is that everyone in the theatre can see what is being done, so it is difficult to have the subtle rest periods that one builds into open surgery. It was always possible in an open operation to lean on a swab for a moment or two and chat about other things, but in minimally invasive surgery, this is impossible and once the operation starts, it has to flow through without a break to the end. I am sure that in time the development of the instrumentation will reach a stage whereby one can sit at a consul and work the instruments in a more user friendly position.

Advantages of minimally invasive surgery

What then are the advantages of minimally invasive surgery for the patient? It was very noticeable that the push for laparoscopic cholecystectomy was almost entirely patient led. I cannot remember during my entire surgical career where a particular technique has been requested by so many patients in such a short time. At the time when one asked what they thought the advantages of this new keyhole technique were to themselves, there was obviously some confusion in people's minds. Because initially the technique was championed by the manufacturers of the laser devices, the two words which seemed to stick in most patients' minds were laser and television. It was clear that the technique was looked upon as a magical manoeuvre, where there would be very little inconvenience to the patient themselves. There is no doubt on closer questioning that it was the absence of a large scar which many people find attractive. Very quickly it became apparent that the second attraction was the short stay in hospital. This latter has certainly been borne out with practice in that, in the majority of units undertaking laparoscopic cholecystectomy, the hospitalization time has been reduced from seven days for the open operation to two days for the laparoscopic procedure. The benefits initially therefore to the patient are that they have a smaller scar and that they have a shorter time in hospital. Of course, the third consideration is that the technique is less painful. It has been suggested that in any form of surgery these days, post-operative pain should no longer exist, but I think this is probably wishful thinking. However, now that the control of post-operative pain is so good, it is difficult to be completely sure whether the pain suffered following laparoscopic surgery is less than open surgery. Certainly the pain is no more and the clinical impression is that the majority of patients suffer far less.

The other consideration following surgery is how quickly the patient can return to normal life, either going back to work or resuming normal social habits. No definitive work has been carried out on this subject as often the control of when a patient returns to work lies not in the hands of the surgeon, but rather the general practitioner. There is also a certain reluctance, certainly amongst some patients to return to work very rapidly. My first 50 cholecystectomies were all performed on private patients and it was noticeable that they had all returned to work within two weeks. I am sure that in time the systems of audit will give a better indication as to how quickly people return to work following minimally invasive surgery. This will be a much better measure than any constructed trial.

Training

It is, of course, an overriding principle that any new technique should be safe for the patient. The problem that laparoscopic surgery has had to face is that its emergence has occurred under the full spotlight of media attention. In the United Kingdom quite suddenly a whole generation of consultant surgeons who had never performed minimally invasive surgery were expected, and indeed encouraged by the Department of Health, to embark on the new technique. It was at this stage that the problems of training became very apparent.

Training for minimally invasive surgery presents some problems. A large number of existing consultant surgeons, often rather set in their ways, have had to learn the technique in a short period of time. They have also had to organize the training of their juniors. The range of learning processes by consultants has been interesting. Some went on courses – usually abroad; some watched the video and started; some were taught by the instrument manufacturers' representatives and some learnt from their registrars. There were no guidelines and no control. Inevitably dreadful mistakes were, and still are, made. There seems to be a reluctance amongst British surgeons to admit technical ignorance and face up to training.

My own training consisted of going to America, Germany and France very early on in the introduction of the technique. I estimate that it cost me about £20,000 for my training. For the first year of laparoscopic surgery I worked in conjunction with a very experienced gynaecologist who taught me the laparoscopic techniques. Along the way I attended pig courses and simulator sessions.

At the end of the day, what is the best way of learning and teaching laparoscopic surgery? I think that the saddest thing that has emerged over the last few years is the appearance of very expensive training courses. In the past one would never dream of charging to teach colleagues, but now almost every centre in the world, often with the barest of track records, advertises one or two day courses with the obligatory dinner and large participant's fee. Attending good courses is all well and good, but often juniors have to pay for part or all of the fee themselves.

From my own experience I think that animal work is of little value. Some of the American centres are superb, providing large numbers of specially bred herniated pigs. Apart from the ethical considerations of animal work, I find that the skills learned are of limited value and can be more easily learnt elsewhere.

Similarly, I find simulators of limited value. Certainly watching young trainees at work, they outgrow the simulator in a very short space of time. Spatial awareness in two dimensions seems to be more easily acquired by the young rather than by the elderly. Now that laparoscopic surgery is so well established in most British hospitals these early skills can be learned as an assistant. I believe, however, that it is essential for trainees to spend as much time as possible handling and playing with the instruments in a non-operative environment. One needs to get to know the instruments – not only how they work, but also how they are balanced – where, instinctively, the end of the instrument is – the subconscious awareness of the relationship of the functioning end of the instrument to the hand. The perennial problem of using a new instrument without reading the instruction book does not apply only to new VCRs! With constant handling of the instruments their use should become as instinctive as the use of the old Colt 45 was to the movie cowboy. He pulled it from his holster, pointed it at the law breaker and fired. Inevitably, however far away his target was, he would hit it; no aiming, no sights, no hesitation, and instinctive awareness as to where the barrel was pointing. So it should be with laparoscopic instruments. I am sure that the best way of learning laparoscopic techniques is to work with someone who is experienced. The age-old apprentice system is the best. Working in tandem with a colleague – holding, grasping, dissecting, cutting, then gradually taking over as the main operative avoids problems. Much was made at first concerning the number of assistants required. People spoke of dedicated camera operatives, first and second assistants and there was a terrible clutter of people. Some surgeons I came across had their own camera nurse who would follow them round wherever they went. Now that the initial hysteria has passed, these practices are disappearing and in good units there is a more relaxed attitude. Personally, I like to work with one assistant and one instrument technician. Because of the intensive and often destructive media interest in any mistakes made in hospitals, I believe that somewhere along the line there should be certification of proficiency in minimally invasive surgery. Probably in the future this will either be not necessary as everyone will be taught or one will need a certificate for every operation performed. The final decision on this must rest in the hands of the Royal Colleges.

Conclusion

Minimally invasive surgery will not go away. It is an attractive technique, both for surgeon and patient. Over the next few years minimally invasive surgery will find its level and become an everday surgical technique. I believe that as a new generation of trained young surgeons come through, laparoscopy will be used more and more and the era of midlines, paramedians, transverse incisions and prolonged hospital stays will be over.

2

The case against minimally invasive colorectal surgery

R.K.S. Phillips

Introduction

This debate should not be in black and white, but rather in various shades of grey. I do not wish to argue against minimally invasive surgery in general as there are very clear benefits to all manner of minimally invasive approaches, especially when it comes to gallbladder surgery and various (particularly upper gastrointestinal) operations, such as Nissen's fundoplication. One should be aware, however, that a frequently applied but less morbid operation might yet kill more patients than an infrequently applied yet more morbid procedure. As cholecystectomy is seen as a less and less invasive procedure for the patient, so the indications for surgery have become relaxed which could yet result overall in more patients dying than when open cholecystectomy was the norm.

What are we trying to achieve?

To some extent, this depends on who is paying. The patient does not want to wait for surgery, would like the neatest possible scar and the least disturbance to work and recreation. At the same time, disastrous complications, even if only in a few patients, might well put the patient off; just as some people are put off flying by their fear of crashing – a most unlikely event.

The purchaser of healthcare in the United Kingdom is Government, whereas in the United States it is for the most part third party insurers. Any Government is looking for the best possible value for money commensurate with a modern and progressive service. If the same amount of care starts to cost more in real terms year on year, then either the economy must expand to accommodate the increased requirement for money, or taxes must go up, or services will need to be cut.

Providers of healthcare, which in the United Kingdom are NHS Trusts (but the point applies equally to private hospitals), need to balance their books, preferably with a small margin in their favour – either for profit or for service development. It is a simple matter for them to decide whether increased cost in the operating theatre, for example when performing a laparoscopically-assisted colonic resection, can be recouped financially through a shorter hospital stay. The increased operating theatre cost can arise through the increased use of disposable equipment, through the need to purchase new and expensive equipment, through longer operating times, which generate higher per case staff operating costs, and so on. If an operation can be done in the same (or a similar) time, as is the case in experienced hands with cholecystectomy, once the costs of equipping the operating theatre have been met the shorter hospital stay and the very obvious patient benefits from a rapid recovery and return to work make laparoscopic cholecystectomy quite clearly the preferred option. Even so, there will be some patients who, fully acquainted with the facts, might still prefer a conventional approach. Common bile duct division is a disaster, revision is difficult, and problems can be ongoing. Some patients might perceive a smaller scar and a quicker return to work a poor prize when set against what many surgeons feel is a small but real increased risk of bile duct injury.

Colorectal operations

Most colorectal surgical operations have now been achieved laparoscopically,[1] although usually a small conventional incision is necessary if a specimen needs to be removed. Where a specimen does not need to be removed, as for example when operating on a rectal prolapse, or when constructing a stoma, there are already conventional ways of performing a minimally invasive operation without recourse to the laparoscope. Thus there are perineal operations for rectal prolapse, such as Delorme's[2] or Altmeier's[3] operations, both of which can be performed under regional rather than general anaesthesia and each of them can be associated with very short hospital stays. Stomas can be constructed by the trephine technique.[4,5]

When we come to assess the relative benefits of laparoscopic colorectal surgery as against conventional, but at times minimally invasive, techniques, we need to take into account the issues that already existed before the laparoscopic revolution. Taking again as an example rectal prolapse surgery, the issues were these:

1. Abdominal rectopexy was tried and trusted. Even the very old tolerated the operation well, so mortality rates were negligible.[6,7]
2. Recurrence was uncommon, say less than 5 per cent in the literature[6,7] (although this author suspects that the true rate is probably higher than that if follow up is extended).[8]
3. In recent times it was found that about 50 per cent of patients became constipated after abdominal rectopexy.[6]

The alternative perineal operations remain an order of magnitude less traumatic than conventional abdominal rectopexy, seem not to be associated with constipation but do suffer from a significantly higher rate of recurrence – of the order of 16 per cent.[1]

Given this background, what we want to know with regard to laparoscopic rectopexy is whether or not it achieves the worst of both worlds: higher recurrence rates than its conventional abdominal counterpart and significant rates of constipation (occasioned perhaps by rectal denervation by the extensive mobilization) compared with the perineal alternatives which are perhaps less invasive. What has been published so far with regard to laparoscopic abdominal rectopexy has small numbers and too short follow-up periods to have any good idea of longer term recurrence rates, and usually ignores any mention of bowel function.[9,10] The issues that have been addressed are 'new' issues, related to time in the operating theatre, time to return of bowel function and length of hospital stay. In addition, there has been a worryingly high rate of significant complications of laparoscopic colorectal operations, such as ureteric injury[11] and major arterial injuries,[12] which would be impossible from Delorme's operation and vanishingly rare with conventional abdominal rectopexy. (Other complications of laparoscopic colorectal operations include accidental small bowel enterotomies,[12] cannula site bowel herniation[13] and even removal of the wrong segment of bowel.[11,14])

Most other colorectal operations require removal of a specimen, and the present evidence suggests that once a significant incision is made in the abdominal wall (such as is necessary to extract most specimens), length of hospital stay, analgesia consumption and perhaps even return to work are not markedly different between patients operated upon conventionally and those having a laparoscopic-assisted operation.[12,15,16] Obviously, the incision is smaller (usually by a significant amount) with the laparoscopic-assisted operations, and this on its own would account for quite marked preference by some patients. There are, of course, occasions when conventional operations can be done through small incisions, particularly right hemicolectomy or sigmoid colectomy in elderly and frail individuals, but there is little doubt that use of the laparoscope significantly increases the proportion of patients who end up with a shorter incision.

The financial dilemma

In some patients a laparoscopically-assisted operation has to be converted to a conventional approach. This arises for all manner of reasons: intra-operative difficulties; confusion over anatomy; and not least, surgeon frustration. Clearly, these operations will take much longer than would have been the case if only the second (conventional) part of the operation had been performed from the outset. Furthermore, the evidence to date is that, unlike the case with cholecystectomy, even after the learning curve has been climbed laparoscopic colorectal operations take significantly longer than their conventional counterparts. This does not matter very much to providers of healthcare as they can very easily work out whether laparoscopic and laparoscopic-assisted colorectal operations are affordable, given other potential savings with regard to length of stay, but the situation is *very* different from the perspective of the purchaser.

A government spends a certain proportion of its gross domestic product on healthcare. The amount of money supplied pays for a given amount of healthcare. If time in the operating theatre increases, then less work can be performed through the same plant by the same staff than before. As the demand for healthcare will not have decreased (and may well have increased, if laparoscopic cholecystectomy is anything to go by), then more operating theatres will need to be built and more surgical teams trained *to do the same amount of work*. This means borrowing large capital sums of money for operating theatre construction, repaying the capital and the interest on the loans, and having persistently higher staff costs than before.

What gains might accrue? Any reduction in hospital stay pales into insignificance when measured against these increased costs. What about earlier return to work? Most colorectal surgical operations are performed on retired people, who make no financial return to the Treasury. Those who are still in work might conceivably return to work an average of two or three weeks earlier than if they had been operated upon conventionally. The sums of money earned for the exchequer by this minority during this time will have no chance of approaching the vast investment by government that would be needed to make it possible, while at the same time not seeing an overall reduction in healthcare.

It is quite clear, therefore, that where significant increases in operating time persist after the learning curve for the procedure has been passed, such procedures will prove significantly more expensive than their conventional counterparts. Nevertheless, there may yet be sound human and clinical reasons for spending this extra money.

The cost analyses that have been done so far with regard to laparoscopic colorectal surgery have ignored the major capital expenses outlined above, but even when they have done this, they have not been able to demonstrate a clear advantage for a laparoscopic approach.[1,13,17]

Potential clinical indications _____

It is entirely possible that laparoscopically-assisted operations may influence the metabolic response to surgery to a lesser extent and immune function may not be as depressed.[18] How such possible advantages might be turned to clinical advantage remains speculative.[19] Set against this are the real possibilities that in some circumstances laparoscopic operations might be dangerous: not only because of the increased chance of iatrogenic error caused by loss of a strategic view, but also through possibly increased rates of pelvic and deep vein thrombosis, occasioned by prolonged periods of positive intra-abdominal pressure;[20,21] and when operating in cancer.

Minimal invasive cancer surgery ——

When considering surgery in a patient with colorectal cancer, there are four issues that should concern both the patient and surgeon:

1. Operative morbidity and death.
2. Local recurrence.
3. Longer term survival.
4. Quality of life.

We have pretty hard measures of quality of life: restorative operation versus stoma; bowel frequency and control; and bladder and sex function. These are an order of magnitude more important than the only one currently demonstrated to be superior for a laparoscopic-assisted approach: the length of the surgical incision!

Longer-term survival depends on adequacy of the primary operation coupled with the presence or absence at the time of surgery of occult metastases elsewhere (usually in the liver), the body's response to all this, and the use and effectiveness of adjuvant therapy. Conceivably the body's response to surgery might be influenced favourably from a cancer-specific point of view by a minimal invasive approach. Offset against this are the real fears that inadequate local surgery might be performed, not simply by performing different (easier) operations laparoscopically, but through the loss of tactile sensation when operating conventionally that cancer is encroaching on the anatomical boundary of dissection. Confronted by this, the surgeon operating conventionally abandons the anatomic plane and excises more widely, but operating laparoscopically may simply be unaware and transgress the tumour.

Of greatest recent interest has been the issue of port site recurrence.[1,22] Wound recurrence operating conventionally is very unusual, so the spate of reports of port site recurrence when operating laparoscopically is worrying. Potential mechanisms are currently being explored, from poor technique through to the effects of anoxia and positive intra-abdominal pressure on the implantability of viable cancer cells, known to be exfoliated from the surface of some tumours. Because of this problem, most surgeons are now reluctant to operate laparoscopically on a curable case of bowel cancer. Such operations as are done should be performed within the confines of a randomized trial.

Conclusions ——————————

Minimally invasive surgery has captured the popular imagination. All of us, confronted by illness, would rather that illness went away with as little disturbance to our routines and lifestyle as possible. Minimally invasive surgery holds out this promise. Where the costs and outcomes are equivalent to or better than conventional approaches, minimal approaches will become the norm. This applies today to cholecystectomy and to a number of other operations, such as transthoracic cervical sympathectomy. There is fierce debate with regard to inguinal hernia surgery, where opponents question how the excellent results of day case tension-free mesh repair under local anaesthetic can be improved upon, particularly when the costs and sometimes bizarre and serious complications of laparoscopic repair become apparent.

Alternatives exist to most laparoscopic colorectal operations and it remains unclear whether at present they show an advantage. Economies that can afford the increased costs of laparoscopic-assisted operations, particularly colorectal operations, will no doubt continue to develop the techniques. It would help us all if these developments were done according to protocols and were strictly audited and compared in a randomized fashion to the conventional alternatives.[23]

References

1. Monson JRT, Hill ADK, Darzi A. Laparoscopic colonic surgery. *Br J Surg* 1995; **82**: 150–157.
2. Senapati A, Nicholls RJ, Thomson JPS, Phillips RKS. Results of Delorme's procedure for rectal prolapse. *Dis Colon Rectum* 1994; **37**: 456–460.
3. Altmeier WA, Culbertson WR, Schowengerdt C, Hunt J. Nineteen years' experience with the one-stage perineal repair of rectal prolapse. *Ann Surg* 1971; **173**: 993–1006.
4. Senapati A, Phillips RKS. The trephine colostomy: a permanent left iliac fossa colostomy without recourse to laparotomy. *Ann R Coll Surg Engl* 1991; **73**: 305–306.
5. Anderson ID, Hill J, Vohra H, Schofield VF, Kiff ES. An improved means of faecal diversion: the trephine stoma. *Br J Surg* 1992; **79**: 1080–1081.
6. Mann CV, Hoffman C. Complete rectal prolapse: the anatomical and functional results of treatment by an extended abdominal rectopexy. *Br J Surg* 1988; **75**: 34–37.
7. Penfold JCB, Hawley PR. Experiences of Ivalon-sponge implant for complete rectal prolapse at St Mark's Hospital 1960–1970. *Br J Surg* 1972; **59**: 846–848.
8. Boulos PB, Stryker SJ, Nicholls RJ. The long-term results of polyvinyl alcohol (Ivalon) sponge for rectal prolapse in young patients. *Br J Surg* 1984; **71**: 213–214.
9. Senagore AJ, Luchtefeld MA, MacKeigan JM. Rectopexy. *J Laparoendosc Surg* 1993; **3**: 339–343.
10. Baker R, Senagore AJ, Luchtefeld MA. Laparoscopic-assisted vs. open resection. Rectopexy offers excellent results. *Dis Colon Rectum* 1995; **38**: 199–201.
11. Larach SW, Salomon MC, Williamson PR, Goldstein E. Laparoscopic assisted colectomy: experience during the learning curve. *Coloproctology* 1993; **1**: 38–41.
12. Wexner SD, Cohen SM, Johansen OB, Nogueras JJ, Jagelman DG. Laparoscopic colorectal surgery: a prospective assessment and current perspective. *Br J Surg* 1993; **80**: 1602–1605.
13. Falk PM, Beart RW Jr, Wexner SD *et al.* Laparoscopic colectomy: a critical appraisal. *Dis Colon Rectum* 1993; **36**: 28–34.
14. Monson JRT, Darzi A, Carey PD, Guillou PJ. Prospective evaluation of laparoscopic assisted colectomy in an unselected group of patients. *Lancet* 1992; **340**: 831–833.
15. Tate JJT, Kwok S, Dawson JW, Lau WY, Li AK. Prospective comparison of laparoscopic and conventional anterior resection. *Br J Surg* 1993; **80**: 1396–1398.
16. Peters WR, Bartels TL. Minimally invasive colectomy: are the potential benefits realized? *Dis Colon Rectum* 1993; **36**: 751–756.
17. Musser DJ, Boorse RC, Madera F, Reed JF III. Laparoscopic colectomy: at what cost? *Surg Laparosc Endosc* 1994; **4**: 1–5.

18. Bessler M, Whelan RL, Halverson A, Treat MR, Nowygrod R. Is immune function better preserved after laparoscopic versus open colon resection? *Surg Endosc* 1994; **8**: 881–883.
19. Baxter, JN, O'Dwyer PJ. Pathophysiology of laparoscopy. *Br J Surg* 1995; **82**: 1–2.
20. Cushieri A, Shimi SM, Van der Velpen G, Banting S, Wood RA. Laparoscopic prosthesis fixation rectopexy for complete rectal prolapse. *Br J Surg* 1994; **81**: 138–139.
21. Guillou PJ, Darzi A, Monson JRT. Experience with laparoscopic colorectal surgery for malignant disease. *Surg Oncol* 1993; **2**(suppl 1): 43–49.
22. O'Rourke NA, Heald RJ. Laparoscopic surgery for colorectal cancer. *Br J Surg* 1993; **80**: 1229–1230.
23. Kmiot WA, Wexner SD. Laparoscopy in colorectal surgery: a call for careful appraisal. *Br J Surg* 1995; **82**: 25–26.

SECTION II

Training in laparoscopic surgery

3

Surgical competence, training and privileges

A. Cuschieri and G.B. Hanna

Introduction

Surgical competence in Western countries is assumed as the inevitable outcome of training through the long-established clinical apprenticeship system. Although the cognitive aspects are asessed by national examinations, technical proficiency in operative work is never tested, even at the time of appointment to the consultant grade when effectively an 'open' licence is issued to the individual for independent practice on humans within a working life span averaging 25 years. In some countries, but not in the UK, a system of credentialling is employed by which privileges to carry out specific operations are granted to the attending surgeons from the hospitals or institutions concerned. This system, though often confused with, is different from 'certification or accreditation'. While the latter indicates that an individual has completed a surgical training programme and can be officially listed as a specialist, the credentialling process entails evidence that the surgeon can actually perform the specified procedures. There is a contrasting situation between the existing conditions governing practice of surgery within the UK and the requirements for licence to operate on animals under the 1986 Animal Act which dictates that both operator and institution require close and continued, often unannounced, inspection by inspectors and detailed audit (returns) on the animals operated upon within a given year. Under the Animal Act, the Secretary of State has the power to revoke the licence on a proven infringement brought to his attention by the Home Office Inspectorate. No such draconian powers are exerted in relation to operations on humans, the assumption being that the system of training and guidelines for safe practice issued by the Royal Colleges ensure that surgical operations are conducted by technically competent surgeons within the NHS and private hospitals. This may be the case in the vast majority of practising surgeons but assured competence is not guaranteed by the existing system.

Surgical competence has attracted media attention in recent years because of the morbidity and mortality encountered with the introduction of Minimal Access Surgery (MAS). This chapter addresses surgical competence, training and conditions for safe practice of surgery. Although special considerations apply to MAS, the underlying principles governing the various issues are the same and it is inappropriate to address MAS as if it were a different discipline.

Components of competence

Even the terminology relating to competence is often used loosely and requires precise definition before meaningful review of the subject.

Ability is the adaptive capacity, trait, attribute or aptitude that a person brings to a given task; whereas *skill* is the result of applying a specific combination of abilities to a given task. *Performance* implies the overall efficiency with which a complex activity is executed. *Competence* is the ability to perform a task safely, to an acceptable standard and within an acceptable time frame. *Proficiency* indicates that competence has been achieved consistently and improved 'to an expert level' over time.[1]

Norman in his methodological review of clinical competence[2] highlighted the following components: clinical skills, knowledge and understanding, interpersonal attitude, problem solving and clinical judgement, and technical skill. There are three major components of surgical competence: cognitive factors, personality and psychomotor skills.

Cognitive factors and surgical performance

Cognitive factors include intelligence, knowledge of surgery and current literature and judgement.[3] Intelligence and knowledge of surgery are objectively evaluated by written and clinical examinations, but, they are only one aspect of the cognitive skill required.[4,5] Decision-making is important for sound clinical practice. Spencer argued that surgery is 75 per cent decision making and 25 per cent dexterity[6] and although this may be an exaggeration, other studies have stressed the importance of decision making.[3,7] In the American residency surgical training programme just over 59 per cent of the reasons reported for non-advancement to chief and/or non-certification have been attributed to deficiency in surgical knowledge or clinical judgement.[8]

Cognition is regarded as the essential first phase in the acquisition of psychomotor skills.[9] The trainee has to understand the nature of the task (what it entails) and then acquire the skill to execute the steps necessary for accomplishing the task. Once the cognitive element has been acquired, the process of integration of this knowledge into the appropriate motor behaviour is initiated.

Cognitive factors are also important in operative surgery. Kopta included cognition by residents in the operating room as a part of evaluation of surgical performance.[10] In this study, two independent observers scored the cognitive element based on whether the surgeon knew by name other personnel, understood the aseptic technique, the surgical anatomy and the nature of the procedure being performed; whether he asked for appropriate instruments and anticipated and dealt effectively with the pathology. In this study an increase in the cognitive scores was found with each additional year of residency but the increment between the third and fourth years was rather small. Thus the cognitive element underlying surgical technical performance is developed early and over a relatively short period of time in most residents.

Personality

Greenburg *et al.* surveyed the views of the faculty members and the residents concerning the personality traits of the surgical residents[7] within six university surgical departments to determine the perceived importance of 35 personality traits on a standard assertiveness scale. Traits with the lowest mean scores and least variance for both groups indicating agreement were: admits errors, is well disciplined, considers all facts, is highly motivated and consistent, and listens. For some general personality traits (decisiveness, fairness, good team participation, flexibility), there was excellent score and rank agreement, whilst disagreement was observed with others (priority setting, independence and purposefulness).

In another study, ideal personality traits for a surgical career were identified as the ability to learn from teaching encounters, willingness to work the extended and/or unusual hours required of a surgeon, emotional stability, completeness and accuracy of histories and physical examination, accurate and updated current record keeping, dependability and punctuality, possession of moral and ethical standards and the ability to assume responsibility.[11] These studies clearly indicate that surgery is a hard and demanding profession requiring a certain personality type capable of commitment and work which is normally considered as excessive. The recent changes concerning the hours of service of surgical trainees may be encouraging individuals who do not possess the necessary reserve to embark on a surgical career.

Kopta assessed the attitude of the surgeons in the operating room.[10] Two independent observers scored each of the following areas: relations with the nursing staff, anaesthetist, patient, attending physician and assistants, ability to integrate with the other members of the surgical team, reaction towards complications and verbal communication. As in cognitive ability, attitude scores improved with each additional year of residency but the maximal gain was obtained between the first and the second years with only a small incremental gain between the third and fourth years.

Psychomotor skills

Surgery is a technical subject[12-14] and its practice largely a craft. The clinical outcome following surgical intervention is mainly determined by the quality of craftsmanship. Pettigrew *et al.* highlighted the importance of surgeon-related variables in the assessment of risk factors and concluded that operative performance was the main factor in the development of post-operative complications.[15] A multicentre study on the anastomotic integrity after operations for large bowel cancer involving 1466 patients identified the surgeon as the most important single factor influencing anastomotic integrity. There was a six-fold range of outcome in respect of the surgeon variable (5–30 per cent) that could not be accounted for by any detectable differences in patient population.[16] Another study of 645 patients treated for colorectal cancer by 13 consultants showed that the hazard rate ratios among individual surgeons ranged from 0.56 to 2.03, from 0.17 to 1.92, and from 0.57 to 1.50 for curative resection, palliative resection, and palliative diversion respectively.[17]

General perceptual and motor abilities

Fleishman and his colleges investigated more than 200 tasks administered to thousands of subjects in a series of interlocking studies. From the patterns of correlation obtained, they were able to account for performance in terms of a relatively small number of abilities[18] the most important being:

- *Control precision*: this factor is common to tasks which require fine, highly controlled, but not overcontrolled muscular adjustments, primarily where large muscle groups are involved.
- *Multilimb co-ordination*: this is the ability to co-ordinate the movements of a number of limbs simultaneously.
- *Response orientation*: this is related to visual discrimination reaction psychomotor tasks involving rapid directional discrimination and orientation of movements patterns. It reflects the ability to select the correct movement in relation to the stimulus, especially under high speed conditions.
- *Reaction time*: this represents the speed with which the individual is able to respond to a stimulus when it appears. There are consistent indications that individual differences are independent of whether the stimulus is auditory or visual and also independent of the type of response which is required.
- *Speed of arm movement*: this concerns the speed with which an individual can make a gross, discrete arm movement where accuracy is not required.
- *Rate control*: this ability involves the performance of continuous anticipatory motor adjustments relative to changes in speed and direction of a continuously moving target or object.
- *Manual dexterity*: this involves skilful, well-directed arm–hand movements in manipulating fairly large objects under speed conditions.

Table 3.1   Tests for perceptual motor abilities – Fleishman and Ellison[19]

Ability	Best tests (highest loadings)
Wrist–finger speed	medium tapping [0.77]
	large tapping [0.75]
	pursuit aiming [0.54]
Finger dexterity	Purdue pegboard – both hands [0.66]
	Purdue pegboard – right hand [0.60]
	Purdue pegboard – assembly [0.59]
	O'Connor finger dexterity [0.59]
Speed of arm movement	Ten-target-aiming-corrects [0.72]
	Ten-target-aiming-errors [0.70]
	Han-precision-aiming-corrects [0.72]
Manual dexterity	Minnesota rate of manipulation-placing [0.53]
	Minnesota rate of manipulation-turning [0.52]
Aiming	Pursuit aiming I [0.63]
	Pursuit aiming II [0.63]

- *Finger dexterity*: this is the ability to make skill-controlled manipulations of tiny objects involving primarily the fingers.
- *Arm–hand steadiness*: this is the ability to make precise arm–hand positioning movements where strength and speed are minimized; the critical factor being the steadiness with which such movements can be made.
- *Wrist, finger speed*: this is also referred to as tapping. It is measured by printed tests requiring rapid tapping of the pencil within relatively large areas.
- *Aiming*: this has been defined as the ability to perform quickly and precisely a series of movements requiring eye–hand co-ordination, but this definition seems much too broad, since many other kinds of psychomotor tests require eye–hand co-ordination.[21]

There are several well-established tests of perceptual motor abilities. Fleishman and Ellison conducted a factor analysis of fine manipulative tests[19] to determine their usefulness as indices of perceptual motor abilities. Their findings are summarized in Table 3.1.

Bourassa and Guion in a factorial study of dexterity tests[20] observed three important factors of perceptual motor ability:

- *Manual dexterity* in terms of the ability to execute skilful and rapid arm–hand movements.
- *Visual sensitivity* defined as the ability to make fine visual discriminations involving acuity and/or depth perception.
- *Visual feedback*, the ability to use visual cues in the manipulation and placing of small objects.

Psychomotor skills in surgery ———

Kaufman *et al.* characterized the factors which contribute to surgical skill as follows: 'surgeons require the integration of muscle strength, speed, precision, dexterity, balance and spatial perception as well as poise and endurance in the execution of surgical procedures'.[21] In otolaryngology, Krespi *et al.* based their research on the development of aptitude tests for psychomotor skills required for this specialty such as purposeful hand direction, tactile discrimination, finger pressure co-ordination, finger strength, speed of movements, fine control precision, finger dexterity, steadiness during movement, steadiness without movement, neatness, finger visual tracking of moving objects, spatial visualization and depth perception.[22]

Two important parameters of psychomotor skills merit further attention: visuo-spatial ability and dexterity.

Visuo-spatial ability

Visuo-spatial ability is defined as the ability to keep in mind a definite configuration so as to identify it in spite of perceptual distractions.[23] Although it is not a manual ability, it does affect the psychomotor aspect of surgery. Several studies have shown a significant correlation between visuo-spatial ability and surgical ratings. Gibbons *et al.* investigated the relationship between a specialized form of spatial ability known as 'field articulation' and technical surgical skill.[24] Field articulation is operationally defined as the ability to differentiate a simple figure from a complex configurational surround. The correlation between hidden figures test scores and average ratings of technical surgical skill of 17 members of the academic surgical faculty in two different institutions was observed to be highly significant. Schueneman *et al.* demonstrated that visuo-spatial organization was statistically unrelated to academic achievement but showed a significant positive correlation ($r = 0.68$) with the surgery ratings.[25] Steele *et al.* also reported a positive correlation ($p < 0.005$) between improvement in performing jejunal anastomosis by junior surgical trainees (as measured by a cumulative error score) and the visuo-spatial ability measured with the hidden figures test.[23]

By contrast, Deary *et al.* failed to establish a significant correlation between visuo-spatial ability and ratings of surgical abilities.[26] Despite using a wide range of spatial ability measures, this study was limited by the small numbers of subjects who were rated by a single consultant for whom they were currently working (i.e., no measure of inter-assessor reliability). Even so the data from this study suggest that those trainees rated as superior tended to have better stereoscopic depth perception.

Visuo-spatial ability is unrelated to overall academic achievement, verbal ability and IQ.[27] In contrast, correlation has been demonstrated between visuo-spatial ability and field articulation testing, school geometry, quantitative thinking, shop mechanics and watch repair.[28] No difference in visuo-spatial ability has been reported between surgical trainees and those of other medical specialisms.[29]

Within individuals, spatial ability is stable over time and does not appear to be influenced by duration of surgical training.[24] Similarly, in diagnostic radiology, the performance on spatial ability test was unaffected by the level of training.[30,31] Furthermore, there is evidence of sex-linked major-gene influence on human spatial visualization ability.[32–34] However, large differences in visuo-spatial ability were observed between the experienced Naval aviators and the Naval flight cadets on performance ratings with the rod-and-frame test.[35] It is not known whether these differences represent an aviation training effect on rod-and-frame test performance or a selection effect within the training programme or constant reinforcement leading to an expert level of performance.

Dexterity

Surgery is traditionally regarded as a profession demanding a high level of dexterity but although this view is self-evident, there have been few objective psychomotor studies in general surgery to support this view. Schueneman *et al.* used a battery of neuropsychological tests and a surgical skill rating scale to evaluate psychomotor skills of 120 general surgical residents.[25] They concluded that 'it appears that contrary to surgical folklore, manual dexterity is not the major dimension distinguishing the proficient surgical performance from the mediocre. Rather, non-verbal, visuo-spatial problem solving abilities and the ability to distinguish essential from non-essential detail even when the signal-to-noise ratio is high appears most crucial to superior technique'. Steele *et al.* found a negative correlation between improvement in performing jejunal anasto-mosis by junior surgical trainees (cumulative error score) and manual dexterity measured with the Crawford test.[23]

Squire *et al.* studied manual dexterity in surgical consultants, and medical/surgical residents and found that surgical consultants performed significantly worse than the residents on tests of manual dexterity (Minnesota manipulation test and Purdue pegboard test).[36] Harris *et al.* found no significant difference in manual dexterity between surgical trainees and different medical specialists.[29]

The effect of age on psychomotor performance was investigated by Schueneman *et al.* in a cohort of 141 general surgical residents.[37] Older residents (age 28 to 42 years) exhibited less motor speed and co-ordination and more caution in avoiding psychomotor errors than did their younger counterparts. No differences were found for visuo-spatial abilities and rated surgical skill.

Minimal access surgery _____

Aside from the assumption that the cognitive factors and personality traits considered desirable for surgery in general are also necessary for endoscopic surgery, the requirements are largely unknown and the subject is further clouded by certain considerations relating to the practice of MAS. In the first instance, endoscopic surgery is a new and developing surgical activity. There is therefore need for time and effort to evaluate the emerging operative techniques and to establish the abilities and skills necessary. Some of these are likely to be the same as for open surgery, but other attributes particularly those related to visual perception and processing of an (indirect) image of the operating field and ambidexterity may be of crucial importance. MAS is technology dependent[38,39] and the surgeon therefore requires additional cognitive skills relating to the physics behind and the safe deployment of the technologies involved.

Advanced MAS is cerebrally-intensive as a great deal of mental processing is involved since surgeons have to reconstruct a three-dimensional interpretation of the anatomy and work space from a two-dimensional indirect image. The perceptual ability and processing required together with the magnified field slows the execution and endoscopic procedures require more time than conventional surgery. Increased concentration and constant mental processing introduces the fatigue factor[40] which may affect judgement, behaviour and dexterity. Studies are needed to investigate and quantify this problem. The optimal personality type, temperament, and perceptual and psychomotor skills for endoscopic surgery also need to be defined.

Restrictions in endoscopic surgery —

With the current technology there are three major restrictions which degrade task performance in endoscopic surgery: kinematic, sensory feedback and impaired visual perception.

Kinematic restriction

The limited degrees of freedom impose a significant kinematic restriction during endoscopic surgical manipulation[39,41] – only 4° of freedom are possible with the access ports and instruments in current use, contrasting sharply with the 20° of freedom with the unrestricted arm–hand combination in open surgery. The human arm–hand combination has 'mechanical redundancy' imparting a high manoeuvrability and control of forces exerted on tissues and the ability to grasp, roll, twist and re-grasp an object between fingers, essential for delicate tasks such as tissue approximation by suturing.

Diminished sensory feedback

Haptic feedback, which is essential for the controlled highly precise movements, is dependent on two sensory input systems. The proprioceptive system records and transmits information on limb joint angles, muscle contraction and tension, thereby enabling the continuous adjustment of forces applied to the tissues. The exterioceptive system provides feedback information on deformation and temperature changes at the contact interface. This affects orientation, manoeuvrability and the ability to identify the nature of component structures and tissue planes. The direct tactile feedback (hand to tissue) is lost and indirect tactile feedback (through the instruments) is considerably diminished during endoscopic surgery.[42] Reaction forces at the tip can be negligible compared to friction at the instrument entry point or forces needed to move the mass of the instrument and the unsupported hand and arm. The fulcrum effect of the long instrument handle can also reduce sensory input.[41]

Impaired visual perception

This is still an inadequately researched area. The following constraints may affect task performance in endoscopic surgery:

- *Loss of normal direct vision*: especially binocular retinal disparity which impairs depth perception.
- *Reduced field of view compared to ordinary unrestricted sight*: results in a decrease in sensory input leading to inaccurate spatial orientation. It is equivalent to tunnel vision.
- *Altered view point* which may result in mismatch between the sensory space (as perceived by the monitor) and motor space (actual work space), and adversely affects spatial judgements by the surgeon.[41]
- *Disturbed display-control correspondence*: the entry points of the instruments do not correspond with the optical axis of the endoscope. Azimuth angle and the elevation angle of the instrument are important for the ease of manipulations by the surgeon.
- *Display location*: leads to improper location of the surgeon's eyes and hands relative to the visual display which may affect task performance in endoscopic surgery.
- *Accommodation and eye movement problems*: inherent to viewing of indirect images on a TV monitor.[43]

Perception of endoscopic images ———

An indirect image is defined as 'an optical image formed by the *apparent* divergence of rays from a point, rather than their *actual* divergence from a point'.[44] This is encountered when an object is viewed through a lens system. Although this may appear to be at a particular distance from the viewer, there is no real object at that site. All telescopes and microscopes present an indirect image to the user whether this is focused directly on the retina or is displayed on a TV screen. The sensory stimulations (visual cues) are in this sense indirect since the photons forming the image reach the retinae from displayed representations rather than real objects. Furthermore, the display structure limitations such as resolution of the system, including the monitor, influence this indirect sensory stimulation since the resolving power of the human eye (1 min. arc on standard Snellen acuity) is automatically degraded to the resolution of the display. Thus there is a varying reduction of visual cues available for interpretation by the brain. In a classic experiment Holloway *et al.*[2] presented an indirect equivalent to the Snellen eye chart to subjects wearing head-mounted displays and showed them to be legally blind!

Accommodation problems have been studied in relation to head-up displays (HUD) and helmet-mounted displays (HMD) by Edgar[43] *et al.* Some individuals focus (accommodate) inappropriately on both HUD and HMD image display. This problem is more pronounced if the user has to mentally process the image as surgeons have to do during endoscopic surgery. The consequences of inappropriate accommodation are:

- Misperceptions of size and distance of objects in the 'real world' which is obviously important in surgical manipulations; and
- Loss of contrast sensitivity so that targets (structures) of low contrast may be missed. Thus in surgery, as in airline pilots, if the accommodation level is

inappropriate to the distance of the object, the image will appear blurred, and if the contrast is low, important anatomical landmarks may be missed.

The level of accommodation (focusing of the lens by the ciliary muscle) is controlled by the dual (sympathetic and parasympathetic) innervation of the ciliary smooth muscle. Accommodation is traditionally expressed in dioptres (D) which is the reciprocal of the focusing distance in metres. The accommodation oculomotor reflex responds to both physical and psychological factors.

Psychic or proximal accommodation

The individual's knowledge of the proximity of an object or scene also affects accommodation to a different extent in different individuals. An extreme example of proximal accommodation is provided by the difficulties which some individuals have with over-accommodating when using optical instruments such as micro-scopes and telescopes. This effect has been well documented and is referred to as *instrument myopia*.[45] Several other studies have demonstrated that knowledge of 'nearness' or 'thinking near' can influence the level of accommodation, at least in some people.[46,47] If subjects are required to process mentally an indirect image, then accommodation shows a strong tendency to lapse towards the subject.[48] This effect is probably very important in endoscopic surgery as the surgeon has to process the complex visual information continuously. However, it has never been studied in this context.

Visual perceptual cues ————————

These include monocular depth (pictorial) cues, distance and stereoscopic cues.

Stereoscopic cues

These are important for near-object perception and consist of retinal disparity and visuomotor cues (accommodation and convergence).

Retinal or binocular disparity: this stems from the fact that the eyes see the world and objects therein from two different positions and refers to the differences in an object-image that exist between corresponding areas of the two retinae. This binocular disparity inevitably follows from the geometry of the physical situation. The disparity becomes more marked, the closer the object viewed is to the observer and becomes less so as the distance increases. Thus beyond 30 feet, the eyes (which are then almost parallel) receive the same image and there is no disparity between the two retinal images. In near vision, binocular disparity is a powerful cue of depth perception.

Convergence: is the horizontal and inward rotation (optical alignment) of the eyes when objects are viewed at close range. It is automatically accompanied by changes in accommodation. The opposite, *divergence*, is the outward rotation of the eyes to an almost parallel alignment when viewing objects at a distance.

Collectively convergence and divergence are sometimes referred to as *vergence* in the literature.

Monocular visual depth cues

Depth can also be perceived by one eye. There are many monocular depth (pictorial) cues which can be interpreted from a single image and these are used by people who have lost sight in one eye and enable these individuals to play sport, drive cars, operate machinery etc. Generally these people are able to judge distances and objects correctly with normal (direct viewing). Indeed there is good evidence that individuals who have been single sighted since birth can and do perceive 3-D. Examples of monocular depth or pictorial cues are perspective, overlapping or interposition, shadows, relative sizes of objects, motion parallax, optic flow, texture gradients and viewpoint variability.

Motion provides added information about the spatial arrangement and this follows from the optical geometry of the situation. As we move our heads from right to left, the images of objects visualized will move across the retina. This provides a powerful depth cue which is known as *motion parallax*. As we move through space (e.g. passenger in a car), objects and scenery seem to move in a direction opposite to us, and objects close to us move much more quickly than those at a distance. Motion parallax has been shown to enhance depth perception in indirect imaging. Another motion-related depth cue is *optic flow* which is experienced when we move towards or away from objects. These appear larger as we get nearer and smaller as we move away from them.

Degradation on monocular depth cues by standard image displays

The same monocular depth cues are captured by the telescope-CCD camera but when displayed as an indirect 2-D image on a CRT, many of these depth cues are lost and the viewer sees a flat image. The reason for this is that perception of these monocular depth cues is grossly impaired or overridden by the *flatness cues* or *anti-cues* imposed by the monitor (display medium). These include the edge of the television set which is on the same plane as the image, reflections from the surface of the screen and degraded resolution.

Abolition of these flatness cues in an image display system will considerably enhance depth perception without the need for binocular depth cues. This can be achieved by three techniques.

- *Considerable enhancement of the resolution.* Digital enhancement acts in this way but degrades colour and luminance. High Definition TV will be much more effective but is unlikely to be a practical proposition in the short term.
- *VISTRAL development.* This involves the creation of a 'frame' consisting of a non-distracting interference pattern around the edge of the image display which appears to float in front or behind the image (although it is actually in the same plane as the image). This 'optical' plane obscures the edge of the television set and dissociates the image from its immediate surroundings.

Although the physics of this phenomenon were described and proven only a few years ago, this effect was known to the renaissance artist Melozzo di Forli whose famous 3-D frescoes at the Church of Loreto clearly exploit this phenomenon.
- *Suspended Image System (SIS)*. This is the most exciting development which eliminates the flatness cues by suspending the image in space. It uses the catadioptric collimator principle involving hemispherical or flat mirrors and advanced beam splitter technology. No screen is required and the image can be positioned over the patient. Although a laboratory version is available, it will require at least two years of further development before, a clinical prototype comes on stream.

Psychomotor skills in endoscopic surgery

Currently there are no data upon which an evaluation of the component cognitive, visuo-spatial, perceptual and psychomotor skills required for efficient and safe execution of endoscopic operations can be defined. On *a priori* grounds which are backed, to some extent, by clinical experience in endoscopic surgery and in the training of surgeons in MAS, the following abilities are likely to be important and certainly require investigation.

- *Manipulative abilities*: steadiness, aiming, two-hands co-ordination (ambidexterity), manual dexterity.
- *Visuo-spatial and perceptual abilities*: with special consideration to depth perception, eye accommodation and vergence for imaging and processing of indirect image information.
- *Eye–hand co-ordination*: in a magnified field.

The level of skill required to perform component surgical tasks is likely to be of a higher order than that for open conventional surgery, since the necessary controlled manipulations are more difficult due to the restrictions referred to earlier. Thus it is much more difficult to suture and tie knots endoscopically than it is by direct vision during open conventional surgery.[49] Undoubtedly, the skills required will include all those recognized as important for open conventional surgery on the assumption that an endoscopic surgeon must be trained to equivalent competence with both approaches. It does seem likely that MAS will require additional skills or enhancement of the level of certain component skills. Thus, for example, ambidexterity may be more important in endoscopic than in open surgery.

Selection, training and evaluation of surgical trainees

The important issues here are selection of candidates for a surgical career, the trainers, the training system itself, assessment of competence and in-service training.

Selection of candidates – aptitude testing

In many Western countries employers use aptitude tests for recruitment to key positions especially when these entail the possession of special cognitive and psychomotor skills. This aptitude-based recruitment is used by industry, the civil service and the armed forces, but not by the medical profession, although it is employed by Dental Schools[50-52] and there has been in recent years a renewed interest in evaluating specific aptitude tests to improve on the current selection of surgical trainees.[53-55] With the implementation of the Calman report and the consequent reduction in the duration of the training programme, the need for more efficient and effective selection of candidates to minimize wastage is obvious.

Within the UK, the need for personality assessment techniques and aptitude testing in the selection of surgical trainees was raised during an Anglo-Dutch symposium held in 1987[56] although no practical development has since ensued. Until a few years ago, the criteria used for the 'short listing' of applicants for surgical training in the Netherlands[57,58] were as follows.

- *Intelligence*: verbal, spatial and numerical.
- *Operative skill*: dexterity, psychomotor ability, and attention and concentration.
- *Stability and organization*: emotional stability (stress tolerance), common sense (sound judgement), organization and planning ability (time management).
- *Work attitude*: motivation (professional/academic), accuracy and carefulness, and energy, drive, stamina.
- *Co-operation*: stability (team spirit), independence (leadership), self-criticism, empathy (patients).

The short listing procedure was based on a structured questionnaire and psychotechnical tests. The *questionnaire* obtained basic information on university career, grades, medical experience, age, stress of surgical training and job, team work and discipline, leisure activities and dexterity. The *psychotechnical tests* were designed to assess cognitive factors by paper and pencil tests. Dexterity and stress tolerance were judged with the aid of computer tracking tests. In a memory task the candidate had to co-ordinate two activities simultaneously.

The applicants were ranked by their performance on this initial assessment by two psychologists and this ranking was used as the basis for short listing candidates for formal interview by the Central Selection Committee composed of a panel of five surgeons and a psychologist.

Although there has not been any published account of the outcome following the adoption of such a system, it appears that this approach to selection of surgical trainees has been given up in the Netherlands. It was an overambitious and rather complex system of selection which stressed the cognitive and intellectual qualities of the prospective trainees unduly and paid insufficient attention to other aspects of psychomotor skill and personality type.

Predictors of clinical competence

Valid prediction of clinical competence has proved to be difficult. Keck investigated the relationship between the clinical performance by physicians of different specialties and the criteria used by the medical school admissions and promotions committees.[59] He utilized a seven-point scale to evaluate the performance of the residents with cognitive and non-cognitive performance measures to predict the competence of medical students. He observed that the combination of cognitive and non-cognitive predictor variables is more valuable than any individual variable or even any specific class of variables in predicting the postgraduate clinical performance of physicians.

Academic achievement should not be the only parameter of surgical competence. Wingard and Williamson found little or no correlation between the undergraduate grades and subsequent career performance in their review of the literature for the period 1955–1972.[5] Furthermore, no correlation was found between the surgical residents' performances in the American Board of Surgery In-Training Examination (ABSITE) and the residents' overall clinical performance.[4] Academic predictors do not correlate with internship performance[60] or surgical ratings.[25]

As the clinical clerkship may be the only surgical experience obtained by many trainees, Schwartz and Gonella argued that Departments of Surgery should identify the knowledge, skills and attitudes germane to that discipline and then make certain that each student achieves the predetermined level of competence that the faculty deems necessary for all physicians regardless of their future career direction.[61] Clinical competence has customarily been measured by two separate parameters: knowledge as measured by objective examination and clinical performance subjectively appraised by the bedside demonstration of applied knowledge and skills. The relatively low correlation between these may represent an independent measurement of the different components of competence.

Assessment of technical skills

Technical skills can be evaluated by a variety of assessment procedures categorized by Watts and Feldman[62] as follows.

- *Procedural lists/log books*: the trainee is required to log those procedures actually performed by him. This allows the training institution some degree of certainty that the trainee has accumulated the necessary experience in performing the required procedures. Although there is some relationship between practice and competence, the simple listing of procedures performed has no training value, and is therefore of low validity.
- *Direct observation without criteria*: this method is more valid than mere log books. However, it requires a substantial manpower (observer) resource and suffers from low inter- and intra-observer variations.
- *Direct observation with checklists*: this is the most useful technique of assessment of technical skills. Each step involved is written down in advance by a group of experts and the trainee is assessed with the checklist at hand to determine whether the trainee enacts the component steps of the procedure in the correct sequence and with the required level of competence. This method has high inter-rater reliability and high validity. In practical terms, such an assessment may be undertaken within a dedicated skills unit.

- *Direct observation using synthetic or animal models with checklists*: there are three reasons for the use of simulation devices: standardization of the technical exercise or assessment problem; avoidance of risks to or lack of availability of real patients; and abolition of ethical problems. The technical exercise simulations, in particular, can permit an additional assessment of outcome rather than process which does not require an observer. This method has high reliability and validity which are, however, related to the realism of the simulated task.
- *Videotape assessment of performance (patients or animals)*: this entails extra costs but has high reliability and validity. When used on procedures performed on animals, both reliability and validity are proportional to the degree of realism. Liu *et al.* used videotapes to evaluate clinical performance in anaesthesia[63] and developed checklists for spinal anaesthesia (49 items) and anaesthetic set-up/machine checkout (43 items). The reliability (using an interclass correlation) was 0.75 for the spinal anaesthesia checklist and 0.83 for the machine set-up checklist.

Winckel *et al.* designed a two-part structured technical skills assessment form.[64] Part I, which is completed while an operation is in progress consists of the essential components of the procedure. Part II, completed at the end of the operation, is a 10-point global rating form. Inter-assessor reliability of both Parts I and II was high (0.78 and 0.73 respectively). Statistically significant differences were noted between senior resident and junior resident performances, suggesting contrast validity.

Training system and trainers ———

Training system

There is a need for revision of the surgical training system and although all are in agreement, views differ on content and nature within the changed time span dictated by the implementation of the Calman report. The clinical apprenticeship system must remain although restructuring is needed to ensure that progress in competence can be better assessed.[65,66] In the training of basic surgical skills (open and endoscopic) '*ex-vivo* standards of proficiency should be demonstrated before *in vivo* performance is sanctioned'.[67] This entails the setting up of regional Skills Centres operating in association with the Royal Colleges and run by a dedicated team of full-time technician tutors. These skills courses should be intercalated within the surgical training programme such that trainees would attend basic (initiation), advanced and specialty-related skills courses at strategic intervals in their training programme. The emphasis in all these courses is on hands-on training. The objectives are to ensure that component surgical tasks are performed to an acceptable standard, and the principles governing the safe use of the ancillary technology used in endoscopic surgery are acquired. It is far better to acquire the skill for performing an anastomosis (endoscopic or open) using animal tissues in the skills laboratory than doing it first time, even under supervision, on a human.

The clinical operative training in MAS is very time consuming and requires special consideration. The pressure on time has proved a disincentive for busy consultants to take their juniors through specific operations on a regular basis. This restriction within NHS Trusts has to be recognized and the introduction of *Training Initiative Lists* by MATTUS has dealt with this problem. Within this scheme, Hospital Trusts with recognized College appointed Tutors in Minimal Access Therapy, can apply for funds to run these operating sessions (up to 80 per year) which are extra to service lists. The undertaking is that the operating sessions concerned are performed by trainees with designated consultants as preceptors and with detailed feedback on each session regarding the trainee's performance and indeed on the preceptor himself by the trainee.

Trainers

Much has been said but little of substance written concerning trainers and the need for 'training the trainers'. The latter exercise is applicable to the teaching of cognitive skills but seems incongruous to training in technical operative skills. In an ideal world one would have the luxury to select trainers, since undoubtedly, as we all know from our training experience, some are better than others and a few should be exempted from this responsibility. The existing system of surgical tutors needs expansion in line with the development initiated by the Minimal Access Therapy Training Unit for Scotland (MATTUS) where all the practising surgeons, interventional endoscopists and interventional radiologists within Scotland were invited to apply for consideration by the Scottish Royal Colleges for honorary appointment as Clinical Tutors in their specialty. Aside from their active involvement in the clinical and operative training in minimal access therapy within their hospitals, this large substantive identified tutoring resource provides the Scottish Royal Colleges and the Chief Executive Group in charge of MATTUS with active and on-going input on the training programme at 'shop-floor' level via the Scottish Training Board for Minimal Access Therapy (STBMAT) made up of two representatives from each specialty and chaired by the Director of MATTUS. Some of the tutors play an additional active role as preceptors to consultants in various hospitals and others contribute to skills training courses in Dundee on a regular basis.

Credentialling, privileges, proctors and preceptors

Credentialling is the process operated at hospital/institution level in North America by which privileges are granted for the performance of specific operations by individual attending surgeons within specific hospitals. Details of the Hospital Credentialling Committees (HCC) vary quite considerably, although the majority operate in accordance with guidelines issued by Specialty Associations and the American College of Surgeons.[68,69] In this respect the Society of American Gastrointestinal Endoscopic Surgeons (SAGES) has been at the forefront in formulating guidelines for safe practice in endoscopic surgery as has the European Association for Endoscopic Surgery (EAES).

It has to be said that 'operating on fellow human beings is never a right but always a privilege' and the granting of privileges in accordance with confirmed specialist training and competence should become the norm within the UK and replace the present ad hoc arrangements. The benefits would include reduced litigation and improve clinical outcome. Concerns have been raised, quite justifiably, regarding the possible abuse of such HCC which have to operate at local Trust level within the Surgical Directorates. Issues relating to composition, precise remit and modus operandi of HCCs require to be addressed nationally. If introduced within the NHS, HCCs would have to be structured such that they accommodate the needs of the surgeons and are prescriptive as well as restrictive, thereby stimulating continuing education and in-service training. In withholding the award of procedure-related privileges for specific operations, endoscopic or otherwise, the HCC would have the responsibility to outline the additional surgical training required before re-application.

The practice of expert-lead induction and assistance of consultant surgeons embarking on new endoscopic procedures safeguards both the surgeons and the patients. The scheme is eminently feasible within the NHS and should be funded at either Trust or National level. Even in this context confusion reigns supreme and the need for 'proctors' and 'preceptors' is voiced in many forums and conferences as if these were synonomous.[70] As a profession we should foster and strive for preceptoring but be very wary of proctoring since the functions of the two are very different. According to the Oxford Dictionary, a preceptor is 'one who instructs; a teacher, tutor' whereas a proctor is identified as a 'syncopated form of procurator'. In Oxford and Cambridge Universities proctors 'are charged with various functions, especially with the discipline of all persons *in statu pupillari*, and the summary punishment of minor offences'. In law proctor is defined 'as one whose profession is to manage the causes of others in a court administering civil or canon law'; the legal implications of these two very diverse activities are obvious. Recognition and appointment of preceptors should be considered by the Royal Colleges and such appointments should be procedure and specialty related.

Following on the reported total of 159 adverse incidents following laparoscopic cholecystectomy between August 1990 and March 1992 to the State's Department of Health (as required by legislation), strict guidelines were issued concerning credentialling, training and competence to all surgeons and institutions within the State of New York. These guidelines refer to the 'institution competence in being able to support endoscopic operations'. This is specified in terms of staff training, caseload, equipment, information systems and quality assurance.[71] The Working Party on Minimal Access Surgery: Implications for the NHS[72] endorsed this view.

Guidelines for safe surgical practice

It is often stated that surgery is both an art and a science. In truth and certainly from the patients' viewpoint 'surgery is a controlled assault on human beings whose consent is obtained under the duress of pain, suffering, disability and fear of death'. Safe practice in both open and endoscopic surgery minimizes the severity of this assault and herein lies the advantage of MAS. Irrespective of the nature of the intervention, strict selection and surgical competence are crucial and reflect the quality of the training and the code of practice. The granting of privileges for special operations, endoscopic or open, a low threshold for elective conversion to the open approach during minimal access surgery, the Achilles heel of this approach,[73] sustained case load to reach and maintain the necessary level of expertise and dedicated facilities for endoscopic surgery will go a long way to reducing morbidity and maximizing benefit following surgical interventions. These considerations together with revision of surgical training programmes and adequate facilities and resources for in-service training and continuing education will steer surgical practice in the right direction as we approach the next century.

References

1. Barnes RW. Surgical handicraft: teaching and learning surgical skills. *Am J Surg* 1987; **153**: 422–427.
2. Norman GR. Defining competence: a methodological review. In: Neufield VR, Norman GR (eds), *Assessing Clinical Competence*, Springer, New York, 1985, pp. 15–35.
3. Spencer RW. Deductive reasoning in the lifelong continuing education of a cardiovascular surgeon. *Arch Surg* 1976; **111**: 1177–1183.
4. Lazar HL, DeLand EC, Tompkins PK. Clinical performance versus in-training examinations as measures of surgical competence. *Surgery* 1980; **87**: 357–362.
5. Wingard JR, Williamson JW. Grades as predictions of physicians' career performance: an evaluative literature Review. *J Med Educ* 1973; **48**: 311–322.
6. Spencer FC. Competence and compassion: two qualities of surgical excellence. *Bull Am Coll Surg* 1979; **64**: 15–22.
7. Greenburg AG, McClure DK, Penn NE. Personality traits of surgical house officer: faculty and resident views. *Surgery* 1982; **92**: 368–372.
8. Anwar RAH, Bosk C, Greenburg AG. Resident evaluation; is it, can it; should it be objective? *J Surg Res* 1981; **30**: 27–41.
9. Kopta JA. The development of motor skills in orthopaedic education. *Clin Orth* 1971; **75**: 80–85.
10. Kopta JA. An approach to the evalution of operative skills. *Surgery* 1971; **70**: 297–303.
11. Albo D, Taylor CW, Page B, Chang FC, Moody FG. Multifactor evaluations of surgical trainees and teaching services. *Surgery* 1976; **80**: 115–121.
12. Russell RCG. Surgical technique. *Br J Surg* 1987; **74**: 763–764.
13. Matheson NA. Surgical technique. *Br J Surg* 1987; **74**: 1190 (letter).
14. McKeown KC. Surgical research in training. *Br J Surg* 1988; **75**: 396.
15. Pettigrew RA, Burns HJG, Carter DC. Evaluating surgical risk: the importance of technical factors in determining the outcome. *Br J Surg* 1987; **74**: 791–794.
16. Fielding LP, Stewart-Brown S, Blesovsky L, Kearney G. Anastomotic integrity after operations for large-bowel cancer: a multicentre study. *Br Med J* 1980; **2**: 411–414.
17. McArdle CS, Hole D. Impact of variability among surgeons on postoperative morbidity and mortality and ultimate survival. *Br Med J* 1991; **302**: 1501–1505.
18. Fleishman EA. Human abilities and the

acquisition of skill. In: Bilodeau EA (ed.), *Acquisition of Skill*, Academic Press, New York, 1966, pp. 147–167.

19. Fleishman EA, Ellison GD. A factor analysis of manipulative tests. *J Appl Psychol* 1962; **46**: 96–105.

20. Bourassa GL, Guion RM. A factorial study of dexterity tests. *J Appl Psychol* 1959; **43**: 199–204.

21. Kaufaman HH, Wiegand RL, Tunick RH. Teaching Surgeons to operate – principles of psychomotor skills training. *Acta Neuochir* 1987; **87**: 1–7.

22. Krepsi YP, Levine TM, Einhorn RK, Mitrani M. Surgical aptitude test for otolaryngology – head and neck surgery resident applicants. *Laryngoscope* 1986; **96**: 1201–1206.

23. Steele RJC, Walder C, Herbert M. Psychomotor testing and the ability to perform an anastomosis in junior surgical trainees. *Br J Surg* 1992; **79**: 1065–1067.

24. Gibbons RD, Baker RJ, Skinner DB. Field articulation testing: a predictor of technical skills in surgical residents. *J Surg Res* 1986; **41**: 53–57.

25. Schuenman AL, Pickleman J, Hesslein R, Freeark RJ. Neuropsychologic predictors of operative skill among general surgery residents. *Surgery* 1984; **96**: 288–295.

26. Deary IJ, Graham KS, Maran AGD. Relationships between surgical ability ratings and spatial abilities and personality. *J R Coll Surg Edin* 1992; **37**: 74–79.

27. Gardner RW, Jackson CN, Messick SJ. Personality organisation in cognitive controls and intellectual abilities. *Psychol Issues* 1960; **2**: 1.

28. Bennet GK, Seashore HG, Wesman AG. *Manual for the Differential Aptitude Test*, New York Psychological Corp: New York, 1966.

29. Harris CJ, Herbert M, Steele RJC. Psychomotor skills of surgical trainees compared with those of different medical specialists. *Br J Surg* 1994; **81**: 382–383.

30. Smoker WRK, Berbaum KS, Luebke NH, Jacoby CG. Spatial perception testing in diagnostic-radiology. *AJR* 1984; **143**: 1105–1109.

31. Berbaum KS, Smoker WRK, Smith WL. Measurement and prediction of diagnostic performance during radiology training. *AJR* 1985; **145**: 1305–1311.

32. Bock RD, Kolakowski D. Further evidence of sex-linked major-gene influence on human spatial visualisation ability. *Am J Hum Genet* 1970; **25**: 1–14.

33. Hartlage LC. Sex linked inheritance of spatial ability. *Percept Motor Skills* 1970; **31**: 610.

34. Stafford RE. Sex differences in spatial visualisation as evidence of sex-linked inheritance. *Percept Motor Skills* 1961; **13**: 428.

35. Long, GM. Rod-and-Frame test performance among naval aviation personnel. *Percept Motor Skills* 1975; **41**: 950.

36. Squire D, Giachino AA, Profitt AW, Heaney C. Objective comparison of manual dexterity in physicians surgeons. *Can J Surg* 1989; **32**: 467–476.

37. Schuenman AL, Pickleman J, Freeark RJ. Age, gender, lateral dominance and prediction of operative skill among general surgery residents. *Surgery* 1985; **98**: 506–515.

38. Treat MR. New technologies and future developments for endoscopic surgery. In: Greene FL, Ponsky JL (eds), *Endoscopic Surgery*, WB Saunders, Philadelphia 1994, pp. 518–528.

39. Patkin M, Isabel L. The ergonomics, engineering and surgery of endoscopical dissection. A paper presented at the Annual Scientific Meeting of the Royal Australasian College of Surgeons, Hobart, May 1994, 1–22.

40. Cuschieri A. Whither minimal access surgery: tribulations and expectations. *Am J Surg* 1995; **169**: 9–19.

41. Tendick F, Jennings RW, Tharp G, Stark L. Sensing and manipulation problems in endoscopic surgery: Experiment, analysis and observation. *Presence* 1993; **2**: 66–81.

42. Cuschieri A. Ergonomics of minimal access surgery. *Surgery* 1993; 526–528.

43. Edgar GK, Pope JCD, Craig IR. Visual accommodation problems with head-up

and helmet-mounted displays? *Displays* 1994; **15**: 68–75.

44. Edgar GK, Neary C, Craig I, Pope JCD. Oculo-motor responses and virtual image displays. *AGARD Conference proceedings*, 1993; 18–1 to 18–8.

45. Hennessy RT. Instrument myopia. *J Opt Soc Am* 1975; **65**: 1114–1120.

46. Rosenfield M, Cuiffreda KJ. Proximal and cognitively induced accommodation. *Ophthalmic Physiol Opt* 1990; **10**: 252–256.

47. Malmstrom FV, Randle RJ. Effects of visual imagery on the accommodation response. *Percept Psychophys* 1976; **19**: 450–453.

48. Holloway R, Fuchs H, Robinett W. Virtual-worlds research at the University of North Carolina at Chapel Hill. *Proceedings of the Computer Graphics Conference*, London 1991, pp. 181–196.

49. Crosthwaite G, Chung T, Dunkley P, Shimi S, Cuschieri A. Comparison of the effect of direct vision and electronic 2-D and 3-D imaging on task efficiency in endoscopic surgery. *Br J Surg* 1995; **82**: 849–851.

50. Thompson GW, Ahlawat K, Buie R. Evaluation of the dental aptitude test components as predictors of dental school performance. *J Canad Dent Assn* 1979; 407–409.

51. Wong AY, Watson JF, Thye RP. Evaluation of Predictor variables for a self-instructional preclinical course. *J Dent Educ* 1979; **43**: 637–640.

52. Deubert LW, Smith MC, Jenkins CB, Berry DC. The selection of dental students: a pilot study of an assessment of potential manual ability by psychometric tests. *Br Dent J* 1975; **139**: 167–170.

53. Graham KS, Deary IJ. A role of aptitude testing in surgery? *J R Coll Surg Edinb* 1991; **36**: 70–74.

54. Gough MH, Bell J. Introducing aptitude testing into medicine. *Br Med J* 1989; **298**: 975–976.

55. Grace DM. Aptitude testing in surgery. *Can J Surg* 1989; **32**: 396–397.

56. Gough MH, Holdsworth R, Keeman JN, Lagaay MB, Van de Loo RPJM, Droog A. Personality assessment technique and aptitude testing as aids to the selection of surgical trainees. *Ann R Coll Surg Engl* 1988; **70**: 265–279.

57. Keeman JN, Lagaay MB. Candidate selection for surgical training in The Netherlands. *Ann R Coll Surg Engl* 1988; **70**: 275–277.

58. Van de Loo RPJM. Selection of trainees in the Netherlands. *Ann R Coll Surg Engl* 1988; **70**: 277–279.

59. Keck JW, Arnold L, Willoughby L, Calkins V. Efficacy of cognitive/non-cognitive measures in predicting resident/physician performance. *J Med Educ* 1979; **54**: 759–765.

60. Korman M, Stubblefield RL. Medical school evaluation and internship performance. *J Med Educ* 1971; **46**: 670–673.

61. Schwartz GF, Gonnella JC. Measurement of clinical competence in the surgical clerkship. *J Med Educ* 1973; **48**: 762–763.

62. Watts J, Feldman WB. Assessment of technical skills. In: Neufield VR, Norman GR (eds), *Assessing clinical competence*, Springer, New York, 1985, pp. 259–274.

63. Liu P, Miller E, Herr G, Hardy C, Sivarajan M, Willenkin R. Videotape reliability: a method of evaluation of a clinical performance examination. *J Med Educ* 1980; **55**: 713–715.

64. Winckel CP, Rezinck RK, Cohen R, Taylor B. Reliability and construct validity of a structured technical skills assessment form. *Am J Surg* 1994; **167**: 423–427.

65. Forde KA. Endosurgical training methods: is it surgical training that is out of hand? *Endosc Surg* 1993; **7**: 71–72.

66. Cuschieri A. Reflections on surgical training. *Surg Endosc* 1993; **7**: 73–74.

67. Walt AJ. New technology: temptations, challenges and educational implications. *Surg Endosc* 1994; **8**: 1375–1379.

68. SAGES Guidelines for granting of privileges for laparoscopic (peritoneoscopic) general surgery. *Surg Endosc* 1993; **7**: 67–68.

69. American College of Surgeons: State-

ments on emerging surgical technologies and the evaluation of credentials. *Surg Endosc* 1995; **9**: 207–208.

70. Satava RM. Proctors, preceptors, and laparoscopic surgery. *Surg Endosc* 1993; **7**: 283–284.

71. State of New York. Department of Health Memorandum, Health Facilities Series H-18; New York 1992.

72. Minimal Access Surgery: Implications for the NHS. HMSO, Edinburgh, 1993.

73. Morgenstern L. Achilles' heel and laparoscopic surgery. *Surg Endosc* 1995; **9**: 383.

4a

Practical aspects of laparoscopic surgery training in the UK

C.G. Fowler

Introduction

With an increase in the number of operations performed endoscopically, and the number of surgeons performing them, surgical training became a matter for public debate in the United Kingdom, with an alleged failure of general surgeons to train properly for laparoscopic surgery. Why has this happened? Has training for laparoscopic surgery been inadequate? If it has, what can we do about it?

The introduction of laparoscopic cholecystectomy in the UK

Almost every article written about the introduction of laparoscopic cholecystectomy uses terms like 'explosive' and 'revolution'. That such intemperate language seems appropriate is due, of course, to the speed at which laparoscopic cholecystectomy became established but it is also a consequence of the overall complexity and surgical hazards of the technique and the low level of existing expertise. The introduction of fibreoptic endoscopy can be seen as revolutionary in retrospect but it caused little public concern at the time, largely because the complications of a failed gastroscopy were usually comparatively minor and patients were generally less well informed about these matters. In the early 1980s, percutaneous renal surgery became part of routine urological practice with similar rapidity but urologists were already skilled in endoscopy. There was little discussion of complications outside the profession and barely a ripple in the collective consciousness. In each case the procedures were rapidly included in the traditional, apprenticeship-style, surgical training.

The development of training in the UK

The introduction of laparoscopic cholecystectomy in the UK[1] coincided with an upheaval in the internal financing of the National Health Service.[2] Surgeons were under pressure to 'run before they could walk'.[3] The major instrument companies responded by organizing courses in laparoscopic surgery and sponsored courses run by enthusiastic pioneers. Many surgeons travelled abroad to learn.

In December 1990, the Royal College of Surgeons of England issued a report welcoming the development of minimal access surgery (MAS).[4] The Colleges' suggest guidelines for training in laparoscopic surgery including attending gynaecological laparoscopic lists and laboratory skills training. The newly founded Society of Minimally Invasive General Surgeons arranged two-day laparoscopic cholecystectomy seminars around the country in an early attempt to standardize course content.[5] These courses included didactic lectures, training on simulators and assisting in the operating theatre.

Because there was no centralized monitoring of these courses, it is difficult to obtain precise information about the take-up of such training in the UK. In December 1993, a questionnaire on laparoscopic cholecystectomy was circulated to all Fellows of The Royal College of Surgeons of England with a request that all those who were performing laparoscopic cholecystectomy should complete and return the form.[6] (Of the 1074 replies received, 709 were from surgeons who were routinely performing laparoscopic cholecystectomies. Some 575 were consultants and 134 were trainees; 79 (24.5 per cent) of the consultants had undertaken more than 100 procedures in the preceding year.

The respondents were asked to state how they had been trained before starting to operate independently: 486 (64.5 per cent) had attended a laparoscopic workshop. Whether these were undertaken in centres abroad was not recorded. Of the consultants, 458 (79.5 per cent) had assisted a colleague already experienced in the technique and 421 (73 per cent) had also been supervised by a trained colleague. Almost all of the 26 (5 per cent) of consultants who had neither attended a workshop nor watched a colleague operating were pioneers of the technique in this country who had travelled abroad to watch the technique. Many of these largely self-taught surgeons were now running courses in this country. Only half the trainees had attended a laparoscopic workshop though all had both assisted and been assisted in procedures.

One must always be circumspect about data from questionnaires, but this survey indicates that most UK surgeons who replied did undergo some special training before attempting to operate independently. There is also evidence from the trainees that the procedure is already being taught by example and assistance in the traditional way. Do we need unusual arrangements for training in laparoscopic surgery? Is it a special case?

Quality and consistency

The main argument for overhauling training in laparoscopic surgery is the difficulty in assessing the quality of the training which is available. Although there are many well-established workshops in the UK, their content is variable. Many are sponsored, at least in part, by instrument manufacturers who have no effective way of controlling the format or faculty. A certificate of attendance on a course whose educational content is unknown is almost worthless both to the surgeon and to those who use his or her services. There is therefore a powerful argument for regularizing the objectives, content and assessment of laparoscopic training.

But the proposition applies equally strongly to other significant surgical innovations which require training. The Senate of The Royal Surgical Colleges of Great Britain and Ireland, a body representing the four Royal Colleges and the Specialist Associations, addresses this point in a recent consensus on Quality Assurance[7] in which the following statement appears:

> . . . the profession has a moral and ethical obligation to address all aspects of surgical practice and to produce a system that encompasses all current and new techniques in all surgical specialties – not just Minimal Access Surgery.

The future of training in laparoscopic surgery therefore needs to be seen within the context of surgical training as a whole.

Changes in the pattern of surgical training

The period of planned surgical training in the UK has become much shorter with the implementation of the recommendations for higher specialist training of the Chief Medical Officer, Kenneth Calman.[8,9] Completion of higher specialist training will be acknowledged by the award of a Certificate of Completion of Specialist Training (CCST) after a total of seven years of surgical training. At the same time, the intensity of training is decreasing because of a welcome reduction in the hours worked by surgeons in training. A consultant-provided service further limits opportunities for trainees to learn practical skills by hands-on experience with patients in the traditional way. These are very powerful constraints to which surgical training must adapt and adapt quickly.

Although the holder of a CCST will be entitled to practice independently as a consultant, new techniques and procedures developed after an individual's training has been completed will be dealt with by the continuing professional education programme. The Senate of the Royal Surgical Colleges makes this explicit:

> We believe that the training (and therefore certification) of consultants in techniques that are developed after they have completed their training can only be effectively ensured, monitored and certified by a controlled system of continuing professional education, audit and recertification.[7]

The Colleges have introduced registration of continuing medical education (CME) with five-yearly certification of participation.

The future of laparoscopic training in the UK

Laparoscopic training represents but one part of a general need for change in surgical education. That the media have treated it as a special case has had a very important benefit. A substantial amount of public and charitable money has been made available to encourage and develop training in minimal access therapies. If this money is spent wisely, the lessons learned will be applicable to surgical training as a whole.

National training units for minimal access therapy

In early 1993, the Wolfson Foundation in partnership with the National Health Service Management Executive (and the Scottish Office in Scotland) invited bids for money to establish an unspecified number of training centres in the UK. Nearly two hundred units applied. As a result of this initiative, funding was granted to three centres.

MATTUS (Minimal Access Therapy Training Unit for Scotland) is based on an established endoscopic skills unit at Ninewells Hospital, Dundee in collaboration with the Royal Colleges of Surgeons of Edinburgh, and of Physicians and Surgeons of Glasgow. The Unit has founded its strategy on skills training by full-time skills tutors and clinical exposure of trainees within designated Units in various Scottish Hospitals. The programme has been initiated, supervised and directed by the Scottish Training Board for Minimal Access Therapy (STBMAT) which is responsible through the Chief Executive Committee to the Scottish Royal Colleges. In addition to basic and advanced skills training, procedure-related courses and specialist courses, MATTUS will sponsor clinical training through the 'Training Initiative Lists' scheme. These lists (40 sessions per annum per unit) will be conducted by preceptors appointed by the Scottish Royal Colleges on the recommendation of STBMAT. They are additional to service operating lists and will allow for the additional time required for hands-on instruction. Detailed feedback on the number of types of operation which trainees perform supervised by appointed clinical tutors will be audited in depth. These developments are in line with recommendations made by an highly respected working group set up to examine the implication of MAS for the NHS.[10]

LIMIT (Leeds Institute for Minimally Invasive Therapy) is also based on an existing establishment founded with independent charitable funds. LIMIT is developing an ambitious portfolio of courses using very extensive audio-visual links with contributing hospitals. The Unit will also co-operate with scientists at the University of Salford in the development of virtual reality training.

The Minimal Access Therapy Training Unit (MATTU) at The Royal College of Surgeons of England (RCS) is by contrast an entirely new venture. However, MATTU has been established as a consortium with The Royal London Hospital and The Royal Surrey County Hospital, Guildford both clinical units with an impressive track record for training in surgical and gynaecological endoscopy. The activities of MATTUS, LIMIT and MATTU are to be scrutinized by an outside academic assessor.

The challenge for these units is to encourage and develop training in minimal access therapy across all disciplines. Each has given laparoscopic surgery priority in its plans since this is the area of immediate public concern but the range of interest will rapidly widen. The Units are committed to working in unison but there will inevitably be differences in methodological approach.

MATTU at the Royal College of Surgeons
As seen from MATTU at the RCS, there are two medium term tasks and an interim problem to be addressed.

1. We need to exploit available and developing technology and up-to-date educational techniques to produce effective and economical instruction in laparoscopic surgery. This instruction must be standardized and assessable and form a part of the relevant programme of higher surgical training leading to CCST.
2. We need to be responsive to the development of new techniques in laparoscopic surgery and be ready to develop and define training requirements as part of CME.

And, in the shorter term:

3. We need to offer guidelines for consultants who wish to take up laparoscopic surgery and have not yet completed a satisfactory training. A related matter is the increasing demand by healthcare users for some means to recognize practitioners with appropriate training.

As a body charged with maintaining standards in surgery it is appropriate that the RCS should take a lead in this. However, nothing effective can be done without the co-operation and consent of the specialist associations which represent surgeons working in the field. Many members of the Association of Surgeons of Great Britain and Ireland (ASGBI) and the new Association of Endoscopic Surgeons of Great Britain and Ireland (AESGBI) already run respected training courses. Some of them have justifiable suspicions[11] of large centralized training units with government funding. Since laparoscopic training depends upon these experts, it is up to the centres to demonstrate the benefits of collaboration.

Laparoscopic surgery as part of higher specialist training

At the time of writing the Specialist Advisory Committee (SAC) in General Surgery is finalizing a detailed curriculum which will include training in laparoscopic surgery. It is already clear that surgical trainees are encountering laparoscopic surgery at an early stage in their career. At this stage the main requirement is for them to be taught the safety aspects and hand–eye skills which are common to all laparoscopic operations. MATTU has therefore used the development of a course on 'Basic Skills for Safe Laparoscopic Surgery' to pilot a possible approach to course development. In this MATTU is to some extent acting as a paradigm for the activities of the Raven Department of Education at The College.

Course development has been seen as a staged process:

1. A working party of experts is convened to set objectives for the courses. The working party identifies potential authors of course materials. For the first course, a handbook has been written and an instructional videotape has been produced. In time, course materials may include interactive videos, computer-led programmes and distance learning packages.
2. A core content for the course is identified and appropriate means of teaching and testing it are agreed. In a basic skills course, exercises in laparoscopic simulators are a central component backed by seminar discussions and demonstrations. Core slides and notes are provided for instructors.
3. The course is piloted and assessed.
4. Potential trainers are identified and offered training as trainers. The 'Training for trainers' courses are given by a professional educationalist working with a surgeon. In future, attendance on such a course could be a requirement for recognition as an instructor.
5. The course is made available for export to other centres to be run by recognized instructors.

Readers familiar with the Advanced Trauma and Life Support (ATLS) course may recognize this format. It provides a means of disseminating courses of known standard and content. It should allow assessment methods to be developed so that successful completion of a course will carry the same credit wherever it is taken.

If this method of course generation proves successful, it can be applied to the production of intermediate and procedure-specific training which should be developed with the relevant specialist associations. An important change in the proposed new scheme for surgical education is that much of the surgical science previously taught and examined at basic level will now be encountered during specialist training. A fundamental decision will have to be made on whether laparoscopic techniques should continue to be taught in isolation. An alternative would be to incorporate MAS into more wide-ranging system-related teaching. Thus laparoscopic cholecystectomy might reasonably be taught as an important component of a 'biliary' course. Perhaps a range of different course formats are needed. In any case, a systematic approach to course design will improve quality, consistency and assessability.

Assessment of teaching technology

As well as acting as agencies to co-ordinate course design, the training centres can also act as foci for the development of training technology. Much of this technology, like computer-assisted learning programmes, is expensive unless produced in bulk and is likely to be increasingly applied to surgical education in all its phases. In the field of laparoscopic training in particular, two developments are under evaluation. Both of them are designed to improve operating skills before the surgeon begins to operate on patients. If successful, they could obviate the need for skills training on animals.

Animal models

Many laparoscopic surgeons believe that training on a living animal model is a valuable component of skills training for laparoscopic surgery.[12] The major instrument manufacturers have set up training centres in European countries which permit animals to be used in this way. In the UK, the use of animals for training in surgical skills is controlled by the Cruelty to Animals Act (1986). The Act does not exclude surgical skills training on animals but the Notes of Guidance which accompany the Act state that 'at the present time (1986), such training is confined to the use of rodents for training in microsurgery'. In 1991, the then Presidents of The Royal Colleges advised the Home Office that training for laparoscopic cholecystectomy on living animals was not necessary on the grounds that the technique was well established and could be taught by assisting and supervised surgery on patients in the traditional way.

It is conceivable that the Home Office could be persuaded of the case for allowing surgeons to train on living animals in the UK. However, the public opprobrium which such a campaign would attract would be considerable and it is unlikely that any Minister would be prepared to take the political risk. It is therefore reasonable to assume that the present effective ban will persist and that alternatives to animal training should be sought.

Plastic body form

Remarkable progress has been made in simulating the abdominal contents using a combination of artistry and materials technology. The result is a body form which looks and behaves in many ways like the real thing. The device is equipped with exchangeable parts which can be replaced when destroyed during a simulated surgical procedure. 'Tissue' can be cut and diathermied and blood vessels can even be made to bleed.

The effectiveness of simulated tissue for laparoscopic training needs to be tested. It is most likely that the body form will be useful in teaching the details of laparoscopic operations rather than basic skills, but this also needs to be demonstrated. The simulation will need to be sufficiently convincing to give the 'feel' of operating on a patient. In the future it would, perhaps, be useful to have simulations of the minor abnormalities of anatomy which are almost routine in real surgery.

Virtual reality

The remarkable advances in computer graphics have made virtual reality training a possible reality. Virtual environments are constructed by a computer to give the user the impression of a world which is indistinguishable from reality other than by its artificial content. Since we use all our senses to sample our environment and the changes which our activities cause to it, true virtual reality involves immersion and full interactivity. In practice this level of virtual reality is not available outside fiction except for some special environments where the real environment is already presented via mechanical or electronic devices. The training simulators used to instruct power station operators are a good example of this. Every new power station has a simulated control room indistinguishable from the real one. The computer presents its version of reality via screens, dials and digital displays identical with those in the real power station. The same applies in the advanced flight trainers used by pilots converting from one airliner to another. In this case the evidence which the trainee is fed from the instruments is supplemented by visual information displayed to mimic the view outside and appropriate motion generated by hydraulic jacks acting on the simulator.

Laparoscopic surgery is potentially suitable for virtual reality training because the surgeon works from visual information from a cathode ray tube (CRT) and limited sensory information from the hand instruments. A number of promising simulations of the abdominal contents have already been produced with the possibility of limited interaction. However, some problems remain. In particular, the computing power needed to control the high quality graphics is very complex and expensive at the present time. There is still a perceptible delay as the computer refreshes the image when the surgeon makes a move. When the system is developed the texture and behaviour of tissue will need to be fully modelled and the biomechanical information needed to do this is not yet available. Most of these technical and hardware problems will probably be overcome within a very few years so long as money is made available to cover the high cost of software development.

If virtual reality does become available it could greatly extend the range of surgical training. A surgeon may be asked to deal with simulated intra-operative disasters as part of the process of recertification. Proposed new techniques could be piloted on the model. It is even possible from the results of imaging a real patient being fed into the electronic patient that pathology could be reproduced. The surgeon could then practice the procedure before performing it on the patient. It is too early to say whether most or all of this will remain fantasy for the foreseeable future. A possible way forward is to focus more closely on the skills which the surgeon must acquire for various procedures. By dissecting surgical activities into part tasks, the computer might be spared the labour of generating exact verisimilitude in the virtual environment.

Laparoscopic training in continuing medical education _____

The Senate of the Royal Surgical Colleges proposed a four part approach to new techniques: [7]

1. New techniques must be detected, through literature, communication and conference reviews, when they are first made public.
2. If a technique is considered by the profession to be sufficiently novel as to require special training and assessment before being introduced into general clinical practice, its initial clinical use should be controlled and limited to a number of specified centres for clinical trial. The Colleges are now devising the mechanisms for achieving such control.

3. During the trial the methods of training and the training requirements should be developed and defined.
4. When its value is proven, all consultants who wish to use it will be required, as part of their CME certification, to show evidence (certification) of learning via the prescribed courses and by working with surgeons in the trial centres already skilled in the technique.

It is clear that the Training Units can play an important part in this process. The first problem is to identify procedures which are truly novel and need special training. This will require collaboration between innovators and trainers which could be mediated by the units. The course development techniques described above for higher surgical training could be applied to the development and definition of training methods for new devices. Prescribed courses could then be recognized and trainers accredited.

The process is similar to that used when a new drug is developed and the simplicity of this proposal is appealing. However, there are difficulties to be overcome and these can be illustrated by considering the interim arrangements which may be needed before the scheme is fully implemented.

Interim guidelines for training in laparoscopic surgery after completion of higher surgical training

By linking training in novel techniques to recertification the Colleges have offered a possible mechanism to compel surgeons to undertake such training. At the present time, the Colleges have no such power. There is, however, pressure from health service purchasers, providers, patients and insurers to offer guidelines for training surgeons who wish to 'convert' to laparoscopic surgery. These would be analogous with those offered by the Society of American Gastrointestinal Endoscopic Surgeons[13] and if agreed would provide a basis for assessing whether the surgeon had trained appropriately. It would then be the responsibility of health-care providers to ensure that the training of their staff conformed to these guidelines and purchasers would be likely to demand this as a quality standard.

The first difficulty is in identifying which procedures have completed the necessary evaluation to warrant guidelines for general training to be issued. Laparoscopic cholecystectomy most nearly fulfils the criteria and it is widely accepted in surgical practice. It therefore seems appropriate to issue guidelines for training in laparoscopic cholecystectomy. However, there is still some doubt about almost all other major laparoscopic procedures. There are difficulties in issuing guidelines for training in laparoscopic hernia repair or surgery for colon cancer when the long-term results are at issue. How are these decisions to be made and who is to make them?

If prescribed courses are to be recognized, their content and quality must be standardized and those who run the courses must also be accredited. A special problem arises with the designation of proctors who are willing to undertake assisted and supervised operating with consultant trainees. In the UK, Hospital Trusts in the National Health Service accept medico-legal responsibility for procedures performed in their operating theatres. It is known that untoward events are more likely to occur when a surgeon is in training for laparoscopic surgery. Will Trusts be willing to accept an increased exposure to liability if an employed surgeon undertakes work as a proctor? There is even a possibility that an instructor will be medico-legally responsible if a surgical accident occurs.

Finally, there may be problems for surgeons who are already performing laparoscopic procedures whose training does not conform with the guidelines.

Who pays?

Training is expensive and there is not enough money to go round. Experts who give their time and expertise to training should be able to see some benefit either for themselves or their unit. On the other hand, should the surgeon who wants to give patients the benefits of a new technique be expected to fund training from his or her own pocket. Without the initiatives mounted by the major instrument companies it is likely that there would have been little provision for laparoscopic training in the UK. These companies are spending a large amount of money because they hope to stimulate sales by building brand loyalty. In the longer term, commercial priorities may change and this money may no longer be available. In any case the money must eventually be recovered by increased charges to the customer. In the UK, the major customer is the NHS.

It is essential that the true cost of training is assessed so that NHS Trusts can be made aware of the provision they need to make for quality laparoscopic training for their staff. It is only in this way that rational, organized and fully integrated training in MAS can be secured.

References

1. Cuschieri A. Minimal access surgery: the birth of a new era. *J R Coll Surg Edinb* 1990; **35**: 345–347.
2. *Working for patients.* Her Majesty's Stationery Office, London, 1989.
3. Cuschieri A. The laparoscopic revolution – walk carefully before we run (Editorial). *J R Coll Surg Edinb* 1989; **34**: 295.
4. *Minimal Access Surgery: laparoscopic cholecystectomy and related gastrontestial procedures.* The Royal College of Surgeons of England, London, 1990.
5. Rosin RD. Video-enhanced telescopic surgical training. In: Rosin RD (ed.) *Minimal access general surgery.* Radcliffe Medical Press, Oxford, 1994, p. 229.
6. *Laparoscopic cholecystectomy.* The Royal College of Surgeons of England, London, 1994 (press release May).
7. *Quality Assurance: The role of training, certification, audit and continuing professional education in the maintenance of the highest possible standards of surgical practice.* The Senate of The Royal Surgical Colleges of Great Britain and Ireland, London, 1994, 1.
8. Calman KC. *Hospital doctors: training for*

the future (PL/CMO(93)3). Health Publications Unit, Department of Health, London, 1993.

9. Calman KC. *Hospital doctors: training for the future* (PL/CMO(94)5). Health Publications Unit, Department of Health, London, 1993.

10. *Minimal access surgery: implications for the NHS. Report of a working group set up by the Department of Health and the Scottish Office Home and Health Department.* Her Majesty's Stationery Office, London, 1993.

11. Royston CMS, Landsdown MRJ, Brough WA. Teaching laparoscopic surgery: the need for guidelines. *BMJ* 1994; **308**: 1023–1025.

12. Asbun JH, Reddick J. Credentialling in laparoscopic surgery: a survey of physicians. *J Laparoendoscopic Surgery* 1992; **2**(1): 27–32.

13. *Guidelines for granting of privileges for laparoscopic (peritoneoscopic) general surgery.* Society of American Gastrointestinal Endoscopic Surgeons, Los Angeles, 1992.

4b

Practical aspects of laparoscopic training outside the UK

E.G. Weiss and S.D. Wexner

Introduction

Surgical training has evolved in the United States from a system of unorganized preceptorships without any formal governing body assuring their adequacy, to a well-organized model of residency training programmes. The ultimate result of any surgical residency training programme is to produce well-trained surgeons capable of providing appropriate, safe, and informed care. Ultimately, this training will allow a physician to become credentialled by some group which assures their competence. However, the introduction of laparoscopy has caused many problems in connection with education, training, and credentialling of surgeons in these techniques. The reader who is not familiar with 'credentialling' should look at the first paragraph of the chapter by Cuschieri and Hanna who put it in the UK context alongside 'accreditation' and 'certification'.

To date there is no uniformly accepted list of prerequisites that a surgeon needs to fulfil in order to be considered competent or credentialled in laparoscopic surgery. There are some guidelines that have been published in the USA and elsewhere in the world, but none have been universally followed. The majority of those responsible for credentialling surgeons do so on an individual basis.

Historically, most surgeons in the USA, except for those involved in obstetrics and gynaecology had little if any laparoscopic experience in their residency training programmes. Similarly most practising surgeons had very little exposure to laparoscopy unless they assisted gynaecologists with diagnostic laparoscopy, laparoscopic tubal ligations, or laparoscopic infertility surgery. There was virtually no application of laparoscopy to general surgery until the introduction of laparoscopic cholecystectomy. Then a new era of laparoscopic surgery, with increasingly sophisticated images and instrumentation, was ushered in and training began.

Traditionally surgical procedures are taught through residency programmes. If a new technique was developed after completion of residency training, a course was regarded as sufficient to achieve proficiency, for example, the application of the laser to standard surgical procedures. Laparoscopic cholecystectomy courses were initially instituted by companies, individuals, or institutions to teach not only laparoscopic cholecystectomy but also laparoscopic technique and basic principles. Many surgeons, however, prior to embarking on these 'weekend' laparoscopic training courses had already scheduled their first laparoscopic procedures for the Monday following the completion of the course. These 'weekend' courses were evidently deemed adequate training under the prevailing circumstances by their hospitals, credentialling bodies, and societies. However, there was no uniformity, and variable requirements were placed upon surgeons to gain privileges. Many questions arose, including should a certain number of cases be performed prior to being granted 'privileges'? and should surgeons be reviewed or proctored and if so by whom and for how long? These questions remain unanswered.

Another problem is that of the increasing complexity of some of the laparoscopic procedures. The techniques involved with laparoscopic cholecystectomy may be very different from those necessary to perform laparoscopic hernia repair, fundoplication, appendicectomy, or colonic resection. Prior training in one use of the laparoscope may not be adequate to perform more difficult procedures. For example, in the case of colonic resection there are at least five identifiable differences, compared to other laparoscopic procedures.[1]

These differences may require further advanced skills that enable the surgeon to perform such a procedure safely.

Firstly, most laparoscopic procedures are performed in essentially one single quadrant of the abdomen (herniorrhaphy, fundoplication and cholecystectomy, for example). Thus, once the ports are placed and the instruments have been inserted, the positions of the personnel, monitors, and equipment are relatively fixed. Conversely laparoscopic colectomy is a multi-quadrant procedure and requires numerous, time-consuming, and often disorienting shifts in position of all of the above components.

Secondly, vascular control is relatively easy in the other procedures mentioned as the vessels are generally small and single. In fact, some of the other procedures do not require any vascular division. Laparoscopic colectomy entails the ligation of numerous vascular pedicles. Although, in other procedures, this step may be rapidly and inexpensively effected with either 'clips', or 'loops', in colectomy multiple applications and combinations may be required. This problem increases both the time and the expense necessary to control safely the vascular supply to the colon. Although stapling devices can expedite this phase of the procedure, the cost of such a venture may be prohibitively high.

Thirdly, most other laparoscopic procedures result in either no specimen (hernia and fundoplication, for example) or a small, easily deliverable specimen (such as the gallbladder or appendix). Colectomy results in a larger specimen that will not be deliverable through a standard port. Thus either a very large port or an incision is required to remove the specimen.

Fourthly, all of the other procedures conclude after repair of the defect or delivery of the small specimen, colectomy requires a well-vascularized, tension free, circumferentially perfect anastamosis. Furthermore, after anastamosis there may be a mesenteric defect to close.

Lastly, most laparoscopic procedures are performed for benign disease; however, colectomy is usually performed for malignancy. The application of laparoscopy for cancer surgery has resulted in significant controversy regarding adequate lymph node harvesting, level of ligation of vascular pedicles, adequacy of margins, and port site recurrences.[2–10] Although recurrence of an inguinal hernia or a hiatal hernia may be troublesome, lengthen hospitalization and increase cost, anastomotic or port site recurrence of malignancy are potentially lethal complications. Therefore, laparoscopic procedures for the cure of malignancy should be performed only within appropriate prospective randomized, controlled trials.[11–13]

The development of a 'laparoscopic surgeon' is unprecedented in the history of surgery. There were no 'electrocautery surgeons' or 'Kelly clamp surgeons'. The closest approximation is endoscopy, but that was naturally incorporated into the practice of surgeons and gastroenterologists. In the case of laparoscopy, new societies and journals have developed to focus upon a technique rather than upon a disease process or organ system. There are two schools of thought. One group demands the ability to diagnose and treat all surgical disorders and endorses the laparoscope as a tool to achieve that end. The other school favours technical expertise with all uses of the tool instead of proficiency in all facets of surgical disease. Thus credentialling groups cannot turn to a national consensus for guidance.

Many questions therefore need to be addressed regarding training and credentialling in laparoscopic surgery:

1. What is considered adequate training in general laparoscopy?
2. Does each specific procedure need to be individually credentialled?
3. Do new applications of laparoscopy to traditionally 'open' procedures need formal training?
4. Is expertise in the management of disorders of the respective area requisite to application of the laparoscope to that area?
5. What are the definitions of 'adequate' and 'expertise'?

In an effort to answer the above questions each will be addressed individually with historic precedents being explored in order to derive a new schema for the credentialling and training in laparoscopic procedures.

What is considered adequate training in laparoscopy?

As mentioned previously several authors have described recommended sequences and criteria for granting privileges in laparoscopic surgery. Dent, Asbun, and The

European Association for Endoscopic Surgery have all published guidelines for training. It is probably simpler to list the basic tenets of those criteria and to discuss each individually. The basic criteria are as follows:

One must have:

1. Privileges for the corresponding open procedure.
2. Privileges for laparoscopy.
3. Taken a formal training course.
4. Completed preceptorship or proctorship including assisting a more advanced surgeon and then being observed at independent performance of the same procedure.

Laparoscopy has the potential for significant morbidity and possible mortality. The technique may be minimally invasive, but the complications described to date are 'maximally lethal'. Therefore all of the inherent risks associated with the open procedure are present as are some risks specific to laparoscopy. The latter group includes trocar injuries and problems with pneumoperitoneum. Certain complications require immediate intracolonic access. Thus the surgeon performing the laparoscopic procedure must be able to perform the open procedure as well.[14,15] No laparoscopic privilege should be granted to anyone who cannot meet the above requirements as the safety of the patient is otherwise in jeopardy.

Proficiency in laparoscopy itself will vary as will the methods by which it is insured. Most surgical residents and fellows currently receive adequate laparoscopic training as part of their overall education. They have become adept with the laparoscope and the endoscope along with scissors, electrocautery and clamps. However, those surgeons who were not formally trained in laparoscopy as part of their general surgery or subspecialty training, must have postgraduate training. This training can be accomplished in several ways. Certification and completion of a course with both didactic and animal laboratories is the first step.[16,17,18] Then the surgeon should undergo a preceptorship or proctorship under another adept at these procedures.[19,20,21] Failure to adhere to such a schema may invite potentially disastrous results. Many anecdotes were recounted of surgeons who, before taking a course, scheduled one or more laparoscopic cholecystectomies to be done the morning after completion of the 'weekend' course. Altman described in graphic detail some of the serious and life-threatening complications which ensued during this period.[22] As a result of such irresponsible policing by the surgeons themselves, the legislature of New York mandated that all surgeons must perform fifteen supervised laparoscopic cholecystectomies before credentialling can be given. Thus a professor of surgery is viewed in the same context as is a non-board certified recent graduate. Hopefully the cautious conservative development of laparoscopic colorectal surgery will obviate the recurrence of such a problem.

See, *et al.* performed a postal survey of urologists who had completed a laparoscopic training course.[23] They looked at complications from laparoscopic urological procedures at both three- and twelve-month intervals with respect to additional laparoscopic training, those with whom they attended the training course, and the type of assistant used during laparoscopic procedures. At the three-month interval, those urologists who had no further training beyond their initial training course were almost three-and-a-half times more likely to have a complication compared with those who sought additional training. At the twelve-month interval surgeons who attended the course alone, were in solo practice, or used a variable assistant, were at least four-and-a-half times more likely to have a complication. Also, they showed a learning curve at both intervals, where the likelihood of complications was inversely related to the number of cases performed. These data can similarly be applied to any laparoscopic procedure.

As mentioned above a formal course is mandatory for those surgeons who have never performed laparoscopic procedures but may not be necessary for those residents and graduates with laparoscopic experience. Should one need a new course for each new application of laparoscopy? Is it necessary for one to take a course in every application that one wants to perform?

Although the precedent is that each new application of laparoscopic surgery should not require specific training or credentialling, an exception may be advanced laparoscopic surgery such as laparoscopic colon resections. For the reasons enumerated earlier the skills are sufficiently different and the potential adverse sequelae significantly large to mandate advanced training.

As with laparoscopic cholecystectomy, training for other advanced laparoscopic procedures should commence with a didactic course, acquiring skills in the porcine or canine model, then observe other surgeons performing the intended procedure(s), and then be observed or assisted by a preceptor during the first several cases. However, the exact number of hours of didactic education or practical 'wet lab' experience and the number of observed or proctored cases is ill-defined. Moreover, it does not appear appropriate to require repetition of the process for each new advanced procedure. The surgeon should be trained for all procedures applicable to a given organ system or disease process. The surgeon must be expert at both the diagnosis and management of all diseases and surgical options as well as the use of the laparoscope.

Eventually some of the heterogeneity of training and credentialling will disappear. To date there are policy statements that have been issued by the American College of Surgeons, the American Society of Colon and Rectal Surgeons and the Society of American Gastrointestinal and Endoscopic Surgeons regarding laparoscopic surgery[14,24,25,26] the common denominator among all of these statements is that they fail to list specific guidelines and are merely philosophic dicta.

After thorough review of the literature we suggest the following guidelines.

1. General knowledge and performance of basic laparoscopic techniques must be obtained by anyone who wishes to perform laparoscopic surgery.[27,28] This training may be obtained in one of two ways:
   (a) Through didactic and practical training courses followed by observing and subsequently being observed by a competent laparoscopic surgeon.
   (b) Through integration into residency training programmes.[29,30] In this latter scenario the residency programme director will attest to the candidates' skills and will verify adequate didactic and practical training. However, the irony of the New York State law is such that a resident may complete several hundred laparoscopic procedures in training. After graduation, if he remains on staff at that same institution, he cannot perform laparoscopic cholecystectomy until he has been observed during an additional 15 cases.

2. The surgeon must be credentialled to perform the open version of the laparoscopic procedure.
3. Advanced training in new applications should be required. Such a requirement should not be organ system or disease process specific and not instrument specific.
4. All data including morbidity and mortality must be kept in a registry for peer review. The registry should be institutional and not private. Access to the data by individuals other than those surgeons who enter the data should be mandatory. When possible such data should be sent to a national registry.

It is hoped that universal adoption of these four recommendations will help ensure the safe applications of the laparoscope. Furthermore universal submission of all data to centralized registries will allow meaningful, prospective accrual of morbidity, mortality, and long-term success. However, until recognition of these recommendations the surgical community must share the common goal of optimal patient outcome rather than either maximal market share or optimal ego gratification.

References

1. Cohen S, Wexner SD. Laparoscopic colectomy and appendectomy. In: *Shackelford's Surgery of the Alimentary Tract*, 4th Edn, Vol. 4, Condon (ed.) WB Saunders, Philadelphia, 1996, pages 164–183.
2. Alexander RJ, Jaques BC. Laparoscopically assisted colectomy and wound recurrence (letter). *Lancet* 1993; **341**: 249–250.
3. O'Rourke N, Price PM, Kelly S, Sikora K. Tumor inoculation during laparoscopy (letter). *Lancet* 1993; **342**: 368.
4. O'Rourke NA, Heald RJ. Laparoscopic surgery for colorectal cancer. *Br J Surg* 1993; **80**(10): 1229–1230.
5. Fusco MA, Paluzzi MW. Abdominal wall recurrence after laparoscopic-assisted colectomy for adenocarcinoma of the colon. Report of a case. *Dis Colon Rectum* 1993; **36**(9) 858–861.
6. Guillou PJ, Darzi A. Monson RT. Experience with laparoscopic colorectal surgery for malignant disease. *Surg Oncol* 1993; **2** (Suppl 1): 3–11.
7. Ngoi SS, Kum CK, Goh PMY, *et al.* Laparoscopic colon resection – the Singapore experience. Poster Presentation (P56). Tripartite Colorectal Meeting, Sydney, Australia, October 1993.
8. Fingerhut A. Laparoscopic colorectal surgery. Presented at the World Congress of Endoscopic Surgery. Kyoto, Japan. June 16–19, 1994.
9. Nduka CC, Monson JRT, Menzies-Gow N, Darzi A. Abdominal wall metastasis following laparoscopy. *Br J Surg* 1994; **81**: 648–652.
10. Wade TP, Comitalo JB, Andrus CH, Goodwin MN, Kaminski DL. Laparoscopic cancer surgery. *Surg Endosc* 1994; **8**: 698–701.
11. ASCRS. Approved Statement of Laparoscopic Colectomy. *Dis Colon Rectum*, 1994; **37**(6): 638.
12. SAGES. Position Statement, 1992.
13. Sackier JM, Berci G, Paz-Partlow M. A new training device for laparoscopic cholecystectomy; technical note. *Surg Endosc* 1991; **5**(3): 158–159.
14. Statement on Laparoscopic and Thoracoscopic Procedures. *Bulletin American College of Surgeons* 1993; **78**(9): 48.
15. Cuschieri A, Berci G, McSherry CK. Laparoscopic cholecystectomy. *Am J Surg* 1990; **159**: 273.
16. Dent TL. Training, credentialing, and evaluation in laparoscopic surgery. *Sur-*

gical Clinics of North America 1992; **72**(5): 1003–1011.

17. Greene FL. Training, credentialing and privileging for minimally invasive surgery. *Problems in General Surgery* 1991; **8**: 502–506.

18. Guillou PJ. Laparoscopic surgery for diseases of the colon and rectum – quo vadis? *Surg Endosc* 1994; **8**: 669–671.

19. Asbun HC, Reddick EJ. Credentialing in laparoscopic surgery: A survey of physicians. *J Laparoendosc Surg* 1992; **2**(1): 27–32.

20. Cuschieri A, Bailey M, Jago R. Report of Working Party to Council of the Royal College of Surgeons of Edinburgh, July 1993.

21. Proctoring and Hospital Endoscopy Privileges (leader). *Gastrointest Endosc* 1991; **37**(6): 667.

22. Altman LK. Surgical injuries lead to new rule. *New York Times*, June 14, 1992, pp. 1 and 47.

23. See WA, Cooper CS, Fisher RJ. Predictors of laparoscopic complications after formal training in laparoscopic surgery. *JAMA* 1993; **270**(22): 2689–2692.

24. Dent TL. Training, Credentialing, and Granting of Clinical Privileges for Laparoscopic General Surgery. *Am J Surg* 1991; **161**(3): 339–403.

25. SAGES. *Guidelines for Granting Privileges for Laparoscopic General Surgery.* SAGES Publication #0014, 1992.

26. EAES. Training and Assessment of Competence. *Surg Endosc* 1994; **8**: 721–722.

27. Cuschieri A. The dust has settled – let's sweep it clean: training in minimal access surgery (Editorial). *J Royal College of Surgeons Edinburgh* 1992; **37**: 213–214.

28. Cuschieri A. The laparoscopic revolution – walk carefully before we run. (Editorial). *J Royal College of Surgeons Edinburgh* 1989; **34**: 295.

29. Bailey RW, Imbembo AL, Zucker KA. Establishment of a laparoscopic cholecystectomy training program. *Amer Surgeon* 1991; **57**(4): 231–236.

30. Laws HI. Credentialing Residents for Laparoscopic Surgery: A matter of opinion. *Current Surg* 1991; 684–686.

5

Ethics and innovative surgery

G. Gillett

Introduction

The introduction of innovations in surgery often bears little relation to the ideal for scientific medicine described by Hippocrates. He remarked of medical knowledge:

> Science and opinion are two different things; science is the father of knowledge but opinion breeds ignorance.[1]

Many surgeons realize that the evaluation of new surgical techniques is often rudimentary and anecdotal compared with the systematic process of investigation and monitoring that is a *sine qua non* of the introduction of a new drug.[2] Our medical colleagues criticize this lack of rigour in surgical innovation but they forget an important feature of real surgical practice. That feature is, perhaps, best illustrated by a paradigm case of effective surgical intervention. Take for instance, the case of an acute extradural haematoma (an example drawn from the queen of the surgical sciences). The patient is rapidly progressing from a conscious state into coma and towards death from raised intra-cranial pressure. The problem is due to an identifiable lesion for which the treatment is both straightforward and dramatic. We do a craniotomy, remove the haematoma, and save the patient's life. Where the treatment is prompt, the patient eats a healthy breakfast the next morning. Such an intervention has an intuitive or obvious rationale and any physician who seriously suggested that it be subject to a randomized controlled trial would not be worth talking to – his mind would have been irretrievably corrupted by 'scientific' brainwashing.

Minimally invasive surgery has something of the same intuitive appeal because it seems simply obvious that the technique offers advantages to all concerned.

However, paradigm cases such as extradural haematoma and, possibly, minimally invasive surgery, often bewitch us into a false perception of what is actually happening in modern surgery. Firstly, in everyday clinical practice our new interventions are often not so dramatic and cannot always be proven to be better than more conservative or traditional measures. Secondly, a technique used safely and effectively by those who developed and gained experience with it may not be quite so safe and effective in other situations. Thus we need carefully to consider, as part of the ethics of innovative surgery, its scientific or clinical credentials. But the perspective of clinical science is only one of the two major perspectives involved in surgical ethics. A more important perspective is provided by the patient.

The values guiding surgical interventions

When we ask whose values should inform surgical decision-making it is clear that the patient's perspective must take pride of place. This conclusion turns on an analysis of the nature of benefit as it applies to medical interventions. Clearly one does not want a purely physiological definition whereby, for instance, one might say 'this regimen is clearly beneficial because it normalizes the patient's electrolytes'; think, for instance, of a patient slipping into uremic coma as the expected final phase of dying with pancreatic carcinoma.[3] Nor would we want a definition solely focused on sustaining life; and here we can think of the unsustainable argument that we ought to withhold opiates in case they suppress the respirations of a patient dying with 80 per cent burns. We need a concept of substantial benefit according to which the aim of our treatment is to produce something like 'An outcome which now or in the future would be regarded by the patient as worthwhile'.[4] But notice that this plausible definition of benefit or worthwhileness of treatment is patient-centred. It is not enough for the surgeon to intend to do what he or she regards as a good or even spectacular operation, it must aim to leave the patient with what the patient regards as a beneficial outcome. We often lose sight of this simple ethical principle when we develop a new and exciting surgical technique. A recent case in point is cavernous sinus surgery.

> Most cases requiring surgery in the cavernous sinus involve benign or very slow-growing lesions and in the latter case the surgery can almost never be regarded as completely curative. The natural history of such lesions is that they will cause slow and progressive cranial nerve palsies including diplopia and possibly blindness. The outcome of surgery also includes, quite commonly, palsies of the same cranial nerves (sudden rather than progressive) and may involve (at a significant level of probability) major disability such as hemiplegia or death.

An interesting question was posed at a meeting where the results of a small series of patients undergoing such surgery were presented: 'Why would any reasonable person agree to such surgery in the light of the evident risks and dubious benefits?' No answer was forthcoming. To most present this indicated that the central importance of substantial benefit to the individual patient was not respected by those carrying out this surgery. This point brings us to the nature and centrality of informed consent in any surgery but particularly in innovative surgery. It also allows us to provide a working definition of innovative surgery.

What defines an innovative treatment?

Innovative surgery is desperately difficult to define. We are, all the time, introducing modifications and improvements into the operations we do. This is very much in accord with Hippocrates' observation that 'The discoveries of medicine are of great importance and are the result of thought and skill on the part of many people.'[1] Thus, in the development of surgical knowledge and expertise, we are faced by a shifting practice rather than a fixed corpus of orthodox surgery. This immediately raises the question as to when an alteration in what we do is major enough to count as innovative.

It is, on reflection, very difficult to formulate a criterion or set of criteria on which to decide when a particular modification counts as innovation. Clear examples of innovative techniques spring to mind: super-selective vagotomy for ulcer; microsurgery; lumpectomy versus mastectomy; and laparoscopic surgery to name but a few. Each, I would suggest, is marked by the fact that the new technique involves a *materially relevant change* from the patient's perspective. A materially relevant change is one that would influence the decision of a reasonable person in the patient's position.[5] So, for instance, in breast cancer treatment, lumpectomy versus mastectomy preserves the breast but runs the theoretical risk of incomplete excision of tumour. This trade-off is clearly a matter of the patient's values: one woman may choose to take the risk, another to sacrifice her breast. The decision depends on the woman's perceptions and the relative value she places on the two options. With other innovations, there is no such relevance for the patient – the technique merely does what we are all trying to do anyway but does it better and more consistently and without introducing countervailing risks. Such changes, as in the use of a microscope for certain procedures, are not materially relevant, although they may still require audit of their effects. Therefore, the ethical tests of consent and information arise from a patient-centred definition of what is at stake in a surgical procedure.

Consent and partnership

This last conclusion is, in fact, highly congenial to a major emphasis of surgical ethics. Surgical care should be seen as a partnership or alliance in which the surgeon and patient do their best together to solve the problem with which the patient presents. In such a partnership each participant has certain legitimate expectations. The patient expects the surgeon to act with due care and skill and in a way that accords with responsible medical opinion. He or she also expects the surgeon to present the options in a way that fairly represents their materially relevant features. The surgeon expects the patient to present true information about his or her problem and make a careful decision based on an honest appraisal of the prospects of the various possible courses of management. In any such joint venture there are uncertainties and particularly where the surgery involved is relatively new and perhaps untried. As long as this is fairly represented and the patient's decision is made in the light of a truthful presentation of those uncertainties, an outcome which realizes one of the uncertain risks should not be a basis for any accusations or damages. Of course, if the possibility of that outcome was concealed or withheld in the information given to the patient then that is a very different matter.

The patient's major assurance in this uncertain process (where the events being discussed are both unfamiliar and alarming) is that the doctor's communications fairly present a reasonable or established body of medical opinion. That is not to say that the surgeon cannot recommend that a new or innovative method be tried but, when he or she does so, must also tell the patient the ways in which this treatment differs from conventional treatment or that which would be endorsed by a more established body of medical opinion. Where the patient is hesitant about putting their faith in the innovative treatment despite the surgeon's recommendation, the surgeon should offer a second opinion.

The second opinion should, indeed must, be independent of the first and is especially important where the new treatment is controversial. The patient has legitimate grounds for complaint if he or she was offered a controversial treatment without being given any clear idea of why and in what respects it was so. The patient also has grounds for complaint if given no opportunity to discuss the options available. Once we accept that the surgeon or medical caregiver is in the same relation to the patient as the captain of a ship is to its owner then these provisions follow, 'domino fashion'. The patient's values and choices guide treatment in the light of medical advice and expertise. That advice should be offered as recommendations supported by reasoning which would be endorsable in terms acceptable to the profession as a whole.

The societal perspective

There is a further perspective on innovative treatment, most evident in those countries where some or all of the health budget is seen as a societal or shared cost. Innovative surgery has resource implications and, in any publically funded system, this is a concern of society in general. In fact, when we look closely at this issue, it is equally relevant if the particular innovative treatment is a private transaction or within a dominantly private system, it will still affect wider budgetary considerations. The innovative use of any procedure, such as MRI scanning, or microsurgery for reanastamosis of the vasa deferentia, results in the production of an opportunity accompanied by more or less accepted medical indications and contra-indications that are of general application. The resulting perception that certain problems, where the procedure is thought to be indicated, are amenable to a certain type of treatment will inevitably affect the management of other individuals including those who depend for their care on publically funded health services.

The resource implications of innovative surgery are not, however, always clear at the outset of the use of a new technique, as was evident in two dramatic cases.

> Dialysis did not benefit any of the first 16 patients in whom it was tried; fewer than half of the first 30 patients receiving replacement heart valves survived the operation.[6]

Jennett goes on to liken new medical and surgical techniques to new born mice in that they are ill-equipped to hold their own in the real world until there has been a period of development and nurture. This is a pervasive feature of the use and development of innovative techniques in real clinical experience (as distinct from the expurgated and semi-Utopian version of the process that appears in print and conference presentations). The hitches and pitfalls vary according to the innovative surgery involved and many of these are not evident until some experience has been gained. This fact, as I have noted, makes it particularly important to obtain adequately informed consent to such procedures.[7,8]

The uncertainties evident in the early development of innovative surgery also mean that our collective assessment of costs and effectiveness of these new techniques requires careful judgement as to the proper phase of development in which that should be done. If we leave assessment too long then some patients may suffer due to inadequate or unnecessarily dangerous treatment but if we begin the assessment of a procedure too soon then we may wrongly reject something, because of the appalling early statistics, that has a similar potential for benefit as did open heart surgery or neurosurgery in general. The only way in which we can do the assessment at all adequately is by ongoing systematic audit and review of what we are doing. This becomes an ethical obligation on the innovator as soon as we heed Hippocrates' warning about the difference between opinion and knowledge as bases for medical practice. In this connection Elwood remarks of New Zealand healthcare research:

> Over the last few years the dominant question has been 'is it ethical to do research?' We also need to ask 'is it ethical not to do research?' Why should a clinical unit providing treatment require ethical approval to ascertain the effects of that treatment? Surely it would be more appropriate to require ethical clearance not to do such studies.[9]

Jennett takes a similar position but notes that the assessment of a surgical procedure can be more difficult than evaluating a drug. He notes the need to develop the requisite skills and that there will always be differences in outcome that result from different skill levels in the use of a procedure. He notes the problem in randomizing patients when the new technique intuitively, and on first reports, just seems obviously to be an improvement over existing methods. Jennett concludes that we may need to discard some of the superstitious reverence with which we view randomized controlled trials and settle for other methods which use retrospective controls when there seems no good reason to reject them in the particular case under consideration. Whatever design methodology is used, it is clear that audit and review of innovative surgery must be systematic and rigorous with stated exclusion and inclusion criteria and uniformly documented measures of key variables. The type of controls used should plausibly take account of significant variations likely to affect the outcome of surgery.

Minimally invasive surgery is an innovation in which the initial indications of safety and outcome, our intuitive appreciation of the advantages it offers, and the resource implications for limited healthcare budgets all seem to be favourable. It should now be clear that these early impressions will have to await a detailed audit before we can make confident and unambiguous statements to patients. Many institutions with an interest in effective, low cost, high turnover health service delivery are in favour of introducing the techniques as widely as possible. To date the procedures do seem to compare favourably with their conventional alternatives with respect to morbidity, in-hospital treatment times, total intervention costs, and so on. However, we should be aware that in units which do not publish their figures and among operators who are untrained there may be a hidden incidence of complications which will not surface unless those patients are referred to an academic or well-recognized centre for corrective treatment. This last consideration highlights an important feature of surgical treatment – the need for training.

The need for training

All techniques must be learned. The administration of a drug requires knowledge and expertise based on clinical acumen but it does not require actual hands-on skills. The famous 'slip of the knife' is more commonly a mismatch between clinical knowledge and its application to an anatomical and pathological situation in front of one's eyes and beneath one's hands. For instance, I may know that the common hepatic artery, the cystic duct, and the common bile duct all, in some cases, run in the same direction and in the same mesentery for a short part of their course, but I may still, down a limited laparoscopic window, ligate the wrong one when removing a gallbladder. Internal medicine specialists do not have this kind of problem. Therefore surgeons need to be trained by actually doing things to human beings in which they apply their theoretical knowledge to real life intra-operative situations. Patients and society in general are well aware of this fact and usually ready to play their part in training and development of surgery and surgeons. Common justice suggests that no already disadvantaged group should be differentially exposed to this kind of risk so that, for instance, publically funded patients are designated as 'resident material'. Therefore residents will and should do operations on a range of patients coming into a hospital no matter what contractual arrangements happen to be in place. The responsibility of the senior surgeon is to ensure that any procedures performed by his or her residents are done with the same safety and competence as their senior would employ. This entails that when a resident is operating, the senior surgeon will attend and assist in person until satisfied that the resident concerned is capable of safely and effectively meeting any contingencies that arise. This judgement can be relativized to the degree of backing that he or she is giving (in the theatre – not assisting, in the theatre suite, in the building, fifteen minutes away, etc.). This is obviously a matter in which firm guidelines cannot be formulated in terms other than those which rely on the judgement of a good practitioner. Of course, this does not mean that the surgeon's word is final, his or her decision is and should be assessed in relation to a standard generally endorsed by the profession. Such a standard is best thought of as:

> that standard of care reasonably expected by a patient of a professional with the relevant knowledge, skills, and experience.

Again the rule should be that the patient knows the circumstances attending the operation and the basis on which responsibility will be delegated.

Conclusion

Innovation is the lifeblood of surgery, and of medicine in general. It should always be subordinate to the real needs of patients. The gold standard for an innovative technique is that it enhances the benefits, in the patient's terms, arising in a situation where there is need for surgical intervention. The principal condition under which any patient should be treated innovatively is that the patient has been adequately informed of the nature of treatment and its innovative status. If the treatment is controversial this should also be conveyed. The further condition that the innovation should be monitored and evaluated is a concern for society and the profession in general as a body of responsible practitioners. Learning new techniques is an ever present aspect of our surgical lives and the provisions for information, consent, and review are, therefore, always with us. The rule is openness about techniques, personnel, and prognoses and the ever present innovative aspects of surgery make the ethical requirements on us as pervasive as they are important for good practice.

References

1. Hippocrates. *Hippocratic Writings.* Lloyd, G. E. R. (ed.) Penguin, Harmondsworth, 1978.
2. Spodick DH. The surgical mystique and the double standard. *American Heart J* 1973; **85**: 579–583.
3. Youngner S. Who defines futility? *JAMA* 1988; **260**: 2094–2095.
4. Campbell AV, Gillett G, Jones DG. *Practical Medical Ethics.* Oxford University Press, Auckland, 1992.
5. Skegg PDG. *Law, Ethics, and Medicine.* Clarendon, Oxford, 1988.
6. Jennett B. *High Technology Medicine.* Oxford University Press, Oxford, 1986.
7. Gillett GR. Informed consent and moral integrity. *Journal of Medical Ethics* 1989; **15**: 117–123.
8. Editorial. Adequately informed consent. *Journal of Medical Ethics* 1985; **11**: 115–116.
9. Elwood M. The operation of Health Research Ethics Committees in New Zealand: a Researcher's view. In: McMillan J. (ed.) *Proceedings of the International Seminar on Bioethics.* Bioethics Research Centre, Dunedin, 1994, p. 53.

6

Quality control

A.V. Pollock

Introduction

Many patients prefer laparoscopic abdominal operations to open operations because long incisions, whether they are vertical, transverse, or oblique, cause a lot of pain and take a long time to heal. The rapid return to work or usual activities after a laparoscopic operation is attractive to some patients (particularly those who are self-employed), and even more to those who pay for the health service and for social security.

To surgeons who have been trained to use the sense of touch as freely as the sense of sight and to dissect with their fingers it is a new experience to operate by looking at a television screen. This requires 'a new form of hand–eye co-ordination', the President of the Royal College of Surgeons of England, Professor Norman Browse was reported as saying, and 'there are a few surgeons who cannot master the ability'.[1] New training is needed for established surgeons, and training in laparoscopic work must be added to traditional training for registrars (residents). Above all, quality must be assured.

The Senate of the Royal Surgical Colleges of Great Britain and Ireland requires that trainee surgeons must obtain a Certificate of Completion of Specialist Training, which will indicate the range of technical procedures that the surgeon has been trained to perform. If a surgeon is going to operate through a laparoscope the training must include these techniques. Established surgeons must undergo additional training before undertaking laparoscopic work.

It is doubtful whether the introduction of minimally invasive surgery will reduce the national expenditure on health. These operations take up a lot of operating theatre time, which is expensive and probably cancels out the savings that are made by keeping the patients in hospital for fewer days. There is also the possibility that patients with gallstones (and other conditions that are suitable for laparoscopic operations) will ask to have the new operation, whereas in the past they have put up with their symptoms rather than have a major operation. This was certainly my experience when I gave up the standard operation for groin hernias under general anaesthesia and offered patients the Shouldice operation under local anaesthesia. Many patients who had been more or less content to make do with a truss now asked for the operation.

It is up to the profession to make sure that the outcome of minimally invasive operations is as good as that of traditional operations, and training schemes must be established to ensure this. The training of registrars (residents) differs from that of established surgeons, but only to the extent that the period of supervision of trainee surgeons is longer. A surgeon should not undertake an operation through a laparoscope until he or she is fully trained in the performance of that operation by a conventional approach. There are problems here: as fewer and fewer laparotomies are done for cholecystectomy there are fewer and fewer opportunities for the trainee surgeon to gain experience in the conventional operation.

The government in the UK has set up three centres for training in minimally invasive surgery, in London, Leeds, and Dundee. The work of these centres will be watched closely by the profession.

Recommendations of the Royal College of Surgeons of Edinburgh ____

In 1993 a working party of the Royal College of Surgeons of Edinburgh reported its recommendations and guidelines for training and safe practice in minimal access (endoscopic) surgery. It is based largely on publications and experience in the USA, where in the state of New York 158 adverse incidents after laparoscopic cholecystectomy were reported in the 20 months from August 1990 to March 1992. Included in this total were 29 bile duct injuries, the incidence of which was 25 times greater than in the previous 10 years. The National Institute of Health recommended, among other things, 'strict guidelines for training in laparoscopic surgery, determination of competence, and monitoring of quality'.

The Edinburgh working party made several recommendations, which I have paraphrased. They made no recommendations about accreditation which must, however, obviously be discussed.

- Minimal access surgery must be practised by surgeons within their own specialty.
- Before embarking on laparoscopic surgery a surgeon must be proficient in diagnostic laparoscopy, must have assisted in endoscopic operations, and visited centres where these procedures are in routine use.
- No surgeon should attempt on his own an endoscopic operation that he has not done previously by the conventional approach.
- Nursing and technical staff in the operating theatre must be trained in assisting at minimal access operations, including handling, maintenance, and care of the equipment.
- Surgeons should become skilled at one operation, such as cholecystectomy, and their proficiency shown by audit before they progress to other endoscopic operations.
- Patients must be fully informed at all times.

- A formal system of proctoring is advisable.
- Consideration should be given to the American system of privileging.

Proctoring

This is accepted without question in the USA, but will need a change of understanding by surgeons in the UK. It means supervision by an experienced colleague of the first few laparoscopic operations that are done by the trainee surgeon after his didactic and simulator learning, and (in certain countries) experience in the animal laboratory. The proctor must be present during each operation; he or she must be assured that all the equipment and staff are to hand, and that the trainee's visual and motor skills are adequate. Every operation must be video-recorded and each recording played back and analysed critically.

The proctor will usually be a colleague at the same hospital, but this is not essential. There are, however, administrative problems attached to the use of proctors from another hospital. It is not only the hospital being visited by the proctor, but also the hospital from which the proctor comes, that may find the financial burden irksome.[2] If the need for proctoring is accepted it will in any case add considerably to the cost of training, but it is thought (although there is no hard evidence to support the belief) that a surgeon who has satisfied a proctor is less likely to cause complications than one who 'learns from his mistakes'.

Privileging

It is accepted without question in the USA and Australia, among other countries, that surgeons who are appointed to the staff of a hospital are subject to restrictions on their practice imposed by the Privileging Committee. There is at present no equivalent in the NHS in the UK; it is only custom and pressure from general practitioners that stops a gynaecologist, for example, from doing laparoscopic cholecystectomies. Private hospitals probably take a more serious view of the competence of their medical staff to undertake laparoscopic operations and are likely to deny operating privileges to surgeons who have not been properly trained. The Edinburgh College working party recommended the establishment of privileging committees in hospitals in the UK, with special reference to minimally invasive surgery.

Hospitals

The Edinburgh working party recommended the following:

- Not all hospitals are suitable for minimal access surgery.
- Surgeons, nurses, and technicians must be specially trained before a hospital should allow minimal access operations to be done.

- There must be adequate resources to provide specialized equipment and backup equipment in case of failure.
- There must be adequate theatre time available; laparoscopic operations take longer than conventional ones.
- The workload should be enough not only to justify the expense of the equipment, but also to give the surgeons sufficient experience.
- The outcome of all laparoscopic operations should be audited and the results of the audit communicated to the surgeons involved.
- Some hospitals should have training facilities for basic and advanced techniques.

Quality control: structure

I want to consider the control of quality in terms of Donabedian's structure and process. Given top quality structure and process, a poor outcome is unusual.

What do we expect to find in a training course for laparoscopic surgery? First of all, there is the equipment: Verres needle, insufflation equipment, telescope, television camera and screen, laparoscopic instruments. Then, the content of the training programme, which should comprise didactic instruction with the help of laparoscopic surgical atlases and videotapes.[3,4] This is followed by working the instruments in a simulator, which encourages the surgeon to appreciate the different (but extremely important) tactile sense that is transmitted from the end of an instrument. The absence of three-dimensional vision is less of an impediment. The simulator can train surgeons in handling tissues, cutting, suturing, tying knots, using diathermy, and applying clips. The acquisition of proficiency in suturing is particularly difficult, and justifies the continued availability in hospitals of a 'skills laboratory'.[5]

'Virtual reality' is much talked about in the computer world these days. It means that real surgical instruments are introduced into a 'phantom' (a fibreglass mould of the body) in which the organs are simulated by computer graphics and interact with the instruments. The resulting 'operation' is viewed on a computer monitor and new images are produced as the dissection proceeds. Tissues and organs can be moved aside by laparoscopic instruments to display other tissues and organs. Trainees can do most of the things that they will have to do in live operations (except, presumably, to arrest haemorrhage). Cine-Med (of 127 Main Street North, Woodbury, CT 06798, USA) has pioneered the use of virtual reality in training for minimally invasive surgery, particularly in relation to neurosurgery, and a simulator applicable to laparoscopic surgery has been developed in Salford, Manchester, by Professor Bob Stone and a company called Advanced Robotic Research.

Three-dimensional images are not hard to generate, but it is probably best for students to become thoroughly familiar with two-dimensional images.

The main difficulties to be overcome by the novice, however, are related to the co-ordination of skills, and in particular the tying of knots, and suturing. The teaching of these processes is helped by having special 'phantoms'. These may be merely boxes into which animal or vegetable structures can be inserted and manipulated by instruments from outside. More sophisticated learning devices are made by Limbs and Things Ltd (of Radnor Business Centre, Bristol BS7 8QS). Special polymer 'patches' are put into a 'body form' which comes complete with all the abdominal organs. The texture of these patches resembles that of natural tissues, and they have 'blood vessels' that 'bleed' when they are cut. The phantom is inflated in the usual way and a telescope and handling instruments are introduced through the 'skin'.

Trainers in France, Ireland[6] and the USA[7] have an advantage in that they are allowed to use animals (with, of course, proper safeguards against causing pain and suffering) to learn how to do operations. This is illegal in the UK. Young pigs are the animals that are usually used. There are, of course, drawbacks in operating on pigs. In the first place, the tissues react differently from human tissues (particularly the peritoneum, which is more friable). Secondly, the organs are healthy and there is a lot of difference between healthy and diseased organs in the proficiency that is needed to dissect them. The trainee may acquire an undeserved sense of competence. Finally, the fact that trainees in the UK cannot practise on animals means that more and more attention is being paid to the development and use of computers and interactive videos. When one considers that a laser videodisc holds 54,000 pictures on each side it is clear that it needs only the insight and industry of computer programmers to produce interactive programs which closely simulate actual operating conditions.

Computer graphics simulation and interactive video technology were first introduced as aids to the teaching of endoscopy[8] and the technology can readily be applied to laparoscopic operations.

Quality control: process

The trainee is by now in a position to assist an established laparoscopic surgeon before embarking on his own practice, at first assisted and then monitored for the first 20 operations.[9] After that, the outcome of all laparoscopic – just as all other – operations should be audited.[10] Videotapes of every operation should be made and kept at least until the patient has recovered completely.

Accreditation

There is at present no scheme in the UK for the accreditation of surgeons in minimal access surgery in addition to their accreditation in general surgery.

Continued quality control of established practitioners

Many people believe that it is in the learning period that disasters occur, and that a surgeon is quite safe once he has done about twenty minimally invasive operations. This may not be so. Wexler *et al.* reported an analysis of a postal survey of laparoscopic cholecystectomy by 736 surgeons in Canada.[11] They found that there was a significant correlation between the number of surgeons who reported complications and the number of laparoscopic cholecystectomies that they had done. The more operations, the more complications. They conclude that 'continued vigilance is necessary'. The implication is that novices take more trouble to avoid trouble (and probably have a higher incidence of conversion to open cholecystectomy). More experienced operators may be tempted to continue with a laparoscopic operation when they should convert. Conversion to open laparotomy should under no circumstances be regarded or called a 'failure'.

I want to discuss quality control after completion of training with reference to four aspects: communication with patients, total quality management, critical incident reporting, and guidelines for conversion to open operation.

Communication with patients ——————

It is important that patients shall be satisfied with both the process and the outcome of their treatment. Above all they must know what options are open to them and must make their own choice of treatment. Surgeons will naturally converse with their patients, but it is worthwhile giving them a printed sheet to take away with them to study in the quiet of their own home.

Total quality management ——————

This is a term that is more easily appreciated by manufacturers but which, nevertheless, summarizes what our surgical endeavours should be. What it means is doing it right first time. The implication is that there are no bad apples among surgeons, only bad structures and processes. The whole team, administrative as well as clinical, has to be involved. If structures and processes are correct it should be possible to achieve top quality performance every time. It is, of course, necessary to develop and monitor measures of performance, to set guidelines or standards, and to establish procedures that result in continual improvement.

Guidelines ————————————————

Guidelines for the proper practice of laparoscopic operations have been published by the Society of American Gastrointestinal Endoscopic Surgeons. If they are to be accepted widely they must include advice on selection of patients, and on the absolute necessity sometimes to abandon a laparoscopic operation and perform a standard laparotomy. This should under no circumstances be regarded as a failure of the laparoscopic operation, and the less experienced the surgeon the more he or she should be encouraged to abandon a difficult dissection rather than run the risk of doing serious damage. The guidelines must include criteria for pre-operative endoscopic cholangiography and sphincterotomy with retrieval of stones from the common bile duct. They must address the question of peroperative cholangiography.

Guidelines and standards are, however, only useful if people abide by them. It is essential that the guidelines should be 'owned' by the surgeons who are doing the operations, and not imposed on them from outside.

Critical incident reporting

The reporting of critical incidents was developed by Flanagan in the 1940s[12] and has been adopted particularly by anaesthetists.[13] It is, however, widely applicable and is much more sensitive than statistical analysis of a surgeon's work.

Troidl introduced the concept of failure analysis.[14] This has five steps:

1. Thorough critical analysis of technique.
2. Definition of failures and complications.
3. Enquiry into the cause of the adverse event: consider patient, surgeon, and environmental factors.
4. Discovery of ways of correcting the failure.
5. Discovery of ways of avoiding the failure in future.

During 14 years at the McGuire Veterans Affairs Medical Center in Richmond, Virginia every complication of a surgical operation was reported every week to the head of department.[15] Once a month a consensus conference was held, at which doctors from all specialties attended. Each complication was classified into one of six categories:

1. Inevitable outcome of a disorder in which some chance of benefit justified an operation.
2. Inherent risk of a necessary and correctly performed operation.
3. Error in surgeon's judgement or technique.
4. Hospital deficit; failure of equipment or ancillary personnel.
5. Coincidental event unrelated to known disease or treatment.
6. Unknown.

After 44,603 consecutive major operations, 2428 patients had 2797 complications, and 749 died. The cause of nearly half these complications was classified as error related to the surgeon's judgement or technique. This contrasted with the annual statistical analyses, which suggested that the performance of surgeons at the Center was acceptable when compared with national norms.

Establishment of a national laparoscopic surgery registry

The Society of Thoracic and Cardiovascular Surgeons of Great Britain showed the way by establishing (in 1977) the Cardiac Surgical Register (of deaths after cardiac operations). There is every reason to believe that surgeons who do minimally invasive operations should be invited to report their complications and deaths to a national registry, possibly established by one of the Royal Colleges of Surgeons. The voluntary confidential audit that has been organized by the Royal College of Surgeons of England has attracted an input from only a few surgeons who are doing laparoscopic operations. Its data are therefore of little validity in relation to the outcome of these operations.

In the USA there are about 16,000 surgeons who practise laparoscopic surgery. A National Laparoscopic Surgery Registry was established and one of the investigations that this organization made was into the training of these surgeons. White analysed the data from about a quarter of the total number and reported that most of the respondents had been trained in general surgery.[16] Nearly 90 per cent had attended a laparoscopic cholecystectomy course, which included practical work. About 16 hours were devoted to acquiring skills by operating in animals, and many surgeons also undertook a further period of training in hospitals.

Conclusions

Training in laparoscopic surgery must take account not only of manual dexterity (which differs from that which is required for traditional general surgery), but also of surgeons' willingness to adhere to guidelines. They must be willing to put aside arrogance and abandon a laparoscopic operation, converting to a standard exposure if the dissection is difficult. They must communicate with their patients in as much detail as each patient wants. Finally, they must audit their work and keep video tapes of all operations, at least temporarily.

References

1. Browse N. Reported by Hawkes N, Surgeons order 'keyhole' training. *The Times*, 2 June 1994, 5: cols 4–7.
2. Royston CMS, Lansdown MRJ, Brough WA. Teaching laparoscopic surgery: the need for guidelines. *Br Med J* 1994; **308**: 1023–1025.
3. Bailey RW, Imbembo AL, Zucker KA. Establishment of a laparoscopic cholecystectomy training program. *Am Surgeon* 1991; **57**: 231–236.
4. Zucker KA, Bailey RW, Graham SM, Scovil W, Imbembo AL. Training for laparoscopic surgery. *World J Surg* 1993; **17**: 3–7.
5. Wolfe BM, Szabo Z, Moran ME, Chan P, Hunter JG. Training for minimally invasive surgery. Need for surgical skills. *Surg Endos* 1993; **7**: 93–95.
6. Kirwan WO, Kaar TK, Waldron R. Starting laparoscopic cholecystectomy – the pig as a training model. *Irish J Med Sci* 1991; **160**: 243–246.
7. Anonymous. Laparoscopic cholecystectomy. *JAMA* 1991; **265**: 1585–1587.
8. Baillie J, Jowell P, Evangelou H, Bickel W, Cotton P. Use of computer graphics simulation for teaching of flexible sigmoidoscopy. *Endosc* 1991; **23**: 126–129.
9. Asbun HJ, Reddick EJ. Credentialing in laparoscopic surgery: a survey of physicians. *J Laparoendosc Surg* 1992; **2**: 27–32.

10. Dent TL. Training, credentialing, and evaluation in laparoscopic surgery. *Surg Clin N Am* 1992; **72**: 1003–1011.
11. Wexler MJ, Hinchey EJ, Sampalis J, Barkun J. Canadian laparoscopic surgery survey. *Can J Surg* 1993; **36**: 217–224.
12. Flanagan JC. The critical incident technique. *Psychol Bull* 1954; **51**: 327–358.
13. Cooper JB, Newbower RS, Long CD, McPeek B. Preventable anesthesia mishaps: a study of human factors. *Anesthesiol* 1978; **49**: 399–406.
14. Troidl H. Failure analysis: evaluation and management of negative events. *Theoret Surg* 1993; **8**: 165.
15. McGuire HH, Horsley JS III, Salter DR, Sobel M. Measuring and managing quality of surgery. Statistical vs incidental approaches. *Arch Surg* 1992; **127**: 733–737.
16. White JV. Registry of laparoscopic cholecystectomy and new and evolving laparoscopic techniques. *Am J Surg* 1993; **165**: 536–540.

7

Economic issues in laparoscopic surgery

K. Kesteloot, F. Penninckx, L. Demoulin,
A. D'Hoore and A. Vleugels

Introduction

Although surgeons, especially those involved in laparoscopic surgery, tend to care more for reputation than for efficiency, there is an urgent need for them to become interested, to acquire some expertise, and to collaborate with hospital administrators and economists in cost-efficient surgical management. Cost containment has become a major issue for healthcare authorities, insurers and hospital administrators because of the runaway healthcare expenses related to the new expensive high-tech medicine in a world with slow economic growth.

No doubt, surgical reputation has to be based on the quality of its product (outcome) and the patient's safety has to be put first. Perfect data on outcome and safety are required to answer the question of cost-effectiveness. Each hospital should know its results and surgeons must be among the first to insist and collaborate on it.

But, if surgeons have to be excellent *performers*, they also have to take their responsibilities for the costs related to surgery. Indeed, the bulk of cost variation is surgeon-specific, relating to technical proficiency and material selection. A tradition of benign neglect can not endure. Both the quality of our product as well as the associated costs are to be audited and measured. This chapter mainly deals with costing methodology.

Economic evaluation in healthcare

Methods

Economic evaluations in healthcare attempt to evaluate and compare costs and effects of medical interventions. Several techniques have been developed.[1]

If the effects are identical, effectiveness measurement can be omitted and only costs are compared in a *cost-minimization analysis*. In this situation, the least cost alternative is to be preferred. In a *cost-effectiveness analysis* the effects are described in appropriate natural or physical units, e.g. days to return to work, and a cost-effectiveness ratio is calculated to compare alternatives. If several health effects have to be taken into account (laparoscopic procedures score better than open procedures, for example in terms of convalescence, but may be worse – at least initially – in terms of risk of injury),[2] all effects can potentially be expressed in monetary terms (cost-benefit analysis) or in 'quality of life' measures (cost-utility analysis). *Cost-benefit analysis* in theory allows an easy comparison between benefits and costs of each intervention, but it remains very difficult and controversial to value certain health effects in monetary terms, for example post-operative complications and mortality, lifelong disability. *Cost-utility analysis* combines quantitative (survival) and qualitative (utility) health effects into an effectiveness measure such as QALYs (quality adjusted life years) or HYEs (health years equivalents).

Comparison of alternatives

Most often one medical intervention is compared with at least one other option, which may be 'doing nothing'. If some of the treatment options are excluded, it should be justified and it should be considered how this may affect the results. Typically, a comparison of an open versus a laparoscopic procedure does not include a comparison with other non-surgical treatment options because they are not considered entirely equivalent, for example as far as definitive cure is concerned.

Viewpoint of the analysis

Ideally, economic evaluations should take the 'societal' perspective because it includes, in principle, all costs and results that are relevant to society. This ideal cannot always be attained because of restrictions on the available data and time limits. Moreover, studies performed by individual institutions will reasonably take their own, narrower perspective, implying that the results may not hold for the society as a whole, for example when healthcare insurers and hospital administrators are speaking about costs they do not mean the same. Insurance organizations are essentially referring to the cost of care as read from the invoices they receive, and eventually also to societal, indirect costs. The hospital administrator considers 'costs' by valuing all resources used in giving care to patients. The distinction is known in the literature as the difference between *charges* and *costs*. Thus, the insurer's *macro*-economic approach of 'What is this care costing to the community?' and the hospital's *micro*-economic approach of 'What is this care costing to our institution?' need not coincide. Hence, studies based on charge data cannot claim to focus on the hospital perspective, since charges are returns for the hospital, rather than costs.

Direct versus indirect costs

A distinction should be made between direct and indirect costs. Direct costs include costs caused directly by the medical intervention and consist of medical (for example equipment, nursing) and non-medical costs (for example overhead for non-medical hospital services, medical or nursing home care). Indirect costs include other 'societal' costs, for example loss of production due to lower productivity after disease/surgery, earlier death, etc. (*cf. infra*).

Opportunity costs and timing of costs

The true economic cost of a medical intervention is its 'opportunity cost'. This is the benefit, expressed in monetary terms, that would have been obtained from deploying these resources in their best alternative use. Often opportunity costs are estimated on the basis of the price of the resource, for example purchase price of equipment, wages of staff. But, prices reflect true economic costs only if markets are perfectly competitive, which is frequently not the case in healthcare.

In order to obtain meaningful financial results, all price and wage data for activities performed within a certain period should apply to the same time period, most often a year.

Costs need not all occur in the same (base) year, that is they have a differential timing. An economically correct evaluation should incorporate this differential timing, which is done by discounting. This problem typically emerges for equipment which is used for several years. While their acquisition costs occur during the first year, not all of these expenses should be conceived of as 'costs' for that year. Economically, it is advisable to attribute part of these expenses to each year that the equipment is in operation (*cf. infra*).

Sensitivity analysis

Since opinions may diverge on the cost or effect of some topic, the degree of reliability of the results of an economic evaluation has to be investigated, that is whether the results would hold in different circumstances. While uncertainty relating to variability in sample data can be dealt with by conventional statistical methods (for example confidence limits), it can also be investigated, like the other causes of uncertainty, through sensitivity analysis. This can take different forms: simple one- or two-way analysis, threshold analysis, analysis of extremes, probabilistic sensitivity analysis.[3] By means of sensitivity analysis, the critical assumptions that drive the results can be identified. If large variations in cost estimates do not lead to significant changes in the results of the economic evaluation, they are judged to be robust.

Estimation of hospital costs _____

Fixed and variable costs

In order to have a good overview of the costs, to facilitate the interpretation of the cost data and to allow easy recalculations of the total costs in case the number of procedures changes, it is advisable to decompose total costs into fixed and variable costs. 'Fixed' costs (*FC*) are that part of total costs that does not change with the number of interventions. They include the costs of buildings and equipment, and sometimes labour. The 'variable' costs (*VC*) are that part of total costs that increases with the number of interventions. They include costs of (consumable) materials and labour time.

On the basis of this distinction, the total costs (*TC*) as well as the average cost per intervention (*AC*) for a varying number of interventions (*Q*) can easily be calculated:

$$TC = FC + (VC \times Q)$$
$$AC = TC/Q = FC/Q + VC$$

Buildings and equipment

These two resources are durable, that is they are to be used for several years. Their acquisition costs, occurring during the first year, have to be attributable to each year that the building/equipment is in operation. Also, the opportunity cost (i) of the capital invested to acquire the inputs, proxied by the cost of loans, should not be ignored. Annuitizing the initial investment (I) over the useful lifetime of the asset in years (n) automatically incorporates the depreciation and the opportunity cost aspect.[4]

The annuity (*A*) due at the end of each year can be calculated as follows:

$$A = I \times i / [1 - 1/(1 + i)^n]$$

where *A* represents the 'annual' capital cost for each input such as buildings or equipment, and i the real market interest rate, for example 5 per cent in the basic scenario with a range from 3 to 10 per cent for sensitivity analysis. For buildings or equipment that are already in place, and which costs need to be attributed to the medical interventions under study, the replacement value (which can be proxied by the actual purchase price) rather than the historical purchase price can be used.

In addition to the acquisition costs, also the operating and maintenance costs must be included. In the absence of a contract with an external firm, maintenance costs are often approximated by a percentage of the purchase price of the equipment, for example 5 to 15 per cent.

Labour

Labour can be considered either as a fixed or as a variable input. If a staff member (or more than one) must be attracted to implement the medical intervention, the labour cost of this (these) person(s) is considered 'fixed' because it does not depend on the number of patients. The implicit assumption is that this person performs only tasks necessary for the intervention under study and nothing else. If labour is regarded as a 'variable' input, only the actual labour time devoted to the medical intervention under study is considered. Care must be taken not to omit any labour time, for example for preparation of the operating theatre, cleaning of reusables, etc. For determining how much labour time is actually devoted to a medical intervention, a sensible combination of primary data collection for the most time consuming activities (for example registration of labour time by an external observer with a stopwatch) and secondary data collection for less time consuming activities can be used in order to avoid delays and waste of research resources during the study.

Not only the labour time, but also the labour cost per time unit must be known, for example average hourly wage cost, which is done by dividing the annual 'gross wage costs for the employer' by the actual number of annual working hours for each person or qualification involved. For activities that are performed during off-business hours, additional wage costs should be incorporated. A further problem may exist with the labour costs of the medical staff. If the MDs affiliated to hospitals are independent, it is really difficult to come up with a good estimate of their labour costs. In contrast, if MDs are salaried, their wage cost can be calculated along the same lines as for the other staff members.

Allocation of overhead costs

It should be noted that the overhead (indirect) cost concept, typical for cost accounting, is different from the 'economic', societal indirect cost concept. Overhead costs indicate the costs of all activities which are supportive for the medical intervention under study and which are shared with other interventions/departments. They include costs of, for example, heating, electricity, hospital kitchen, patient administration, general management. Although many different methods can be applied,[1] it is well recognized in the literature that there is no unequivocal way to allocate these costs to the different departments that employ them, nor to the different interventions. Thus, the impact of the overhead costs on the final results has to be evaluated by means of sensitivity analysis.

Cost comparison of laparoscopic cholecystectomy (LC) and open cholecystectomy (OC) as an example

As could be expected, in terms of clinical effects the symptomatic outcome after LC and OC was found to be similar with identical indications.[5,6] Cost-utility analysis showed that LC dominates OC in terms of QALY.[7,8] The difference is not substantial since laparoscopic surgery affects quality of life only during a short-term life period and since there is no impact on expected life time except in case of, very rare, serious complications.

Data from our study[9] are summarized in Table 7.1. This study aimed at

Table 7.1   Additional hospital costs after open cholecystectomy (OC) and laparoscopic cholecystectomy (LC) (in BF of 1992*)

	OC	LC
Annual fixed costs	163,000	958,000
Operating theatre equipment°	163,000	795,000
Conversion	–	163,000
Average variable costs	80,521	67,384
(including overheads)		
Operating theatre	23,238	37,892
Post-operative stay	57,283	25,658
Conversion (5 per cent)	–	3,834

* 1 ECU = BF 37.5, £1 = BF 45, DM 1 = BF 20, US$ 1 = BF 28 (as of 1 June 1995)
° equipment lifetime 5 yr (OC), 3 yr (LC), 10 per cent maintenance and 5 per cent opportunity costs included

comparing the hospital costs of OC and LC, and thereby all common costs for both procedures were excluded. Both the capital investment cost, expressed as the annual fixed cost (AFC) and the average variable cost for the operating theatre are higher in the case of LC. Only the variable cost for post-operative care is smaller, but enough to bring the variable costs below the level of those of OC. The possibility of conversion to open surgery has also been taken into account. In this example a 5 per cent conversion rate was used for calculation but a sensitivity analysis of what would be the effect of a lower or higher rate can easily be made.

Although it is possible to reduce the variable cost for a LC below the level of the cost for open surgery, the gain per operation is small in comparison to the annual extra-cost for the equipment. In practical terms, this means that to make both techniques of equal value from a financial viewpoint a minimum number of laparoscopic procedures must be performed. At this *critical number* the sum of the AFC and the VC × number of interventions will be equal for both procedures. From this formula the critical number to reach financial equilibrium can be deduced, which illustrates the importance of distinguishing fixed and variable costs. Taking into account our data, this minimal number is 60 LC/yr for the base line scenario.

A *minimum case load* is not only important from an economic point of view. It is also qualitatively important as it constitutes a precondition for the acquisition and retention of a sufficient level of expertise and skill.[10] In addition it will increase the speed of the learning process which also has direct economic advantages (that is lower variable costs). The necessity of a minimum case load, however, also has its disadvantages. If it is achieved through overconsumption or inappropriate use neither the patient nor society are being served. A marked increase in the frequency of cholecystectomy has been observed in the US as well as in Europe after the introduction of LC.[11–14] It seems that this could *not* be explained by large numbers of asymptomatic patients being operated. Thus, it is expected that the cholecystectomy rate will fall back to historical levels, but that remains to be confirmed.

Finally, the cost composition (share in costs of different activities) yields information through which activities costs can most easily be contained. More efficient organization of activities that only account for a small percentage of the total costs will never yield significant cost reductions. For instance, the procedure takes up a large amount of the variable costs. Thus, organizing the operating theatre more efficiently may result in substantial savings.

It should be noted that the same conclusion need not hold for other laparo-scopic techniques, nor for other hospitals, even in the same country. It all depends on routine practice (variations) and unit cost differentials between hospitals. Therefore, in reporting cost calculations it is strongly recommended to report unit prices (for example wage cost per hour) and volumes of resources used (for example labour time per procedure) separately, in order to facilitate cost compar-ison across procedures, hospitals and countries.

Towards more cost efficient management

With the hospital financing, changing from an open ended cost-based financing to a budgetized product financing, any hospital management and therefore also surgical management should give increased attention to several aspects of *man-agerial efficiency.*

One must invest in a product and not in a particular technology or procedure. Often the latter approach is favoured: the procedure is attractive for scientific, clinical, technical or other reasons, the surgeon enjoys it, the image of the surgeon and/or the hospital is enhanced improving their competitive position, etc. Invest-ing in technology for technology's sake without the framework of a structured programme has the dangers of financial collapse, as well as that of overuse or inappropriate use.

When making investment decisions (i.e. which equipment to install) the sub-sequent running costs arising from the asset acquisition must also be taken into account. Investing in equipment for laparoscopic surgery carries with it the fact that operation times will increase – at least initially – and that the use of disposable materials may/will rise. Also, in view of the particular demands on the expertise of both medical and non-medical staff, the cost of teaching and training should be incorporated. They are mostly forgotten.

Waiting time affects the efficient use of personnel in the operating theatre. People have to wait for several reasons and at several moments of the day. The pinnacle of inefficiency is, of course, if, at the end of the day, overtime is created by time wasted during the normal working day. Time is money, but waiting time is even more money! Surveillance of the procedure line time is very relevant. Time spent between two consecutive patients should not be forgotten. It is evident that not only surgeons but also anaesthesiologists, nurses and maintenance personnel can improve efficiency and have to be involved in the study and interpretation of procedure line surveys. *Team work* is a necessity in order to be most effective. Teaching hospitals certainly have a handicap in this respect.

Materials, especially disposable laparoscopic instruments, make up a high percentage of the total running costs of an operating theatre. It is a fact that many surgeons prefer disposables, but this preference most probably has more to do with industry-based laparoscopic training, creating brand loyalty, than with higher cost-efficiency. Most of the advantages claimed for disposables are not evidenced in the scientific literature. The purchase price of disposable instruments is high, they need stock management and there is a cost of disposal, for example by incineration. In contrast, reusables have a higher purchase price, their lifetime has to be assumed, they need maintenance and repair, backup instruments are needed, they have to be cleaned, sterilized, packed and redistributed. We performed a market study (list prices) and cost comparison of disposables and reusables in the Belgian market. The cost of *reusables* was calculated, including the purchase price, assuming a three year lifetime, a 5 per cent interest rate and 100 procedures/year, as well as the variable costs (*cf. supra*). The cost per procedure amounts to about BF 2000–2500. As far as a comparable set of *disposables* is concerned, the cost of all activities except stock management was included. A full set of one brand of disposables costs between BF 45,000 and BF 50,000 per procedure. The cheapest combination of several brands costs BF 38,000 which is considerably less, indicating that price comparisons and negotiations are very useful when making purchase deals. In view of these high costs, surgeons may be tempted to re-use instruments designed for single use. This practice cannot be defended since reusables remain much cheaper than re-used disposables. All reports comparing disposables and reusables conclude that the latter significantly reduce the cost of LC.[15–21] Also, the use of expensive energy sources such as laser cannot be justified, even when used in combination with other departments.[9]

The variable cost may additionally be diminished by reducing the length of stay following laparoscopic surgery. The available data seem to suggest that it is possible to reduce the average post-operative hospital stay after LC to two days. This could be further reduced by day case surgery, and some have already reported that this sort of surgery can even be carried out on an out-patient basis in selected patients, provided adequate, but cheaper non-hospital nursing care is made available.[22–24] Furthermore, such savings could also be realized after OC.

Societal implications: indirect costs

One of the major benefits of laparoscopic surgery (LS) is the faster return to normal activity than after open surgery (OS). This has been well documented for several procedures but most of all for cholecystectomy (Fig. 7.1). Incapacity to work after LC is about half that after OC. There are quite big differences not only between, but also within some countries. Sick leave, indeed, is not only related to the type of procedure, but also to disease state, the personal bias of the physicians,[30] patient motivation and his/her professional status[5,21,30] and the social policy regarding sick leave.[31] No doubt, norms will change as these issues are not missed by budget-conscious corporate reviewers and industry will be quick to reduce paid sick leave periods. In this process, surgeons have to play a role in better education of patients and GPs in order to change their ingrained attitudes and perceptions.

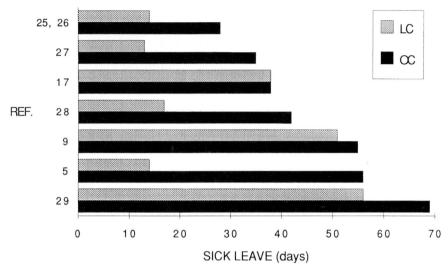

Fig. 7.1 Duration of sick leave after laparoscopic (LC) and open cholecystectomy (OC) as reported in European comparative studies. (REF. = reference number.)

It is often suggested that the total societal gains from moving to laparoscopic interventions are substantial. However, it is difficult to come up with precise estimates of these indirect costs. In the traditional 'human capital' approach, the value of production that would have been realized had the patient not been ill is often approached by the wage cost of the patient during the illness period. This may grossly overestimate indirect costs since the actual production loss may be much lower. It may also underestimate indirect costs, since faster recovery of non-employed people, such as housewives and retired people, is considered of 'no value' for society.[32]

Therefore, the 'friction cost method', which argues that the actual production loss is restricted to the duration of the vacancy to replace the employee, at least during periods of non-negligible unemployment, has been suggested recently.[32] This approach requires even more tedious calculations and is open to further research.

Whatsoever, societal gains, both in terms of lower health insurance expenditures and lower indirect costs, would disappear quickly if the laparoscopic evolution leads to increased treatment rates, for example of asymptomatic gallstones.

Lessons from the laparoscopic evolution for policy makers ⎯⎯⎯⎯

Rapid diffusion

Laparoscopic surgery diffused into routine practice very rapidly despite the absence of scientific evidence of its superiority over comparable open surgery.

This quick diffusion can be explained by consumer-driven demand, absence of major investment in equipment implying that diffusion is difficult to control for healthcare regulators, surgical enthusiasm, the absence of guidelines and control mechanisms on required training, and the competition for patients between institutions.[33] Such rapid diffusion should be avoided with laparoscopic procedures in more controversial and complex areas. However, it is not evident how to do so. Perhaps by reimbursing the new technique only if the surgeon can give proof of sufficient training? If no scientific evidence can be collected through randomized controlled clinical trials because of the impossibility of recruiting and randomizing patients, at least complete and correct data on the incidence and type of complications could be collected through a large scale audit system.[34]

Financing healthcare interventions

If laparoscopic surgery proves to be more cost effective than comparable open surgery (for example cholecystectomy), policy makers can encourage the switch to laparoscopic surgery through the healthcare financing system. If they are not willing to follow this avenue, they should at least make sure that 'perverse' effects are not created. A number of studies have compared the hospital charges (bills) for elective LC and OC. The income from LC is significantly lower in all European reports mainly due to a decreased length of hospital stay. However, the reduction of income may be more substantial than the cost decrease (*cf. supra*), implying that hospital administrators will ask for cost containment (*cf. supra*) or will not insist on the early discharge of 'laparoscopic patients': the income from a sufficient number of patient days is needed to cover the higher equipment and operating theatre costs. This strategy would imply foregoing savings in healthcare expenses. A similar argument could be made for other welfare measures, such as allowances in case of sick leave. In those countries where medical activities and associated material costs are reimbursed through a fee-for-service system while hospitals are financed separately, the switch from open to laparoscopic surgery will require a shift from part of the hospital budget (since patient days are reduced) to the medical sector (higher equipment and operating theatre costs). If this shift is not realized, surgeons may be somewhat reluctant to switch to laparoscopic surgery, or they may be tempted to re-use disposables in order to save on material costs.

Conclusions

Indications for surgery have to remain adequate. The laparoscopic evolution has to be monitored closely in order to avoid unnecessary cost increases or cost increases that are not accompanied by improved outcomes. Conversion from laparoscopic to open surgery has to be performed when judged necessary; however, the rate has to be limited by appropriate training and growing experience. Advanced laparoscopic surgery should be performed by experienced surgeons. Hospital costs can be reduced and have to be kept low by optimizing and surveying the operation time as well as the time-flow in the operating theatre.

The market prices of laparoscopic instruments should be followed closely. If appropriate reusable instruments are available, they are to be preferred above disposables, at least for routine laparoscopic procedures. The post-operative hospital stay can eventually be further reduced and day case surgery or even ambulatory surgery has to be considered in well-selected patients. Post-operative outcome has to be audited. Finally, patients as well as medical doctors have to be educated in order to limit post-operative sick leave.

It is clear that every administrator and doctor wants the hospital to practise good medicine and patients to receive good quality of care, based on current medical knowledge and expertise. If doctors and administrators start to move towards a more appropriate, effective and efficient use of resources, they also start taking up a substantial part of their accountability towards the community which makes available these resources for healthcare.

References

1. Drummond MF, Stoddart GL, Torrance GW. *Methods for the economic evaluation of health care programmes.* Oxford University Press, Oxford, 1987.
2. McMahon AJ, Fullarton G, Baxter JN, O'Dwyer PJ. Bile duct injury and bile leakage in laparoscopic cholecystectomy. *Br J Surg* 1995; **82**: 307–313.
3. Briggs A, Sculpher M, Buxton M. Uncertainty in the economic evaluation of health care technologies: the role of sensitivity analysis. *Health Econ* 1994: **3**: 95–104.
4. Richardson AW, Gafni A. Treatment of capital costs in evaluating health care programmes. *Cost and Management* 1983; **Nov–Dec**: 26–30.
5. Vandervelpen GC, Shimi SM, Cuschieri A. Outcome after cholecystectomy for symptomatic gall stone disease and effect of surgical access: laparoscopic v. open approach. *Gut* 1993; **34**: 1448–1451.
6. Ure BM, Troidl H, Spangenberger W, Lefering R, Dietrich A, Eypasch EP, Neugebauer E. Long-term results after laparoscopic cholecystectomy. *Br J Surg* 1995; **82**: 267–270.
7. Bass EB, Pitt HA, Lillemoe KD. Cost-effectiveness of laparoscopic cholecystectomy versus open cholecystectomy. *Am J Surg* 1993; **165**: 466–471.
8. Cook J, Richardson J, Street A. A cost utility analysis of treatment options for gallstone disease: methodological issues and results. *Health Econ* 1994; **3**: 157–168.
9. Kesteloot K, Penninckx F. The costs and effects of open versus laparoscopic cholecystectomies. *Health Econ* 1993; **2**: 303–312.
10. Segal HE, Rummel L, Wu B. The utility of PRO data on surgical volume: the example of carotid endarterectomy. *Qual Rev Bull* 1993; **19**: 152–157.
11. Legoretta AP, Silber JH, Costantino GN, Kobylinski RW, Zatz SL. Increased cholecystectomy rate after the introduction of laparoscopic cholecystectomy. *J Am Med Assoc* 1993; **270**: 1429–1432.
12. Orlando R III, Russell JC, Lynch J, Mattie A. Laparoscopic cholecystectomy, a state-wide experience. *Arch Surg* 1993; **128**: 494–499.
13. Steiner CA, Bass EB, Talamini MA, Pitt HA, Steinberg EP. Surgical rates and operative mortality for open and laparoscopic cholecystectomy in Maryland. *N Engl J Med* 1994; **330**: 403–408.
14. Passani S, Grieve A, Thelwall-Jones H. The effects of introducing a laparoscopic cholecystectomy in a stable population of British privately insured patients with regards to consumption of

health resources for gall bladder disease. Paper presented at the 10th ISTAHC Conference, Baltimore, 1994.

15. Apelgren KN, Blank ML, Slomski CA, Hadjis NS. Reusable instruments are more cost-effective than disposable instruments for laparoscopic cholecystomy. *Surg Endosc* 1994; **8**: 32–34.

16. Fullarton GM, Darling K, Williams J, McMillan R, Bell G. Evaluation of the cost of laparoscopic and open cholecystectomy. *Br J Surg* 1994; **81**: 124–126.

17. McMahon AJ, Russell IT, Baxter JN, Ross S, Anderson JR, Morran CG, Sunderland G, Galloway D, Ramsay G, O'Dwyer PJ. Laparoscopic versus minilaparotomy cholecystectomy: a randomised trial. *Lancet* 1994; **343**: 135–138.

18. Laporte E, Semeraro C, Alerany C, Babe M, Puig J. Economic study on the use of trocars in laparoscopic surgery. *Surg Endosc* 1994; **8**: 970.

19. Lefering R, Troidl H, Ure BM. Entscheiden die Kosten? Einweg- oder wiederverwendbare Instrumente bei der laparoskopischen Cholecystektomie? *Chirurg* 1994; **65**: 317–325.

20. Prasad A, Foley RJE. Evaluation of the cost of laparoscopic and open cholecystectomy. *Br J Surg* 1994; **81**: 777.

21. Ure BM, Lefering R, Troidl H. Costs of laparoscopic cholecystectomy. Analysis of potential savings. *Surg Endosc* 1995; **9**: 401–406.

22. Reddick EJ, Olsen DO. Outpatient laparoscopic laser cholecystectomy. *Am J Surg* 1990; **160**: 485–489.

23. Llorente J. Laparoscopic cholecystectomy in the ambulatory surgery setting. *J Lap Surg* 1992; **2**: 23–26.

24. Martin IG, Dexter SPL, McMahon MJ. Day case laparoscopic cholecystectomy. *Surgical Endoscopy* 1994; **8**: 478.

25. Lill H, Sitter H, Klotter HJ, Nies C, Güntert-Gömann K, Rothmund M. Was kostet die laparoskopische Cholecystektomie? *Chirurg* 1992; **63**: 1041–1044.

26. Kunz R, Beger D, Beger HG. Laparoscopic cholecystectomy versus minilap-cholecystectomy: a prospectively randomized trial. *Surg Endosc* 1994; **8**: 504.

27. Stevens HPJD, vd Berg M, Ruseler CH, Wereldsma JCJ. Clinical and financial aspects of cholecystectomy, open contra laparoscopic techniques. *Surg Endosc* 1994; **8**: 936.

28. Rasic Z, Cala Z, Cvitanovic B, Kosuta D. The advantages of laparoscopy in relation to the open standard cholecystectomy. *Surg Endosc* 1994; **8**: 995.

29. Ingelmo A, Ansorena L, Alonso J, Palazuelos CM, De La Torre F, Alonso JL, Escalante CF. Economist evaluation of laparoscopic cholecystectomy. *Surg Endosc* 1994; **8**: 1000.

30. McLauchlan GJ, Macintyre IMC. Return to work after laparoscopic cholecystectomy. *Br J Surg* 1995; **82**: 239–241.

31. Vanek VW, Bourguet CC. The cost of laparoscopic versus open cholecystectomy in a community hospital. *Surg Endosc* 1995; **9**: 314–323.

32. Koopmanschap MA. *Complementary analyses in economic evaluation of health care.* Erasmus University, Rotterdam, 1994.

33. Menon D, Marshall D. Diffusion of laparoscopic cholecystectomy in Canada. *Internat J Tech Assess Health Care* 1994; **10**: 287–292.

34. Royston CMS, Landsdown MRJ, Brough WA. Teaching laparoscopic surgery: the need for guidelines. *Br Med J* 1994; **308**: 1023–1025.

8

The negative effects on junior surgical training

S. Sarkar

Contemporary surgical trainees come from the first generation for whom familiarity with digital electronics, fibre optics and remote control systems has been widespread in both the domestic and educational environments. Minimally invasive techniques cause few apprehensions with regard either to the manipulation or reliability of complex equipment or the abandoning of established concepts or techniques.

The foremost apprehensions of trainees remain unchanged from previous generations. That is, fears about immediate and long-term career prospects, concerns about errors of judgement which will affect individuals' lives and doubts about their own ability to master the appropriate skills to complete their training. The adoption of minimally invasive surgery increases concerns about the quality of training and the potential loss of opportunities in the acquisition of practical skills.

In the past junior trainees would have participated closely in laparotomies performed for common surgical conditions such as cholelithiasis, perforations of peptic ulcers, inguinal herniae and appendicitis. Surgical trainees are at risk of losing opportunities to perform simple laparotomies. In the second year of a programme to introduce a teaching programme for laparoscopic appendicectomy there were eleven laparoscopic appendicectomies performed and only one open procedure by participating trainees.[1] This situation is likely to be more common as laparoscopic training programmes increase in number. In particular, basic surgical trainees will lose the opportunity of becoming familiar and comfortable performing simple laparotomies. Those who go on to higher surgical training programmes in general surgery will, of course, be taught advanced open procedures. However those, who enter other surgical specialties, which may require occasional intra-peritoneal procedures, will lose this learning opportunity indefinitely.

The application of minimally invasive techniques is, naturally, not uniform. A survey of one British Regional Health Authority found that over 50 per cent of consultants performed laparoscopic procedures whereas only 14 per cent of their trainees did so. While the management of abdominal pain is largely performed by trainees only 10 per cent used diagnostic or therapeutic laparoscopy in these circumstances.[2] Presumably the proportion of trainees using laparoscopy will increase with time and with a concomitant rise in the proportion of consultants also. While there is debate regarding the value of individual therapeutic procedures in the management of the acute abdomen the value of diagnostic laparoscopy is not in doubt. An increase in the proportion of trainees initially performing diagnostic laparoscopy in emergencies will be of benefit to patients.

Junior trainees have resented losing the role of operating surgeon or first assistant in cases that were customarily theirs. This anxiety has been minimized by involving junior trainees as camera operators from the beginning and by commencing trainees as operating surgeon at a progressively earlier stage as the training programme has matured.[1] Some units have non-medically trained staff as dedicated camera operators. This move is likely to increase resentment further.

Competition between trainees and consultants for the limited time of laparoscopic trainers has been noted and it has been suggested that the order of priority should be stated when an institution introduces a training programme.[3] One programme has reported that trainees acted as supervised operating surgeon in 59 per cent of laparoscopic cholecystectomies within a unit and that there was no difference in rates of complications between trainers and trainees.[4]

The potential loss of skill in performing open procedures has been of concern. The loss of manual palpation while performing laparoscopic procedures has been commented upon.[1] One training programme has reported that laparoscopic experience has improved overall training in biliary surgery because of improved visualization of the porta hepatis and performing the fine dissection required with the laparoscopic procedure and has reported no problems in relation to conversion to open operation.[5] Competition between junior and senior trainees presents a problem. A significant increase in the proportion of open cholecystectomies performed by senior trainees at the expense of juniors has been reported after the introduction of laparoscopic cholecystectomy.[6]

In the United States there has been debate on the criteria for granting clinical privileges for trained surgeons who have converted to laparoscopic surgery. However, less emphasis has been placed on the equivalent assessment of trainees and it has been assumed that laparoscopic surgery would be assimilated into training programmes and assessed in the traditional manner.[7]

Surgical trainees are faced with the problem of limited theatre time during which teaching can take place. Service commitments often override teaching opportunities and the pressure on theatre time is exacerbated by increasing economic constraints. It is often suggested that procedures performed by trainees take considerably longer than those performed by consultants and that laparoscopic operations are especially prolonged. One series reported of laparoscopic cholecystectomy found no difference in mean operating time between trainee performed procedures and the mean time for all operators (although consideration was given to the likelihood that the more difficult cases were performed by consultants).[8]

Several authors have emphasized the value of structured training courses and the use of simulators. The variation in the quality of courses has been mentioned.[5,9] The Royal College of Surgeons of England has set up a Minimal Access Therapy Training Unit which will provide basic courses including the use of simulators and live transmissions of operations.[10] However, one training programme has questioned the necessity of attending formal instructional courses and has found the traditional method of learning through the assistant's role successful.[4]

The introduction of laparoscopic surgery has brought new uncertainties for trainees. Initially the difficulties have been aggravated by need for trainers to become fully experienced in the new techniques. During this period there is inconsistency in the quality of training and there is competition for the opportunity of performing cases. However, after the initial phase of adoption of minimal access surgery by consultants has been completed the position of trainees is very much the traditional role of apprentice with the unusual feature that trainees are often more comfortable with the technology involved than their trainers.

References

1. Scott-Conner CE, Hall TJ, Anglin BL, Muakassa FF. Laparoscopic Appendicectomy. Initial experience in a teaching programme. *Ann Surg* 1992; **215**(6): 660–667.
2. Collier St J, Pollard SG, Morris GE, Dunn DC. Laparoscopy in the management of acute abdominal pain. *Min Invas Ther* 1993; **2**: 93–95.
3. Sigman HH, Fried GM, Hinchey EJ, Mamazza J, Wexler MJ, Garzon J, Meakins JL. Role of the teaching hospital in the development of a laparoscopic teaching program. *Can J Surg* 1992; **35**(1): 49–54.
4. Schirmer BD, Edge SB, Dix J, Miller AD. Incorporation of laparoscopy into a surgical endoscopy training program. *Am J Surg* 1992; **163**(1): 46–50.
5. Zucker KA, Bailey RW, Graham SM, Scovil W, Imbembo AL. Training for laparoscopic surgery. *World J Surg* 1993; **17**: 3–7.
6. Deziel DJ, Milikan KW, Staren ED, Doolas A, Economou SG. The impact of laparoscopic cholecystectomy on the operative experience of surgical residents. *Surg Endosc* 1993; **7**(1): 17–21.
7. Dent TL. Training, credentialing and the granting of clinical privileges for laparoscopic general surgery. *Am J Surg* 1991; **161**(3): 399–403.
8. Bailey RW, Imbembo AL, Zucker KA. Establishment of a laparoscopic cholecystectomy training program. *Am Surg* 1991; **57**(4): 231–236.
9. Bailey RW, Zucker KA, Flowers JL, Scovill WA, Graham SM, Imbembo AL. Laparoscopic cholecystectomy. Experience with 375 consecutive patients. *Ann Surg* 1991; **214**(4): 531–540.
10. Fowler C. Report from the tutor in minimal access therapy. *Ann Royal Coll Surg Engl* (Supplement) 1994; **76**: 145.

SECTION III

Surgical applications of laparoscopy

9

Operative laparoscopy in gynaecology

R.E. Richardson and A.L. Magos

Introduction

Laparoscopy was initially used for diagnostic purposes and it is the physicians who must take the credit for much of the early development of the technique. The earliest attempts at operative laparoscopy were again not by gynaecologists but general surgeons who performed adhesiolysis. In gynaecology two major landmarks have been the descriptions of the laparoscopic diagnosis of ectopic pregnancy by Hope in 1937[1] and laparoscopic sterilization by Power and Barnes in 1941.[2] In the late 1940s Raould Palmer, a gynaecologist, was the main promoter of the laparoscope in Europe but its use remained restricted to diagnostic procedures and female sterilization until the early 1970s when Semm described numerous gynaecological operations using 'pelviscopy'.[3] At that time his instruments and techniques received little positive attention in the United States but attitudes gradually changed and in 1985 it was an American, DeCherney,[4] who wrote 'The obituary of the laparotomy for pelvic reconstructive surgery has been written . . . the use of the endoscope will revolutionize gynaecological surgery'. Since that time the use of operative laparoscopy has increased enormously, not only in gynaecology but across all the surgical specialities. The development of better optics for the laparoscope, the miniaturization of video cameras and improved instrument design have allowed surgeons to attempt more complex procedures and assistants to help as they can see the operation on a television monitor. As technology has caught up with the aspirations of surgeons almost all gynaecological procedures can, and have been, performed laparoscopically, but it must be appreciated that technology is no substitute for ability.

Technique

In our unit, a video chip camera (Supercam 9050PB, Storz, Germany) is attached to a 10 mm 30° forward oblique laparoscope, the image is viewed on a monitor, and the theatre is arranged as in Fig. 9.1. The use of a 30° laparoscope helps the surgeon with perspective as it enables an area to be viewed from more than one angle and allows the surgeon to look at, rather than across, the anterior abdominal wall and pelvic side walls. The latter point is important when introducing secondary trocars and during advanced surgery when exact clarification of the position of the ureter is necessary or if pelvic side wall dissection is being performed.

Surgery is usually performed using a triple puncture approach. The laparoscope is introduced into the abdomen through an infra-umbilical incision. Safe placement of the secondary ports, usually 5.5 mm, is then performed under direct vision. The inferior epigastric arteries are avoided by first locating them lateral to the obliterated umbilical artery and then introducing the trocar tip just medially. Cosmetically, trocar placement in the pubic hairline is desirable, but if necessary the secondary trocars are placed higher and lateral to the epigastric arteries and a fourth cannula used if additional manipulation is required in difficult cases such as neosalpingostomy. Bipolar electrosurgical desiccation (ESD) is employed as our principal mechanism for achieving haemostasis; we prefer scissors for dissection although titanium clips, multifire staplers, laser and suturing techniques are all available.

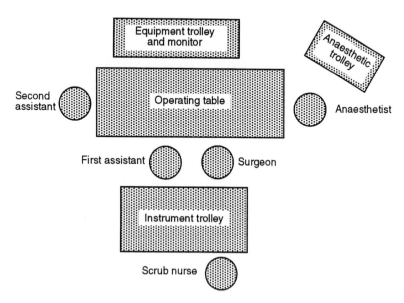

Fig. 9.1   Arrangement of equipment and personnel in the theatre suite.

Applications

Despite ultrasonography, laparoscopy remains the gold standard conservative investigation of acute abdominal pain in young women. Many of the conditions encountered, such as ectopic pregnancy or ovarian cyst accidents, can be treated laparoscopically at the time of diagnosis and are those most likely to be encountered by a general surgeon. Operative laparoscopy also has a major role in the investigation and treatment of subfertility – procedures include adhesiolysis, tubal surgery, ablation of endometriosis and myomectomy. More recently laparoscopic techniques have been used to perform hysterectomy and laparoscopic lymphadenectomy, and in the future laparoscopic surgery will become a routine part of the management of patients with gynaecological cancer.

Ectopic pregnancy

Laparoscopy was first used for the treatment of ectopic pregnancy (EP) in 1973[5] and is now the route of choice. Sensitive assays for the β subunit of human chorionic gonadotrophin (βhCG), vaginal ultrasonography, and early laparoscopy enables EP to be diagnosed before rupture allowing surgery to be conservative. After careful adhesiolysis, salpingotomy is accomplished with grasping forceps to stabilize the tube while using a monopolar needle or laser to make a linear incision about two-thirds of the length of the EP on its antimesenteric surface. The trophoblastic tissue is then removed through the incision with spoon forceps, the lumen rinsed, and bleeding points cauterized using bipolar diathermy. The incision heals spontaneously and suturing the defect is unnecessary especially as enthusiastic suturing may cause a stricture. Bleeding from the salpingotomy incision or bed of the EP can be a problem and vasoconstrictors such as vasopressin or adrenaline may be used.[6,7] Coagulating vessels in the mesosalpinx leading to the site of the ectopic reduces blood loss and is helpful in avoiding excessive diathermy of the tube and the use of vasopressin.

Tubal rupture is not a contraindication to laparoscopic management provided the patient is haemodynamically stable, although salpingectomy is usually necessary. This may be performed using Semm's triple loop technique where the affected tube is pulled through suture loops and the slipknots tightened with a pushrod (Fig. 9.2). Once three loops have been placed over the tube it is resected and removed. Alternatively, salpingectomy can be performed using bipolar diathermy and scissors. The fallopian tube proximal to the ectopic is first desiccated and cut and then the mesosalpinx is sequentially cauterized and cut until the tube containing the ectopic is free. A linear stapler can also be used, but this is an expensive option.

Tubal patency after conservative surgery is high[7,8] and does not appear to predispose to an increased risk of further EP,[9] but preservation of the affected tube does carry a risk of persistent active trophoblast. Persistent trophoblast after laparoscopic salpingotomy is significantly higher than after salpingectomy at laparotomy[10] but is typically less than 10 per cent. The incidence is highest when the pre-operative βhCG value is above 3000 IU/L, consistent with a large

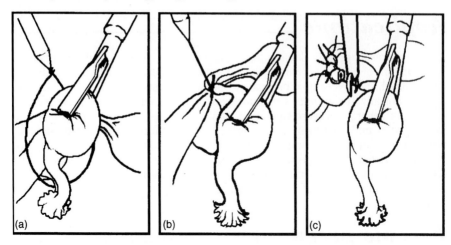

Fig. 9.2   Radical surgical treatment of tubal pregnancy using the triple loop
technique. (a) The fallopian tube containing the ectopic pregnancy is passed
through the Roeder loop. (b) The loop is closed by advancing the Roeder
knot: this is achieved by pushing down on the plastic tube whilst pulling on
the free end of the suture. The plastic tube is then withdrawn allowing the
suture to be cut. (c) Once three loops are in place the fallopian tube
containing the ectopic can be excised. (Reproduced with permission.[63])

well implanted ectopic pregnancy. Symptoms of residual trophoblast, such as
acute abdominal pain, acute intra-abdominal haemorrhage, or pelvic mass appear
one to four weeks after surgery but post-operative βhCG measurements can
detect persistent trophoblast before symptoms develop. The risk of delayed
complications is very low in patients with levels below 1000 IU/L two days after
surgery, but patients with levels above 1000 IU/L at seven days are at risk.[11]

Local injection of methotrexate,[12] prostaglandins[13] and hyperosmolar glucose
solutions[14] have been used to treat unruptured ectopic pregnancies and are
successful in 80–90 per cent of cases. Unfortunately success declines as the
mass of viable trophoblast increases and thus these techniques are limited to
the smaller unruptured cases without active bleeding.

The intrauterine pregnancy rate is higher after conservative treatment than
after salpingectomy,[15–17] and as the latter does not decrease the chance of further
EP salpingotomy is the operation of choice.[16,17] Laparoscopic treatment of EP
costs less, and there is lower patient morbidity when compared with laparotomy.[18]
This is achieved without compromising outcome as laparoscopic treatment is
associated with similar or better subsequent fertility,[15] and therefore conservative
laparoscopic treatment of EP is the best surgical option in the majority of patients.

Ovarian cysts

Careful selection of patients for laparoscopic ovarian surgery is necessary due to
the risk of treating an unsuspected ovarian malignancy.[19] Prior assessment

typically includes ultrasonography, the measurement of tumour markers such as Ca 125, and colour flow Doppler. Magnetic resonance imaging offers significant advantages over ultrasound and computed tomography in terms of diagnostic accuracy but its availability and expense limit its usefulness at present. When an ovarian cyst is the suspected cause of acute pelvic pain ultrasound examination may reveal only free fluid in the pelvis following cyst rupture. The presence of echoes throughout the fluid contained within the cyst frequently indicates that blood is present; this may be due to haemorrhage into the cyst or endometriosis, suggesting either a cyst accident or an endometrioma. Bilateral, multilocular cysts, particularly if they contain solid areas or the septae are thick, are at risk of being malignant,[20] but as many benign cysts have some adverse features, laparoscopic inspection provides the gold standard investigation.

In the case of suspected adnexal torsion prompt diagnosis and treatment is indicated.[21] Torsion is usually due to an abnormality of the adnexa such as an ovarian or para-ovarian cyst which has stretched the utero-ovarian ligament, and after untwisting the ovary or adnexum the causal factor should be treated. Conservative treatment is preferred in pre-menopausal women and the trend has been away from radical surgery except in extreme cases as the ovary appears to have remarkable powers of recovery after ischaemic insults.

If an ovarian cyst is found at laparoscopy the pelvic and abdominal peritoneal surfaces and both ovaries should be inspected, and any fluid in the Pouch of Douglas collected and sent for cytological assessment. Features suggestive of malignancy contraindicate operative laparoscopy while lesions such as endometriotic implants may provide a clue as to the origin of the cyst. Additional diagnostic procedures on an ovarian cyst involve aspiration, allowing differentiation between dermoid, endometrioma and simple cyst, and visualizing the internal surface of the cyst for any excrescence with possible biopsy for frozen section. The intention of these procedures is to exclude malignancy and using a cautious pre-operative and intra-operative protocol Bruhat's[22] group were able to diagnose 7 of 9 cancers out of 508 cysts by visual assessment. The other two were diagnosed after opening and viewing the inner aspect of the cyst. They were incorrectly suspicious of cancer in another 10 women, and in all 19 laparotomies were performed.

Besides oophorectomy, which can be performed using bipolar diathermy, stapling techniques, or Semms' triple loop technique,[23] the other options for treating ovarian cysts include, puncture and aspiration, fenestration or cystectomy. Although aspiration is simple and will relieve acute pain it is unsatisfactory as the nature of the lesion cannot be confirmed and recurrence is common. Cyst fenestration, whereby a small window is cut in the cyst wall, is a simple procedure, provides tissue for histological diagnosis, allows inspection of the inner lining of the cyst and ensures continued drainage.[24] Recurrence following this procedure is infrequent but it is not suitable for endometriomas unless the lining of the cyst is ablated,[25] or dermoid cysts because of chemical peritonitis associated with spillage of their contents.

Cystectomy is technically more demanding especially if removal of an intact cyst is attempted. After incising the tunica albuginea over the cyst on the antimesenteric portion of the ovary the crucial part of the operation is the initial separation of the tunica from the cyst wall. Once separation has begun the cyst lining is gently stripped from the ovary using two atraumatic forceps, one pair on the tunica the other on the cyst.

If there is concern that a cyst might be malignant and oophorectomy has been performed, the adnexal mass can be transferred to a collecting bag. The mouth of the bag is then removed from the abdomen and only then is the cyst deflated, reducing its size without the risk of intra-abdominal spill of cyst contents[26] (Fig. 9.3). The bag may then be removed trans-abdominally, or the bag can be sealed, passed back into the abdomen and then removed by way of a posterior colpotomy. This containment technique can also be used for dermoid cysts as it reduces the risk of spillage of cyst contents and avoids track deposits.

The role of laparoscopy in the management of sub-fertility

Hysteroscopy, hysterosalpingography, salpingoscopy and laparoscopy are complementary methods of assessing causes of infertility. The advantages of an initial hysterosalpingogram (HSG) include screening for uterine abnormality, identification of both proximal and distal tubal occlusion and the assessment of intratubal architecture. Hysteroscopy at the time of laparoscopy allows confirmation of a normal uterine cavity, or in the presence of an HSG abnormality hysteroscopic treatment may be performed. To supplement the HSG findings salpingoscopy, where the mucosal lining of the fallopian tube is visualized using a small endoscope, can be performed during the laparoscopy. Although there is a strong correlation between the degree of intratubal damage and the extent of pelvic adhesions when the underlying aetiology is pelvic inflammatory disease this is not the case with endometriosis.[27] Therefore if an appropriate decision between tubal surgery and *in vitro* fertilization (IVF) is to be made intraluminal assessment is required in all patients in whom adhesiolysis is considered to assess accurately the extent of tubal damage.

With advances in equipment and technique salpingo-ovariolysis, fimbrioplasty and neosalpingotomy may now be performed laparoscopically employing microsurgical principles. The laparoscope provides the magnification, frequent irrigation prevents tissue drying and lasers, bipolar diathermy and monopolar scissors allow haemostatic dissection and minimize tissue trauma. Microsurgical techniques only reduce adhesion formation, and even after laparoscopic surgery, although *de novo* adhesion formation is lower than after laparotomy, it remains a major problem.[28,29] Physical barriers such as Gore-Tex and Interceed, and solutions such as Dextran 70, physiological saline and Hartmann's solution have been used to prevent adhesion formation by limiting tissue apposition during the critical stage of mesothelial repair[30] with variable success. Non-steroidal anti-inflammatory drugs have been shown to reduce adhesion formation in animal models and although clinical efficacy is uncertain[30] it gives this class of drugs a potential advantage when selecting peri-operative analgesia.

If the tube and ovary are involved in adhesions, adhesiolysis may be performed using scissors, electrodiathermy or lasers, restoring the mobility between them. The carbon dioxide laser offers great precision with minimal collateral tissue

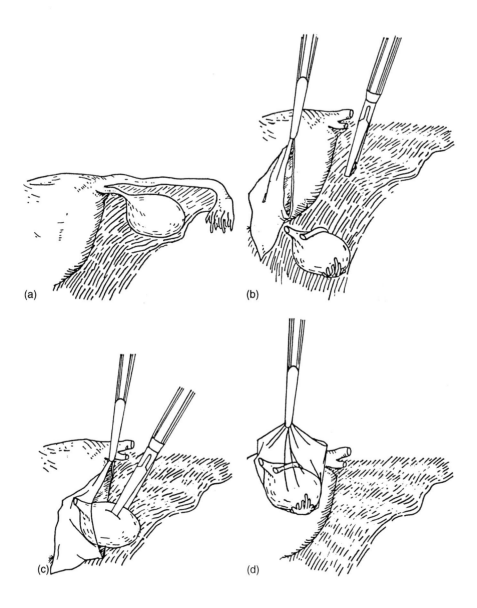

Fig. 9.3 Laparoscopic 'oophorectomy-in-a-bag' for removal of ovarian tumours of uncertain origin. (a) Ovarian cyst and fallopian tube. (b) The fallopian tube and ovary have been excised and the mouth of the bag is ready to receive them. (c) The ovary and tube are placed into the bag. (d) The bag and its contents being lifted up towards the anterior abdominal wall. (Reproduced with permission of Blackwell Science Ltd.[26])

damage and may be safer than electrodiathermy during laparoscopy but at laparotomy the two methods produce similar results in terms of pregnancies.[31]

The chance of pregnancy following this type of surgery is good as the fallopian tubes are patent and endotubal anatomy is usually normal. Pregnancy rates as high as 78 per cent can be achieved:[32] success is not dependent on the surgical modality used and results are similar to those achieved after laparotomy.[32,33]

If the fallopian tube is closed by adhesions the technique of neosalpingotomy can be used to open the hydrosalpinx. Before surgery is planned an HSG should confirm proximal tubal patency. Prior hysteroscopic falloposcopy, where the tubal lumen is assessed transcervically, or salpingoscopy at the time of laparoscopy, can also be performed. These techniques allow tubal damage to be graded which gives an indication about the likely success of surgery.[34,35]

The principal steps of neosalpingotomy include adhesiolysis to restore tubal and ovarian mobility followed by opening of the terminal hydrosalpinx. To facilitate identification of the scars on the terminal end of the damaged tube it is distended by fluid introduced transcervically. The scars usually extend radially from a central dimple which is entered, and after salpingoscopy incisions are made along the avascular scars radiating from it. The edges of the opened tube may be everted using sutures or by gentle electrocoagulation of the serosa. This latter technique leads to shrinkage of the serosa which everts the mucosal lining of the tube and is an effect which can also be achieved using a defocused carbon dioxide laser beam.

Pregnancy rates after neosalpingotomy are much poorer than after simple division of tubal adhesions with intra-uterine pregnancy rates of about 30–35 per cent.[36] This is because there is usually underlying tubal disease and the chance of pregnancy decreases with increasing mucosal damage.[34,35,37,38] As the prognosis for pregnancy is poor and the results after laparoscopy are similar to those after laparotomy it is logical to perform the least invasive form of surgery.

Polycystic ovarian syndrome _____

The surgical treatment of polycystic ovarian syndrome (PCOS) was first reported by Stein and Leventhal in 1935 who performed bilateral ovarian wedge resection at laparotomy. This technique can be complicated by infertility from adhesions, and with the availability of the drug clomiphene, was relegated as a treatment option. However, some patients remain anovulatory despite medical treatment and are suitable for laparoscopic surgical treatment which essentially involves drilling holes in the ovary rather than removing part of it. The measurable falls in androgens and luteinizing hormone levels are similar to those reported after wedge resection, as are the rates of ovulation achieved (52–93 per cent). Both ESD and lasers have been used with comparable results and pregnancy rates of 56–80 per cent have been reported.[39,40] Second look laparoscopy after ovarian drilling has been performed in a few patients and it appears that ovarian adhesions are not a major problem, and certainly less than after laparotomy. The major procedure-related problem after such treatment is ovarian atrophy from excessive drilling and thus it is advisable not to cauterize near the hilum of the ovary and to limit the number of holes depending on ovarian size.[41]

Endometriosis and pelvic pain ⸻

There is a long history of effective laparoscopic treatment of endometriosis for both pain relief and the enhancement of fertility. The standard system for categorizing the extent of endometriosis is the modified American Fertility Society classification,[42] giving the AFS score. The four broad categories are minimal, mild, moderate and severe (stages I, II, III, and IV) depending on the anatomical extent of the disease within the pelvis.

The main reasons for treating endometriosis are symptoms such as pain or subfertility, and the risk of disease progression. The appearance of endometriosis is quite diverse ranging from very subtle lesions which are difficult to visualize to typical black puckered, powderburn lesions.[43] The subtle lesions may well represent early, active disease and thus recognition and treatment of these lesions may prevent progression, stop deep infiltration, fibrosis, peritoneal contraction, and the formation of adhesions and endometriomas. Controversy continues as to whether minimal to mild endometriosis contributes to subfertility and if so whether treatment actually helps. Nevertheless the ablation of endometrial deposits laparoscopically with either electrocautery or laser has been well documented, with pregnancy rates ranging from 40–75 per cent.[44] Bipolar diathermy, although effective, lacks the precision and accuracy for ablating ectopic endometrial implants, especially if they are situated over vital structures such as bladder, bowel or ureter. Of the lasers available, the carbon dioxide laser is the most versatile as it is more accurate than fibre lasers (Nd-YAG, KTP) and tissue damage beyond the zone of vaporization is extremely limited so that healing is not complicated by fibrosis, scarring or contracture. Minimal and mild endometriosis can also be treated medically, however, non-surgical therapy delays attempts at conception and may well only suppress rather than eradicate implants.[45] The treatment of minimal and mild endometriosis surgically at the time of diagnosis prevents or delays progression, and as it is quick and does not postpone attempts at conception it is the logical approach to the management of endometriosis.[46]

Severe forms of endometriosis causing anatomical distortion should be treated surgically. Endometriomas have been treated successfully using laparoscopic techniques which have included excision of the endometriotic cyst or fulguration or laser vaporization of the lining after fenestration.[25] Pregnancy rates following treatment of advanced endometriosis are good and approach those after less severe disease.[47] When compared with treatment at laparotomy, the results and complications of laparoscopic treatment of endometriosis are similar, with savings in hospital expenses and time off work.[48]

Pelvic pain and dysmenorrhoea are immense problems causing periodic absenteeism. In as many as 20 per cent drug treatment will fail and surgery either by pre-sacral neurectomy or laparoscopic uterosacral nerve ablation (LUNA) may be indicated.[49,50] LUNA is simpler and in a prospective double blind comparative study laparoscopic transection of the uterosacral ligaments close to the insertion on the posterior part of the cervix has been shown to be an effective treatment for dysmenorrhoea unresponsive to drug therapy.[49] Transection can be performed using electrocautery or various lasers, care being taken to avoid the ureters and pelvic veins laterally and vessels in the depths of the ligament. Success rates of over 80 per cent have been achieved in most series with few complications, it is a procedure which can be combined with ablation of endometriosis or division of adhesions. Laparoscopic ablation or excision of endometriosis alone gives excellent relief from pelvic pain in the majority of women although as yet there have been no randomized controlled trials to confirm the clinical efficacy of laparoscopic ablation of symptomatic endometriosis.

Laparoscopic hysterectomy ─────────

Laparoscopic hysterectomy (LH) was first described by Reich[51] in 1989. The patient had a fibroid uterus and extensive adhesions secondary to endometriosis and without doubt an abdominal hysterectomy was avoided. Advanced laparoscopic techniques allowed the ovaries and uterus to be dissected free, the vascular pedicles isolated and secured with bipolar electrosurgery, and the uterus and left ovary to be delivered vaginally. Several modifications of Reich's original technique have subsequently been described using suturing,[52,53] linear staplers,[54] and lasers.[55]

The generally accepted indication for LH is to convert an abdominal hysterectomy into a laparoscopic/vaginal procedure and thereby reduce the trauma and morbidity for the patient. While this is a desirable aim, there is little doubt that far too many unnecessary abdominal hysterectomies are performed, which could be carried out vaginally.[56] Therefore, although LH has been shown to be superior to abdominal hysterectomy in terms of recovery and discomfort,[54] the choice for most women should be between laparoscopic and vaginal hysterectomy. Prospective randomized controlled trials have not revealed any advantage in laparoscopic hysterectomy in terms of post-operative discomfort, complications, hospital stay or recovery but there is the disadvantage that in the majority of patients LH takes significantly longer to carry out.[57,58] The only clear advantage of LH compared with vaginal hysterectomy is in allowing pelvic surgery that cannot be completed vaginally to be performed without laparotomy. The indications for the procedure should therefore reflect this. The further investigation and laparoscopic treatment of suspicious pelvic masses, the division of adhesions preventing vaginal hysterectomy, ablation of symptomatic endometriosis and the need for lymphadenectomy are all good indications for a combined approach. However, it is unnecessary to continue with laparoscopic dissection once the procedure can be completed vaginally, as recovery is similar irrespective of how much laparoscopic dissection is performed and laparoscopic dissection takes considerably longer.[59,60]

Laparoscopic lymph node dissection (LLND) and the treatment of gynaecological malignancy

Progress in laparoscopic surgery has made laparoscopic pelvic lymphadenectomy possible and surgically satisfactory in experienced hands. Experience of laparoscopic para-aortic lymphadenectomy is at present limited.

In cervical carcinoma total lymphadenectomy with excision of the parametrial tissue is of therapeutic value, but such radical surgery is not appropriate for all patients. The disease is staged surgically and provides an excellent indication for laparoscopic lymphadenectomy allowing those who are not suitable for radical surgery to avoid laparotomy and commence radiotherapy earlier. Querleu et al.[61] have performed laparoscopic pelvic lymphadenectomy in 39 patients to stage early (IB–IIB) carcinoma of the cervix. The procedure typically lasted 90 minutes and between 3 and 22 lymph nodes were removed without significant morbidity. Five patients had metastatic nodes and were treated with radiation treatment alone while the remainder underwent radical surgery, either vaginally (Schauta–Amreich) or abdominally (Wertheim's). No unexpected metastatic nodes were observed at laparotomy giving a sensitivity of 100 per cent and indicating the accuracy of laparoscopic lymphadenectomy in their hands.

The value of laparoscopic pre-therapeutic staging of stage I endometrial carcinoma by laparoscopic lymph node sampling is limited as surgery is required whatever the nodal status. However, pelvic laparoscopic lymphadenectomy can be combined with laparoscopic hysterectomy for surgical treatment of patients with low risk stage I disease. Such patients may be considered as inadequately staged without para-aortic sampling; however, the level of understaging in node negative patients would be minimal in this group.

In cases of apparently early ovarian cancer pelvic nodes may remain negative despite the presence of positive aortic nodes, and so without adequate infra-renal para-aortic sampling laparoscopic treatment of early ovarian carcinoma, even with containment techniques which isolate the ovarian mass from the peritoneal cavity, are surgically inadequate. The laparoscopic approach using containment techniques remains a valid extension of diagnostic techniques in the management of a suspicious adnexal mass as the vast majority of such cysts are benign.

In a case report of laparoscopic para-aortic node sampling Querleu combined laparoscopic hysterectomy with laparoscopic pelvic and infra-renal para-aortic lymph node sampling and infra-colic omentectomy in a patient presenting with borderline serous ovarian carcinoma.[62] Twelve pelvic nodes and 9 para-aortic nodes were obtained in a procedure lasting 270 minutes. All nodal tissue was tumour-free and the patient was discharged home the day following surgery.

Case reports have shown that almost any surgical procedure can be achieved laparoscopically by experienced surgeons. The expansion of laparoscopy into the field of gynaecological oncology, from second look procedures to staging and treatment, must not be at the expense of standards and these reports must be followed by prospective trials to assess their value and safety in the treatment of patients with early malignancy.

Conclusions

The foundation of operative laparoscopy in gynaecology is a broad base of surgical skills in all aspects of gynaecological surgery, both abdominal and vaginal, combined with a co-ordinated approach from a well-trained and motivated team of surgeons, anaesthetists and nurses. Most suitable gynaecological procedures have been attempted laparoscopically and the reported evidence is adequate to support the use of many of them in routine practice. Unfortunately the conversion of an operation from laparotomy to laparoscopy takes longer than reading this chapter or watching the latest endoscopic video. Operative laparoscopy demands complex hand–eye co-ordination and the three-dimensional perspective of open surgery is missing; surgeons require patience and manual dexterity to gain good hand–eye co-ordination, enabling them to relearn their operating skills. There are no overnight conversion courses and as inexperience may quickly be translated into complications, surgeons must be properly grounded in the basics before attempting more complicated procedures. This is essential to ensure that laparoscopic surgery is used effectively and safely without needless complications.

References

1. Hope R. The differential diagnosis of ectopic pregnancy by peritoneoscopy. *Surg, Gynaecol Obstet* 1937; **64**: 229–234.
2. Power FH, Barnes AC. Sterilization by means of peritoneoscopic fulguration: a preliminary report. *Am J Obstet Gynecol* 1941; **41**: 1038–1043.
3. Semm K. *Atlas of Laparoscopy and Hysteroscopy.* Saunders, Philadelphia, 1977.
4. DeCherney AH. The leader of the band is tired. *Fertil Steril* 1985; **44**: 299–302.
5. Shapiro HI, Adler DH. Excision of an ectopic pregnancy through the laparoscope. *Am J Obstet Gynecol* 1973; **117**: 290–291.
6. Pouly JL, Manhes H, Canis M, Bruhat MA. Conservative laparoscopic treatment of 321 ectopic pregnancies. *Fertil Steril* 1986; **46**: 1093–1097.
7. Phipps JH, John M, Lewis V. Laparoscopic treatment of tubal ectopic pregnancy – a series of 62 cases. *Gynaecol Endosc* 1992; **1**: 191–194.
8. Keckstein J, Hepp S, Schneider V, Sasse V, Steiner R. The contact Nd-YAG laser: a new technique for conservation of the fallopian tube in unruptured ectopic pregnancy. *Br J Obstet Gynaecol* 1990; **97**: 352–356.
9. Hallet JG. Tubal conservation in ectopic pregnancy: a study of 200 cases. *Am J Obstet Gynecol* 1990; **154**: 1216–1221.
10. Seifer DB, Gutmann JM, Grant WD, Kamps CA, DeCherney AH. Comparison of persistent ectopic pregnancy after laparoscopic salpingotomy versus salpingotomy at laparotomy for ectopic pregnancy. *Obstet Gynecol* 1993; **81**: 378–382.
11. Lundorff P, Hahlin M, Sjoblom P, Lindblom BO. Persistent trophoblast after conservative treatment of tubal pregnancy: prediction and detection. *Obstet Gynecol* 1991; **77**: 129–133.
12. Pansky M, Bukovsky J, Golan A, Langer R, Schneider D, Arieli S. Local meth-

otrexate injection: a nonsurgical treatment of ectopic pregnancy. *Am J Obstet Gynecol* 1989; **161**: 393–396.

13. Lang PF, Weiss PAM, Mayer HO, Haas JG, Honigl W. Conservative treatment of ectopic pregnancy with local injection of prostaglandin-F2alpha: a prospective randomised study. *Lancet* 1990; **336**: 78–81.

14. Lang PF, Tamussino K, Honigl W, Ralph G. Treatment of unruptured tubal pregnancy by laparoscopic instillation of hyperosmolarglucose solution. *Am J Obstet Gynecol* 1992; **166**: 1378–1381.

15. Koninckx PR, Witters K, Brosens J, Stemers N, Oosterlynck D, Meuleman C. Conservative laparoscopic treatment of ectopic pregnancies using the CO_2-laser. *Br J Obstet Gynaecol* 1991; **98**: 1254–1259.

16. Dubuisson JB, Aubriot FX, Foulet H, Bruel D, de Jolinere JB, Mandelbrot L. Reproductive outcome after laparoscopic salpingectomy for tubal pregnancy. *Fertil Steril* 1990; **53**: 1004–1005.

17. Pouly JL, Chapron C, Manhes H, Canis M, Wattiez A, Bruhat MA. Multifactorial analysis of fertility after conservative laparoscopic treatment of ectopic pregnancy in a series of 223 patients. *Fertil Steril* 1991; **56**: 453–460.

18. Baumann R, Magos AL, Turnbull A. Prospective comparison of videopelviscopy with laparotomy for ectopic pregnancy. *Br J Obstet Gynaecol* 1991; **98**: 765–771.

19. Maiman M, Seltzer V, Boyce J. Laparoscopic excision of ovarian neoplasms subsequently found to be malignant. *Obstet Gynecol* 1991; **77**: 563–565.

20. Meire HB, Farrant P, Guha T. Distinction of benign from malignant ovarian cysts by ultrasound. *Br J Obstet Gynaecol* 1978; **85**: 893–899.

21. Manhes H, Canis M, Mage G, Pouly JL, Bruhat MA. Place de la coelioscopie dans le diagnostic et le traitement des torsions d'annexes. *J Gynecologie, Obstetrique et Biologie de la Reproduction* 1984; **13**: 825–829.

22. Mage G, Canis M, Manhes H, Pouly JL, Wattiez A, Bruhat MA. Laparoscopic management of adnexal cystic masses. *J Gynecol Surg* 1990; **6**(2): 71–79.

23. Daniell JF, Kurtz BR, Lee J. Laparoscopic oophorectomy: comparative study of ligatures, bipolar coagulation, and automatic stapling devices. *Obstet Gynecol* 1992; **80**: 325–328.

24. Larsen JF, Pedersen OD, Gregersen E. Ovarian fenestration through the laparoscope. *Acta Obstetricia et Gynecologica Scand* 1986; **65**: 539–542.

25. Fayez JA, Vogel MF. Comparison of different treatment methods of endometriomas by laparoscopy. *Obstet Gynecol* 1991; **78**: 660–665.

26. Amso NN, Broadbent JAM, Hill NCW, Magos AL. Laparoscopic 'oophorectomy-in-a-bag' for removal of ovarian tumours of uncertain origin. *Gynaecol Endosc* 1992; **1**: 85–89.

27. Bowman MC, Cooke ID. Comparison of fallopian tube intraluminal pathology as assessed by salpingoscopy with pelvic adhesions. *Fertil Steril* 1994; **61**: 464–469.

28. Diamond MP, Daniell JF, Feste J, Vaughn WK, Martin DC. Adhesion reformation and de novo adhesion formation after reproductive pelvic surgery. *Fertil Steril* 1987; **47**: 864–866.

29. Operative Laparoscopy Study Group. Postoperative adhesion development after operative laparoscopy: evaluation at early second look procedures. *Fertil Steril* 1991; **55**: 700–704.

30. diZerega GS. Contemporary adhesion prevention. *Fertil Steril* 1994; **61**: 219–235.

31. Tulandi T. Salpingo-ovariolysis: a comparison between laser surgery and electrosurgery. *Fertil Steril* 1986; **45**: 489–491.

32. Reich H. Laparoscopic treatment of extensive pelvic adhesions, including hydrosalpinx. *J Repro Med* 1987; **32**: 736–742.

33. Donnez J, Casanas-Roux F. Prognostic factors of fimbrial microsurgery. *Fertil Steril* 1986; **46**: 200–204.

34. Kerin JF, Williams DB, San Roman GA,

Pearlstone AC, Grundfest WS. Fallopo-scopic classification and treatment of fallopian tube lumen disease. *Fertil Steril* 1992; **57**: 731–741.

35. Dubuisson JB, Chapron C, Morice P, Aubriot FX, Foulet H, Bouquet de Joli-nière J. Laparoscopic salpingotomy: fer-tility results according to tubal mucosal appearance. *Hum Reprod* 1994; **9**: 334–339.

36. Chapron C, Dubuisson JB, Chavet X, Morice P. Treatment and causes of female infertility. *Lancet* 1994; **344**: 333–334.

37. Canis M, Mage G, Manhes H, Wattiez A, Bruhat MA. Laparoscopic distal tubo-plasty: report of 87 cases and a 4-year experience. *Fertil Steril* 1991; **56**: 616–621.

38. Marana R, Quagliarello J. Distal tube occlusion: microsurgery versus in vitro fertilization – a review. *Int J Fertil* 1988; **33**: 107–115.

39. Gjonnaess H. Polycystic ovarian syn-drome treated by ovarian cautery through the laparoscope. *Fertil Steril* 1984; **21**: 20–25.

40. Daniell JF, Miller W. Polycystic ovaries treated by laparoscopic laser vaporization. *Fertil Steril* 1989; **51** 232–236.

41. Daniell JF. Complications of laparo-scopic ovarian cauterization. *Fertil Steril* 1989; **52**: 879.

42. American Fertility Society. Revised American Fertility Society classifica-tion of endometriosis. *Fertil Steril* 1985; **43**: 351–352.

43. Jansen R, Russell P. Non-pigmented endometriosis: clinical laparoscopic and pathological definition. *Am J Obstet Gynecol* 1986; **155**: 1154–1159.

44. Cook AS, Rock JA. The role of laparo-scopy in the treatment of endo-metriosis. *Fertil Steril* 1991; **55**: 663–680.

45. Evers J. The second look laparoscopy for the evaluation of the results of med-ical treatment of endometriosis should not be performed during ovarian suppression. *Fertil Steril* 1987; **45**: 502–504.

46. Lassey AT, Garry R. Simultaneous diagnosis and treatment of early stage endometriosis. *Gynaecol Endosc* 1994; **3**: 97–99.

47. Nezhat C, Crowgey S, Nezhat F. Video-laseroscopy for the treatment of endo-metriosis associated with infertility. *Fertil Steril* 1989; **51**: 237.

48. Gant NF. Infertility and endometriosis: comparison of pregnancy outcomes with laparotomy versus laparoscopic techniques. *Am J Obstet Gynecol* 1992; **166**: 1072–1081.

49. Lichten EM, Bombard J. Surgical treat-ment of dysmenorrhoea with laparo-scopic uterine nerve ablation. *J Repro Med* 1987; **32**: 37–42.

50. Tjaden B, Schlaff WD, Kimball A, Rock JA. The efficacy of presacral neurect-omy for the relief of mid-line dysmenorrhoea. *Obstet Gynecol* 1990; **76**: 89–91.

51. Reich H, DeCaprio J, McGlynn F. Laparoscopic hysterectomy. *J Gynecol Surg* 1989; **5**: 213–216.

52. Semm K. Hysterectomy via laparotomy or pelviscopy. A new CASH method without colpotomy [German]. *Geburt-shilfe und Frauenheilkunde* 1991; **51**: 996–1003.

53. Reich H. Laparoscopic Hysterectomy. *Surg Laparosc Endosc* 1992; **2**(1): 85–88.

54. Nezhat F, Nezhat C, Gordon S, Wilkins E. Laparoscopic versus abdominal hysterectomy. *J Repro Med* 1992; **37**: 247–250.

55. Ewen S, Sutton CJG. Initial experience with supracervical laparoscopic hyster-ectomy and removal of the cervical transformation zone. *Br J Obstet Gynae-col* 1994; **101**: 225–228.

56. Kovac SR, Cruikshank SH, Retto HF. Laparoscopy-assisted vaginal hysterec-tomy. *J Gynecol Surg* 1990; **6**: 185–193.

57. Summitt Jr RL, Stovall TG, Lipscomb GH, Ling FW. Randomized comparison of laparoscopy-assisted vaginal hyster-ectomy with standard vaginal hyster-ectomy in an outpatient setting. *Obstet Gynecol* 1992; **80**: 895–901.

58. Richardson R, Bournas N, Magos AL. Is Laparoscopic hysterectomy a waste of

time? *Lancet* 1995 Jan 7; **345**(8941): 36–41.

59. Richardson RE, Broadbent JAM, Bournas NG, Magos AL. Post-operative recovery following laparoscopically assisted vaginal hysterectomy. *Gynaecol Endos* 1994; **3**: 45 (Abstract).

60. Richardson RE, Broadbent JAM, Bournas NG, Magos AL. What factors influence operating time at laparoscopically assisted hysterectomy? *Gynaecol Endosc* 1994; **3**: 45–46. (Abstract).

61. Querleu D. Laparoscopic para-aortic node sampling in gynecologic oncology: a preliminary experience. *Gynecol Oncol* 1993; **49**: 24–29.

62. Querleu D, Leblanc E, Castelain B. Laparoscopic pelvic lymphadenectomy in the staging of early carcinoma of the cervix. *Am J Obstet Gynecol* 1991; **164**: 579–581.

63. Semm K. Endoscopic intra abdominal surgery. Karl Storz GMBH & Co. Tuttlingen 1984, Figure 27, p. 30.

10a

Biliary tract and gallbladder: laparoscopic cholecystectomy

N. Gallegos

Introduction

Since the description of the first cholecystectomy by Langenbuch in 1882 surgery has retained its place as the principal modality for the treatment of gallstones. The traditional open operation, performed through an incised abdominal wound, has now been superseded by the minimally invasive laparoscopic approach.

This article reviews the indications and contraindications for laparoscopic cholecystectomy, describes the technique of the operation and looks at the results.

Indications and contraindications

The indications for laparoscopic cholecystectomy remain broadly similar to those of the open operation. Chronic symptoms from gallstones is the commonest reason for surgery. There is, however, some indication that the technique is being applied to patients who might not otherwise have undergone the open operation; certainly cholecystectomy rates appear to have risen in the United States.[1] Patients with asymptomatic stones and those without stones but with symptoms considered to be of biliary origin are undergoing laparoscopic surgery with increasing frequency.

Unfitness for general anaesthesia remains the only absolute contraindication to laparoscopic cholecystectomy. There are, however, relative contraindications to the procedure, see Table 10a.1. What importance should be given to each of these in deciding to operate will depend on several factors, including the clinical

Table 10a.1   Relative contraindications to performing
laparoscopic cholecystectomy

Coagulopathy
Portal hypertension
Prior intra-abdominal surgery
Pregnancy
Carcinoma of the gallbladder
Cholecysto-enteric fistulae
Morbid obesity
Acute cholecystitis

circumstances of the patient, the experience of the surgeon, the available equipment and whether or not the condition is recognized pre- or peroperatively.

The risk of haemorrhage is present in all surgical procedures. Under laparoscopic conditions the control of bleeding is difficult and frequently cited as the reason for conversion to an open operation. Laparoscopic cholecystectomy should therefore be considered carefully in patients with a coagulopathy or portal hypertension in whom the risk of bleeding will be increased.[2,3]

The presence of acute cholecystitis was thought to militate against laparoscopic cholecystectomy.[4] Series have now been reported that show the operation to be feasible under acute inflammatory conditions although between a quarter and a third of patients may have their operation converted to an open procedure.[5,6] Where an empyema is present or the gallbladder is gangrenous the conversion rate to open operation is even greater, 83 and 50 per cent respectively.[7] Laparoscopic cholecystectomy is more likely to succeed if the interval from the onset of symptoms to operation is less than five days.[8]

Prior intra-abdominal surgery has been cited as a relative contraindication to laparoscopic cholecystectomy. Wongworawat *et al*, however, recorded a completion rate of 95.6 per cent in 175 patients who had had a previous operation.[9]

Although laparoscopic cholecystectomy has been reported to be safe during all trimesters of pregnancy[10] it should still be considered that pregnancy is a strong contraindication to the procedure as relatively few cases (41) have been recorded in the literature.

There are several case reports of abdominal wall metastases following the laparoscopic removal of a gallbladder containing adenocarcinoma.[11,12] In the unusual event that this diagnosis is made pre-operatively, laparoscopic surgery should be avoided.

Although successful transection of fistulous tracks between the gallbladder and the common bile duct (Mirrizi's syndrome) and the gallbladder and the gut have been described,[13,14] these conditions should still be regarded with caution.

It can be difficult to gain laparoscopic access in the morbidly obese patient. This has now been overcome by the availability of longer instruments. Furthermore, there is evidence that in obese patients the risk of major complications, e.g. thromboembolism is no greater with laparoscopic cholecystectomy than with open cholecystectomy.[15]

The operation of laparoscopic cholecystectomy

Pre-operative preparation

Aside from the general measures required to prepare a patient for operation under general anaesthetic the following points should be considered.

1. In obtaining informed consent for laparoscopic cholecystectomy mention must be made of the increased incidence of bile duct injury, which may be up to five times that seen with the open operation.[16]
2. The patient should be warned that it may not be possible to complete the operation laparoscopically and that resort to open operation may be required. The frequency with which this occurs varies between different series but is of the order of 5 per cent.[17,19]
3. As yet there is no evidence to suggest that the risk of thromboembolic disease is increased in patients undergoing laparoscopic cholecystectomy. However, the use of the reverse Trendelenberg position coupled with a positive pressure pneumoperitoneum may encourage deep venous thrombi to form. Thromboprophylaxis should therefore be used, and subcutaneous heparin and compression stockings are both appropriate.[19,20]
4. There is a paucity of data on the value of prophylactic antibiotics in laparoscopic cholecystectomy. Their use in patients undergoing operation for acute cholecystitis or an empyema of the gallbladder is appropriate, but in the absence of these risk factors meticulous antiseptic skin preparation is seen by some as adequate for the prevention of post-surgical infection.[21]
5. Where there is a history of jaundice or the ultrasound scan suggests stones in or dilation of the common bile duct, performance of a pre-operative ERCP (endoscopic retrograde cholangio pancreatography) should be considered.

The operation

Although numerous and varied descriptions of laparoscopic cholecystectomy exist the general principles regarding the performance of a safe operation remain constant.

The patient lies in the supine position on the operating table. The surgeon must have a comfortable view of the TV monitor and ideally he should work along the line of sight of the laparoscope so that the necessity to reorientate the image is minimized.

A Verres needle has conventionally been used to establish the pneumoperitoneum. This method risks visceral and vascular injury, and as an alternative, the direct puncture technique is probably safer.[22] The skin and peritoneum lie closest together at the umbilicus. If the umbilicus is everted, using a Lane's tissue holding forceps, and then incised the peritoneum is easily penetrated. Passage of an artery forceps into the peritoneal cavity will confirm that the peritoneum has been breached. A 10 mm port loaded with a blunt tipped trocar can then be safely advanced through the defect and the laparoscope introduced. Visualization of omentum or gut provides further confirmation that the peritoneal cavity has been entered before the pneumoperitoneum is established. The three other ports required, one 10 mm and two 5 mm ports, are inserted under direct vision. The 10 mm port is in the midline just below the xiphisternum; the two 5 mm ports are just below the right costal margin, one in the midlavicular line, the other in the anterior axillary line.

Either a 0° or 30° laparoscope is suitable although the latter provides greater flexibility in the field of vision obtained and may provide better views of Calot's triangle. A forceps placed through the most lateral of the 5 mm ports grasps the fundus of the gallbladder and retracts it up over the liver. Another grasping forceps, passed through the second 5 mm port, is applied to Hartmann's pouch, which is retracted laterally. This manoeuvre places the cystic duct under tension and facilitates the dissection of Calot's triangle. A hook diathermy may be used for the dissection but care must be taken to avoid inadvertent burns to the duodenum, common bile duct or hepatic artery. The author prefers to use blunt dissection, separating the tissues with curved forceps and always dissecting away from the gallbladder while keeping close to its wall. Once the cystic artery and cystic duct have been clearly identified each is severed between ligaclips placed proximal and distal to the point of division. If peroperative cholangiography is to be performed the cystic duct is only partially divided. A variety of commercially designed cannulas, ports and forceps are available for performing cholangiograms. A more accessible alternative is to introduce an umbilical catheter into the abdomen via a large bore intravenous cannula placed just below the costal margin and to the right of the midline. The catheter is grasped by a pair of dissecting forceps (most easily those introduced through the epigastric port) and directed through the partially opened cystic duct. Here the cannula is secured with a ligaclip applied with sufficient pressure to hold its position while still allowing the injection of contrast. The use of an image intensifier allows immediate access to the views of the biliary tree. Once the examination is complete the catheter is removed and the cystic duct clipped and divided. The gallbladder is then dissected from the liver bed. The neck of the freed gallbladder is grasped with heavy forceps, drawn into one of the 10 mm ports and ultimately through the abdominal wall. This manoeuvre is easiest through the epigastric port as the work takes place along the line of sight of the laparoscope. Where extension of the wound is required a better cosmetic result is obtained if the umbilical port is used. The ports are then withdrawn and the wounds sutured. Many reports now exist of port site hernias and as a result several methods have been developed to ensure their more secure closure. Of these the crochet hook technique is perhaps the best. The hook, loaded with the suture, is passed through the full thickness of the abdominal wall on one side of the port site wound; the suture is released using laparoscopic instruments and the hook withdrawn. The hook is then reinserted on the other side of the wound, the suture remounted, drawn through the abdominal wall and tied.

Peroperative cholangiography?

The value of peroperative cholangiography in laparoscopic cholecystectomy continues to be debated. Those who do not practise it report no increase in morbidity either from missed common bile duct stones or through injuries to the biliary tree.[23] On the other hand surgeons in favour of peroperative cholangiography suggest that anatomical anomalies can be elucidated and damage to the biliary tree either averted or recognized early, enabling a prompt repair to be effected.[24]

The difficult operation

Each stage of laparoscopic cholecystectomy, from establishing the pneumoperitoneum to extraction of the gallbladder, may be marked by difficulties.

Loops of bowel, adherent to the undersurface of abdominal scars, are clearly at risk of injury during the introduction of a Verres needle. Puncture of the abdominal wall should therefore take place through 'virgin territory' or be abandoned altogether in favour of introducing the cannula under direct vision by the Hasson technique.[25] Should bowel have been injured and the defect recognized then repair can be effected either by intracorporeal suturing or conversion to an open procedure.

Blood vessels in the abdominal wall, particularly the subcostal, superior and inferior epigastric arteries, may be injured as trocars are inserted. A hand-held Doppler may aid their identification and avert this complication.[26]

Severe inflammation obscuring Calot's triangle poses the greatest risk to the patient and challenge to the skill of the surgeon. A useful dissecting tool in these circumstances is the combined suction/irrigation instrument which allows for relatively safe, blunt dissection while at the same time permitting blood to be cleared from the operative field. However, where the anatomy cannot be defined the laparoscopic approach should be abandoned; it remains a matter of judgement for each surgeon as to how much time should be spent on dissection before this decision is made and the conversion rates for different series vary as a result. In a series of 746 laparoscopic cholecystectomies Peters *et al.* recorded a conversion rate of 14 per cent;[27] difficult dissection due to dense adhesions and the need to treat common bile duct stones were the most frequent reasons for conversion. Schrenk *et al.* had a conversion rate of 4.3 per cent.[28] Using a logistic regression analysis they identified the following features to be associated with a higher risk of conversion: pain or rigidity in the right upper quadrant, thickening of the gallbladder wall on pre-operative ultrasound, dense adhesions around the gallbladder and acute cholecystitis.

A cystic duct which cannot be safely closed with ligaclips should be encircled with an Endoloop ligature (Ethicon). If the gallbladder is very adherent to the liver bed a partial cholecystectomy, in which the posterior wall of the gallbladder is left behind, may prove easier to accomplish.[29] When the gallbladder is friable and liable to fragment it should be placed in a retrieval bag before attempting to extract it through a port wound.

Complications associated with laparoscopic cholecystectomy ————

Death, bile duct injury, leakage of bile and haemorrhage are the most important complications associated with laparoscopic cholecystectomy. However, as the number of laparoscopic cholecystectomies has increased, so too has the variety of other complications associated with the procedure.

Death following laparoscopic cholecystectomy is rare and less than that recorded for the open operation, with an incidence of about 0.1 per cent. In an analysis of all cholecystectomies, both open and laparoscopic, performed in the 54 acute care hospitals in Maryland, USA over the period 1990–1992, the operative mortality was 80 per cent lower for laparoscopic cholecystectomy.[30]

One of the most serious complications of laparoscopic cholecystectomy is bile duct injury. In the Royal College of Surgeons audit[16] bile duct injury was reported in 4 of 8035 (0.06 per cent) open cholecystectomies. By comparison, in the same audit, there was a significant increase in the number of bile duct injuries associated with laparoscopic cholecystectomy; 11 were reported in 3319 cases (0.33 per cent; Fisher's exact test, p. = 0.0005). In a review of multicentre audits of laparoscopic cholecystectomy involving 136,816 patients there were 634 bile duct injuries (0.5 per cent).[31] From a consecutive series of 2427 patients Morgenstern *et al.* report seven bile duct injuries (0.58 per cent) in their first 1284 cases of laparoscopic cholecystectomy and six injuries in the subsequent 1143 cases (0.5 per cent).[32] These latter figures suggest that even with increasing experience the higher risk of bile duct injury associated with laparoscopic cholecystectomy may not be eliminated. Using a regression model based on the results from 8839 laparoscopic cholecystectomies, Moore and Bennett predicted that a surgeon had a 1.7 per cent chance of a bile duct injury in his first case and a 0.17 per cent chance of such an injury by the 50th case.[33]

The leakage of bile, especially from the cystic duct, appears to be a problem particularly associated with laparoscopic cholecystectomy as compared to the open operation.[34] The incidence of this complication lies between 1 and 3 per cent.[34,35] The leaks may be due to dislodgement of clips used to seal the cystic duct, failure of the clip to occlude the lumen of the duct, or delayed tissue necrosis following diathermy injury.[36] Patients usually present some days after surgery with abdominal pain, nausea and vomiting. Once a bile leak is suspected ERCP should be carried out as soon as possible and if appropriate a biliary endoprosthesis inserted.[37]

Primary haemorrhage is an important reason for conversion to the open operation but reactionary haemorrhage may also precipitate a return to theatre. Chen *et al* record 4 out of 1475 (0.2 per cent) patients undergoing laparoscopic cholecystectomy as requiring a laparotomy for post-operative bleeding.[38] However, a survey from Norway, conducted while laparoscopic cholecystectomy was being introduced, reports a much higher incidence of bleeding with 12 of 527 patients (2.3 per cent) requiring re-operation.[39]

Other, rarer, complications include: fatal CO_2 embolism;[40] the migration into the common bile duct of surgical clips which subsequently act as a nidus for further stone formation;[41] haemobilia;[42] and liver infarction due to unrecognized right hepatic artery ligation.[43] Reports exist of intra-abdominal sepsis associated with gallstones spilled at the time of operation.[44,45] While every effort should be made to recover these stones their loss should not be regarded as reason to convert to an open procedure. Animal studies suggest that spilled stones are unlikely to be a cause of significantly increased morbidity in laparoscopic cholecystectomy.[46]

Laparoscopic cholecystectomy vs *open or mini-cholecystectomy* ─────

The widespread adoption of laparoscopic cholecystectomy as the treatment of choice for gallstones has outpaced the implementation of prospective clinical trials designed to test its superiority over the open operation. It can be argued that such trials are no longer required. The very large number of observational studies now available on the results of laparoscopic cholecystectomy appear to confirm its acceptance amongst surgeons and patients alike. The increased incidence of bile duct injuries is considered to be compensated for by other perceived benefits of laparoscopic surgery, e.g. less post-operative pain, earlier discharge from hospital and an earlier return to normal activities and work. However, in an extensive review of the literature pertaining to laparoscopic cholecystectomy it was concluded that these benefits may not be markedly different from those observed after mini-cholecystectomy.[47] Accordingly this study recommended that surgeons should not be encouraged to replace mini-cholecystectomy with laparoscopic cholecystectomy.

References ──────────────────

1. Legorreta AP, Silber JH, Constantino GN et al. *JAMA* 1994; **271**: 500.
2. Yerdel MA, Tsuge H, Mimura H et al. Laparoscopic cholecystectomy in cirrhotic patients: expanding indications. *Surg Laparosc Endosc* 1993; **3**: 180–183.
3. Soper NJ. Effect of non-biliary problems on laparoscopic cholecystectomy. *Am J Surg* 1993; **165**: 522–526.
4. Cuschieri A, Berci G, McSherry CK. Laparoscopic cholecystectomy. *Am J Surg* 1990; **159**: 273.
5. Zucker KA, Flowers JL, Bailey RW et al. Laparoscopic management of acute cholecystitis. *Am J Surg* 1993; **165**: 508–514.
6. Kum CK, Goh PM, Isaac JR et al. Laparoscopic cholecystectomy for acute cholecystitis. *Br J Surg* 1994; **81**: 1651–1654.
7. Cox MR, Wilson TG, Luck AJ et al. Laparoscopic cholecystectomy for acute inflammation of the gallbladder. *Ann Surg* 1993; **218**: 630–634.
8. Rattner DW, Ferguson C, Warshaw AL. Factors associated with successful laparoscopic cholecystectomy for acute cholecystitis. *Ann Surg* 1993; **217**: 233–236.
9. Wongworawat MD, Aitkin DR, Robles AE, Garberoglio C. The impact of prior abdominal surgery on laparoscopic cholecystectomy. *Am Surg* 1994; **60**: 763–766.
10. Lanzafame RJ. Laparoscopic cholecystectomy during pregnancy. *Surgery* 1995; **118**: 627–631.

11. Pezet D, Fondrinier E, Rotman *et al.* Parietal seeding of carcinoma of the gallbladder after laparoscopic cholecystectomy. *Br J Surg* 1992; **79**: 230.

12. Clair DG, Lautz DB, Brooks DC. Rapid development of umbilical metastases after laparoscopic cholecystectomy for unsuspected gallbladder carcinoma. *Surgery* 1993; **113**: 355–358.

13. Nixon SJ, Mirghani MM. Laparoscopic management of cholecystenteric fistula. *Br J Surg* 1995; **82**: 675.

14. Binnie NR, Nixon SJ, Palmer KR. Mirizzi syndrome managed by endoscopic stenting and laparoscopic cholecystectomy. *Br J Surg* 1992; **79**: 647.

15. Phillips EH, Carroll BJ, Fallas MJ, Pearlstein AR. Comparison of laparoscopic cholecystectomy in obese and non-obese patients. *Am Surg* 1994; **60**: 316–321.

16. Dunn D, Nair R, Fowler S, McCloy R. Laparoscopic cholecystectomy in England and Wales: results of an audit by The Royal College of Surgeons of England. *Ann R Coll Surg Engl* 1994; **76**: 269–275.

17. Scott TR, Zucker KA, Bailey RW. Laparoscopic cholecystectomy: a review of 12397 patients. *Surg Laparosc Endosc* 1992; **2**: 191–198.

18. Croce E, Azzola M, Golia M *et al.* Laparocholecystectomy. 6865 cases from Italian institutions. *Surg Endosc* 1994; **8**: 1088–1091.

19. Coventry DM. Anaesthesia for laparoscopic surgery. *J R Coll Surg Edinb* 1995; **40**: 151–160.

20. Mayol J, Vincent-Hamelin E, Sarmiento JM. Pulmonary embolism following laparoscopic cholecystectomy: report of two cases and review of the literature. *Surg Endosc* 1994; **8**: 214–217.

21. Frantzides CT, Sykes A. A reevaluation of antibiotic prophylaxis in laparoscopic cholecystectomy. *J Laparoendosc Surg* 1994; **4**: 375–378.

22. Motson RW. Direct puncture technique for laparoscopy. *Ann R Coll Surg Engl* 1994; **76**: 346–347.

23. Madhavan KK, MacIntyre IM, Wilson RG *et al.* Role of intraoperative cholangiography in laparoscopic cholecystectomy. *Br J Surg* 1995; **82**: 249–252.

24. Rosenthal RJ, Steigerwald SD, Imig R. Role of intraoperative cholangiography during endoscopic cholecystectomy. *Surg Laparosc Endosc* 1994; **4**: 171–174.

25. Ballem RV, Rudomanski J. Techniques of pneumoperitoneum. *Surg Laparosc Endosc* 1993; **3**: 42–43.

26. Whiteley MS, Laws SAM, Wise MH. Use of a hand-held Doppler to avoid abdominal wall vessels in laparoscopic surgery. *Ann R Coll Surg Engl* 1994; **76**: 348–350.

27. Peters JH, Krailadsiri W, Incarbone R *et al.* Reasons for conversion from laparoscopic to open cholecystectomy in an urban teaching hospital. *Am J Surg* 1994; **168**: 555–558.

28. Schrenk P, Woisetschlager R, Wayand WU. Laparoscopic cholecystectomy. Cause of conversions in 1,300 patients and analysis of risk factors. *Surg Endosc* 1995; **9**: 25–28.

29. Crosthwaite G, McKay C, Anderson JR. Laparoscopic subtotal cholecystectomy. *J R Coll Surg Edinb* 1995; **40**: 20–21.

30. Steiner CA, Bass EB, Talamini MA *et al.* Surgical rates and operative mortality for open and laparoscopic cholecystectomy in Maryland. *N Engl J Med* 1994; **330**: 403–408.

31. McMahon AJ, Fullerton G, Baxter JN, O'Dwyer PJ. Bile duct injury and bile leakage in laparoscopic cholecystectomy. *Br J Surg* 1995; **82**: 307–313.

32. Morgenstern L, McGrath MF, Carroll BJ *et al.* Continuing hazards of the learning curve in laparoscopic cholecystectomy. *Am Surg* 1995; **61**: 914–918.

33. Moore MJ, Bennett CL. The learning curve for laparoscopic cholecystectomy. The Southern Surgeons Club. *Am J Surg* 1995; **170**: 55–59.

34. Wolfe BM, Gardiner BN, Leary BF *et al.* Endoscopic cholecystectomy. An analysis of complications. *Arch Surg* 1991; **126**: 1192–1198.

35. Walker AT, Shapiro AW, Brooks DC *et al.* Bile duct disruption and biloma after

laparoscopic cholecystectomy: imaging evaluation. *AJR Am J Roentgenol* 1992; **158**: 785–789.

36. Woods MS, Shellito JL, Santoscoy GS *et al.* Cystic duct leaks in laparoscopic cholecystectomy. *Am J Surg* 1994; **168**: 560–563.

37. Barton JR, Russell RCG, Hatfield ARW. Management of bile leaks after laparoscopic cholecystectomy. *Br J Surg* 1995; **82**: 980–984.

38. Chen X, Mao J, Wang S *et al.* A two year experience with laparoscopic cholecystectomy – a report of 1475 cases from Kunming, China. *Ann Acad Med Singapore* 1995; **24**: 312–315.

39. Trondsen E, Rudd TE, Nilsen BH. Complications during the introduction of laparoscopic cholecystectomy in Norway. *Eur J Surg* 1994; **160**: 145–151.

40. Lantz PE, Smith MD. Fatal carbon dioxide embolism complicating attempted laparoscopic cholecystectomy – case report and literature review. *J Forens Sci* 1994; **39**: 1468–1480.

41. Martinez J, Combs W, Brady PG. Surgical clips as a nidus for biliary stone formation: diagnosis and therapy. *Am J Gastroenterol* 1995; **90**: 1521–1524.

42. Zilberstein B, Cecconello I, Ramos AC. Hemobilia as a complication of laparoscopic cholecystectomy. *Surg Laparosc Endosc* 1994; **4**: 301–303.

43. Wachsberg RH, Cho KC, Raina S. Liver infarction following unrecognized right hepatic artery ligation at laparoscopic cholecystectomy. *Abdom Imaging* 1994; **19**: 53–54.

44. Shocket E. Abdominal abscess from gallstones spilled at laparoscopic cholecystectomy. Case report and review of the literature. *Surg Endosc* 1995; **9**: 344–347.

45. Carlin CB, Kent RB, Laws HL. Spilled gallstones – complications of abdominal wall abscesses. Case report and review of the literature. *Surg Endosc* 1995; **9**: 341–343.

46. Zisman A, Loshkov G, Negri M *et al.* The fate of long-standing intraperitoneal gallstone in the rat. *Surg Endosc* 1995; **9**: 509–511.

47. Downs SH, Black NA, Devlin HB *et al.* A systematic review of the effectiveness and safety of laparoscopic cholecystectomy. *Ann R Coll Surg Engl* 1996; **78**: 241–323.

10b

Biliary tract and gallbladder: common bile duct stones

R. Nair and R.F. McCloy

Introduction

The introduction of laparoscopic cholecystectomy has reopened the debate on whether common bile duct stones should be managed surgically or endoscopically – this has been the subject of several recent articles.[1-9] Inextricably linked with this are issues relating to imaging of the bile ducts – the need for imaging, the modalities available and the timing of imaging, before, during or after the operation. Algorithms have been devised for the management of bile duct stones based upon the availability of endoscopic sphincterotomy and choledocholithotomy.[2,5-7] At present, the decision to use one modality or the other depends on the likely risks and benefits of that procedure in a given patient, but also upon the availability of a clinician experienced in ERCP (endoscopic retrograde cholangio pancreatography) and/or a surgeon at a given centre. Therefore, no single algorithm for the management of bile duct stones is likely to be appropriate for every hospital. In the early days of laparoscopic cholecystectomy, the presence of a known or suspected common bile duct stone was regarded as a contraindication to the laparoscopic approach.[10] Now that successful laparoscopic bile duct clearance has been reported from several centres,[11-20] the scene is set to change, with more surgeons becoming proficient in this technique. In the laparoscopic era, management of bile duct stones is no longer a 'black and white' choice between endoscopic and surgical methods. Innovative laparoscopic techniques such as peroperative fluoroscopic-guided stone removal,[21] peroperative endoscopic sphincterotomy or electrohydraulic lithotripsy,[22] and laparoscopic transcystic balloon dilatation of the sphincter of Oddi[23] have shown that the services of a good interventional radiologist can be another string in the laparoscopic surgeon's bow. In the future, it is likely that removal of bile duct stones will be accomplished by one of three different modalities – open surgery, endoscopic methods and laparoscopic and laparoscopic-based techniques, the latter being the simultaneous deployment of laparoscopic and interventional radiological or endoscopic techniques.[21–23] The choice of procedure will be as much dependent on patient- and stone-related factors as on the availability of skilled exponents of the techniques in question.

Results of different modalities for the clearance of bile duct stones ____

Open choledocholithotomy

The common bile duct is explored in approximately 15 per cent of all cholecystectomies and stones are removed in approximately 65 per cent of these explorations.[24] In large series of open choledocholithotomy without choledochoscopy,[25–31] retained stones are detected in 1.3–9 per cent of cases. The use of operative choledochoscopy has reduced the retained stone rate to 0–3 per cent[24,32–37] (see Tables 10b.1 and 10b.2). The overall mortality rate of open choledocholithotomy is 1–5 per cent.[25,26,28–31] In patients aged less than 50 years, elective open choledocholithotomy has a mortality of 0.3 per cent and a morbidity of 10 per cent.[24] Two series reported zero mortality in young patients undergoing open choledocholithotomy.[27,38] Common bile duct exploration is necessary in 34–55 per cent of patients aged more than 65 undergoing cholecystectomy.[39–41] Above the age of 70 years, elective open choledocholithotomy carries a mortality rate of 5–13 per cent[25,39–41] and a morbidity of 19–34 per cent.[24,39–41] Apart from age, factors increasing the mortality of bile duct exploration include the presence of cholangitis, pancreatitis, jaundice and concomitant cardiorespiratory problems.[26,29,39–41] Indeed, more than half the deaths in patients over 65 were due to cardiac causes in one series.[40] In the presence of acute suppurative cholangitis, open choledocholithotomy carries a mortality of 19–21 per cent.[41,42]

Table 10b.1   Results of open common bile duct exploration without choledochoscopy ECBD: exploration of the common bile duct

Author (reference no.)	Cases	ECBD	Mortality (%)	Morbidity (%)	Retained stones (%)
Larson[25]	NA	500	10 (5%)	NA	8 (1.6%)
Magee[26]	1000	204	10 (4.7%)	10 (1%)	NA
Pappas[27]	NA	100	0 (0%)	15 (15%)	5 (5%)
Davies[28]	722	92	1 (1.1%)	30 (32%)	8 (9%)
Morgenstern[29]	1200	220	9 (4.1%)	18 (8%)	16 (1.3%)
Kramling[30]	3365	420	8 (1.9%)	38 (9%)	23 (5.5%)
Rogers[31]	1142	100	3 (3%)	NA	9 (9%)

Table 10b.2   Results of open choledocholithotomy with choledochoscopy

Author (reference no.)	No. of patients who had operative choledochoscopy	Percentage with retained stones
Girard and Legros[24]	102	1%
Finnis[32]	83	0%
Nora[33]	300	1%
Berci[34]	120	3%
Jakimowicz[35]	320	2%
Markowitz[36]	102	0%
Yap[37]	149	1.3%

Table 10b.3   Results of endoscopic sphincterotomy for common bile duct stones

Author (reference no.)	Cases	CBD clearance	Complications	Mortality
Seifert[41]	955	92.1%	7.3%	1.7%
Geenen[42]	1250	89%	8.7%	1.2%
Cotton[43]	679	87%	8.5%	1%
Vaira[44]	1000	87.3%	6.9%	1.2%
Lambert[45]	602	81.6%*	10.5%	2.2%†

* average 1.9 ERCPs per patient for clearance
† 1.2% procedure-related mortality

Endoscopic sphincterotomy

Endoscopic sphincterotomy has been in use for the last 20 years, and is now well established as a method of removal of bile duct stones. Several large series from expert centres have reported bile duct clearance rates of 81–92 per cent[43–47] (see Table 10b.3). It is important to realize that these data fall considerably short of the duct clearance rates for surgical techniques (Tables 10b.1 and 10b.2). More than one session may be required to clear some bile ducts.[47] Morbidity rates of 7–10 per cent and mortality rates of 1–1.7 per cent have been recorded in these series.[43–47] The mortality and morbidity of endoscopic sphincterotomy are independent of age of the patient.[48] It is agreed that the bile duct clearance rate increases and the complication rate falls with increasing experience of the endoscopist.[2,48,49] In contrast to choledochotomy, the complications of endoscopic sphincterotomy – cholangitis, pancreatitis, haemorrhage and perforation – are mainly procedure-related, and can have disastrous consequences.[49] Furthermore, significant bacterial contamination of bile is found in 60–70 per cent of patients on long-term follow-up, although this does not correlate with symptoms.[50,51] The long-term consequences of loss of function of the ampullary sphincter are not known, and therefore some experts restrict endoscopic sphincterotomy for choledocholithiasis to patients older than 50 years.[52] Long-term follow-up of 1050 patients in 25 (formerly West) German centres showed recurrent choledocholithiasis in 5.7 per cent and ampullary stenosis in 3.4 per cent of patients who had undergone endoscopic sphincterotomy.[53]

Comparisons of open surgery and endoscopic sphincterotomy for common bile duct stones in patients matched for clinical features and biochemical and medical risk factors have shown no advantage for the endoscopic method.[54–56] In these three studies, the incidence of complications, mortality and bile duct clearance rates were not significantly different between endoscopically and surgically treated patients. It is relevant to note that in patients aged less than 50, the combination of open choledochotomy with intra-operative choledochoscopy can result in complete bile duct clearance in 97 per cent or more patients with one-third the mortality of the endoscopic approach. Above the age of 50, the mortality of open choledocholithotomy exceeds that of endoscopic sphincterotomy, and above the age of 70, the mortality of surgery is five times greater (see Fig. 10b.2).

Laparoscopic approaches to common bile duct stones

Several series of laparoscopic exploration of the bile ducts have been published from major laparoscopic centres[11–20] and the results of those reporting 20 or more cases are shown in Table 10b.4. Bile duct clearance rates of 85–96 per cent have been achieved,[11,13,15,18–20] averaging 94 per cent in the series listed – a figure that compares well with the results of an expert endoscopist. The low mortality in these series probably reflects the fact that 'good-risk' patients have undergone laparoscopic bile duct exploration early on in each author's experience. Laparoscopic manipulations inside the common bile duct are among the most difficult procedures being attempted by laparoscopic surgeons and the good results obtained in the series quoted above may not be expected of the average laparoscopic cholecystectomist. As surgeons become more confident of their technique, fewer patients with suspected stones will have pre-operative ERCPs and more will have laparoscopic bile duct exploration. This has been well illustrated in a recent series of 1050 cases[57] in which the pre-operative ERCP rate fell from 60 per cent in the first year to 30 per cent in the third year of the study while the percentage of

Table 10b.4   Major world series of laparoscopic bile duct exploration

Author (reference no.)	Total LC	Abnormal POC	Attempt LCBDE	Success	Con-verted	Post-operative ES	Compli-cations	Deaths
Petelin[11]	1000	95 (9%)	77	74	5	18	10.4%	1.3%
Carroll[15]	910	105 (12%)	88	82	5	6	5.6%	1.1%
Swanstrom[18]	526	51 (9.7%)	50	47	3	0	NA	0%
Ferzli[19]	NA	NA	24	22	0	2	29%	0%
Franklin[20]	857	86 (10.4%)	60	58	2	23	1.7%	1.7%
Sackier[14]	516	35 (7%)	NA	21	8	5	NA	0%
Hunter[13]	252	20 (8%)	20	17	3	0	10%	NA

LC: laparoscopic cholecystectomy, POC: peroperative cholangiogram, ECBD: exploration of common bile duct, ES: endoscopic sphincterotomy patients with choledocholithiasis having laparoscopic bile duct exploration rose from 5 to 33 per cent during the same period.

Laparoscopic bile duct exploration presupposes that peroperative cholangiography has been performed. In the United States, 81 per cent of surgeons are performing laparoscopic peroperative cholangiography on either a routine or selective basis,[58] while in Europe only 15–30 per cent are doing so.[10,59] A detailed discussion of peroperative cholangiography and laparoscopic bile duct injuries is beyond the remit of this article. However, it must be pointed out that evidence is now accumulating that though routine peroperative cholangiography may not prevent bile duct injuries, it does enable intra-operative recognition and repair of such injuries in significantly more cases than if cholangiography was not performed.[60,61] Furthermore, where peroperative cholangiography has been performed, the injuries are usually Bismuth type I, which are easier to repair than those associated with failure to perform cholangiography in which almost the whole extrahepatic biliary tree can be excised.[60,61,62]

Transcystic duct approach

The transcystic duct approach has been the choice of most authors, with fluoroscopically-guided stone removal[11,13,14,19] and transcystic duct choledochoscopy[11,15,18] being used for clearing the bile duct. Duct clearance rates of 93–96 per cent have been achieved by the experts.[11,15] Transcystic duct balloon dilatation and intra-operative electrohydraulic lithotripsy (via transcystic duct choledochoscopy) and intra-operative ERCP[22] have been employed as additional measures to aid clearance of the ducts. Intra-operative ERCP during laparoscopic cholecystectomy is not recommended because intraluminal gas from the endoscope produces distended loops of bowel and the supine position of the patient renders ERCP difficult.[63,64] The transcystic approach is recommended for stones no greater than 8 mm in diameter and should a stone prove impossible to remove by this approach, Perissat *et al.* recommend that a transcystic–transpapillary drain (TTT, tuteur transcystique–transpapillaire) be placed.[4] This will avoid the potential risk of an obstructed bile duct and will enable easy access to the bile duct for post-operative ERCP. Stones lying above the cystic duct–common hepatic duct junction are very difficult to remove by the transcystic route and usually require a formal laparoscopic choledochotomy.

Laparoscopic choledochotomy

Formal laparoscopic choledochotomy is technically more demanding than the transcystic duct approach, since intracorporeal suturing and knot-tying techniques are required.[11,14,20] Techniques for laparoscopic choledochotomy and suturing techniques for closure with and without a T-tube have been described in detail.[65,66] As with open surgery, laparoscopic choledochotomy should not be performed unless the common bile duct measures at least 10 mm in diameter.[10] Franklin *et al.* have reported successful clearance of the bile duct in 58 out of 60 (96 per cent) patients by laparoscopic choledochotomy, choledochoscopy and balloon catheter removal of stones followed by T-tube placement.[20] In this series, there was only one major complication requiring re-laparotomy and one death in 60 patients, and the post-operative stay ranged from 1–11 days (average 1.8 days for patients with suspected stones and 2.8 days for those with unsuspected stones).

The future – endoscopic sphincterotomy or laparoscopic bile duct exploration?

In the early days of laparoscopic cholecystectomy, the limitations of laparoscopic manoeuvres in the common bile duct led to extensive use of pre-operative ERCP for imaging the bile ducts and sphincterotomy for clearance of common bile duct stones. At the time, the compelling argument for pre-operative clearance of the bile duct was the avoidance of the 'three stage sequence':

- Failed (or inability to perform) laparoscopic common bile duct exploration.
- Failed post-operative endoscopic sphincterotomy.
- Open common bile duct exploration.

The days of routine pre-operative ERCP prior to laparoscopic cholecystectomy should be over now, with current evidence suggesting if such a policy is followed, 86 per cent of such examinations will be normal, 11 per cent will have bile duct stones detected and 2.5 per cent will develop pancreatitis.[67] This pancreatitis rate is equal to the rate of unsuspected stones detected on peroperative cholangiography.[68] The only prospective randomized trial of pre-operative endoscopic sphincterotomy versus open surgery alone for common bile duct stones[55] concluded that there was no advantage for pre-operative endoscopic clearance. Complications and mortality were not significantly different between the two groups. The only advantage for those who had pre-operative endoscopic clearance was a reduction in the duration of hospital stay, and that is no longer an issue with laparoscopic bile duct clearance when choledochoscopy is performed to verify clearance and T-tubes are not placed.

Comparisons of endoscopic sphincterotomy, which is an established procedure, and laparoscopic bile duct exploration, which is still being developed, are difficult to make at this stage. The former is available widely while the latter is being performed at only a few centres in each country where laparoscopic surgery is being performed. Long-term (11–15 year) follow-up data are available for endoscopic sphincterotomy, but similar data on laparoscopic bile duct exploration will take at least another decade to accrue. At the present moment, algorithms for the management of bile duct stones have to be interpreted according to whether a given centre does or does not have expert laparoscopic surgical or endoscopic facilities.[2,5–7] As surgeons develop their laparoscopic skills, the ERCP rate falls and the rate of laparoscopic bile duct exploration increases.[57] The algorithms for the early 1990s will have to be rewritten by the turn of the century, incorporating a range of laparoscopic techniques which will, it is hoped, be more widely available. The present authors share the view of Swanstrom[18] that laparoscopic bile duct exploration is the way forward. Considerations of overall success rates, cost effectiveness and convenience, and morbidity and mortality should influence the decision whether to use endoscopic sphincterotomy or laparoscopic bile duct exploration. The data presented in Table 10b.4 are convincing evidence of the potential of the laparoscopic approach to bile duct stones, with clearance rates at least as good as those obtained by experts in ERCP. Swanstrom[18] and Berci[69] argue for laparoscopic bile duct exploration at the time of laparoscopic cholecystectomy, stressing the convenience and comfort to the patient of having both gallbladder and common bile duct stones tackled in one procedure. It is hard to find fault with such an approach. Cost-benefit analysis favours one therapeutic procedure (laparoscopic cholecystectomy and bile duct exploration) rather than two (laparoscopic cholecystectomy plus ERCP). In one study[70] the cost of surgery alone was estimated at $2,740 while endoscopic sphincterotomy followed by surgery cost $2,952. Furthermore, the use of pre-operative endoscopic sphincterotomy adds to the morbidity of the treatment.[71] Post-sphincterotomy pancreatitis or cholangitis can result in postponement of surgery.

The authors have devised algorithms for the management of expected and unexpected common bile duct stones in patients undergoing laparoscopic cholecystectomy, given the availability of ERCP and laparoscopic bile duct exploration[5] (see Fig. 10b.1 and 10b.3).

'Expected choledocholithiasis' (Fig. 10b.1)

In patients with stones suspected on the basis of a history of jaundice, abnormal liver function tests or a dilated common bile duct on ultrasound, ERCP has been traditionally recommended. A 'selective' approach to ERCP results in this procedure being performed pre-operatively in about 3–5 per cent of patients[11,57,68] and about 33–47 per cent of these 'high risk' patients will have proven common bile

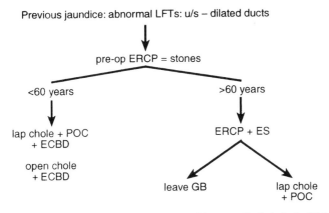

Fig. 10b.1   Algorithm for the management of 'expected' choledocholithiasis, given the availability of ERCP and laparoscopic bile duct exploration (from Nair *et al.*[5]). (LFTs: liver function tests; u/s: ultrasound; POC: peroperative cholangiogram; ECBD: common bile duct exploration; GB: gallbladder.)

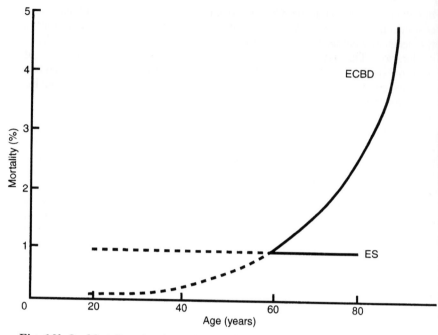

Fig. 10b.2   Mortality of endoscopic sphincterotomy versus open choledocholithotomy (from Nair *et al.*[5]). (ES: endoscopic sphincterotomy, ECBD: common bile duct exploration.)

duct stones[57,68] Thus, when selective pre-operative ERCP is performed, between one-third and one-half of the procedures are unnecessary. *Pre-operative endoscopic sphincterotomy should be performed only in patients aged more than 60.* Below this age, the mortality of bile duct exploration is less than that of endoscopic sphincterotomy (see Figure 10b.2). Even when pre-operative ERCP has been performed, peroperative cholangiography should still be undertaken in all patients for delineation of biliary anatomy. Bile duct stones are removed laparoscopically, and should this fail, or the expertise be unavailable, the operation is converted to an open procedure. *Those older than 60 may undergo post-operative endoscopic sphincterotomy and stone extraction.*

'Unexpected choledocholithiasis' (Fig. 10b.3)

When patients with no pre-operative 'risk factors' for bile duct stones undergo routine peroperative cholangiography, about 2.5 per cent of them will have unsuspected stones.[68] If such patients are young and fit, the surgeon can proceed with laparoscopic bile duct exploration and immediately convert to an open procedure should this fail. Post-operative endoscopic sphincterotomy should be reserved for patients above the age of 60. Small stones (less than 5 mm in diameter) in normal calibre ducts should be left to pass out on their own. One

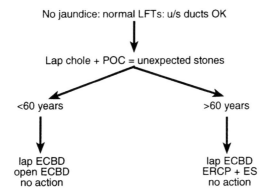

No jaundice: normal LFTs: u/s ducts OK

Lap chole + POC = unexpected stones

<60 years   >60 years

lap ECBD   lap ECBD
open ECBD   ERCP + ES
no action   no action

Fig. 10b.3   Algorithm for the management of 'unexpected' choledocholithiasis, given the availability of ERCP and laparoscopic common bile duct exploration (from Nair *et al.*[5]). (LFTs: liver function tests; u/s: ultrasound; lap chole: laparoscopic cholecystectomy; POC: peroperative cholangiogram; ECBD: common bile duct exploration; ES: endoscopic sphincterotomy.)

study[72] has demonstrated a higher mortality for endoscopic sphincterotomy in patients with normal calibre ducts, but this has been refuted in another study.[73]

Choledocholithiasis in the elderly unfit patient

Following endoscopic clearance of the bile ducts, there is still the option to leave the gallbladder *in situ*. One- to six-year follow-up of elderly unfit patients undergoing endoscopic sphincterotomy for choledocholithiasis has shown that only 5–18 per cent will subsequently require a cholecystectomy for symptomatic gallstones.[74–82] Most patients required cholecystectomy within one year of endoscopic sphincterotomy.[79–81] Attempts have been made to identify risk factors predicting the need for cholecystectomy in such patients, but no clear conclusions can be made at this point. Cystic duct obstruction has been suggested as one risk factor[76,82] but other studies contradict this.[74,81] Cholangitis at presentation has been also suggested as a risk factor in one study,[74] but another study failed to confirm this.[81]

Retained and recurrent common bile duct stones

The retained stone rate following laparoscopic cholecystectomy has not been accurately defined yet. A national audit of 3319 laparoscopic cholecystectomies performed in England and Wales during 1990–1991[83] reported a retained stone rate of 6/3319 (0.18 per cent) and a review of 21 major world series of laparoscopic cholecystectomy published in the same paper put this figure at 0.53 per cent. With the follow-up in all the above studies being very short, these figures are likely to be underestimates: the true figure is not likely to emerge for some years.

Following open choledocholithotomy with choledochoscopy, retained common bile duct stones are found in 0–3 per cent of cases[31–37] Endoscopic clearance is successful in 85–93 per cent of cases,[41–45] with 7–15 per cent requiring further treatment for retained stones.

Management options for retained and recurrent common bile duct stones depend on the presence or absence of a T-tube, the size and type of the recurrent stone and the medical fitness of the patient.

T-tube instrumentation and perfusion

This should be performed no sooner than six weeks after the primary operation, and has a success rate of 95 per cent with a morbidity of 5 per cent.[84,85] Burhenne[84] reported no deaths in 661 patients undergoing T-tube instrumentation, while Mazzarielo[85] reported one death due to pancreatitis in 1086 patients with surgery being required to correct complications in three patients (0.2 per cent). T-tube perfusion with mono-octanoin and methyl-*tert*-butyl-ether (MTBE) is another method. In a review of 343 patients undergoing T-tube dissolution therapy,[86] common bile duct stones disappeared on treatment in 26 per cent of patients, diminished in size to become retrievable in 29 per cent and remained unchanged in the remainder. The procedure had to be terminated in 9 per cent of patients because of side-effects. In the laparoscopic era, with more and more bile duct explorations being performed through the transcystic duct route, T-tube instrumentation and perfusion are going to become rarer.

Lithotripsy (electrohydraulic, laser and mechanical)

Electrohydraulic shock wave lithotripsy has been employed for breaking up common bile duct stones, with the energy being delivered either by extracorporeal means or by the peroral endoscopic route.[87–90] Laser lithotripsy is another method.[91,92] The results of these methods are presented in Table 10b.5. These methods are used as 'third-line' methods in the management of bile duct stones, with endoscopic sphincterotomy and surgery being the first and second line treatments respectively.

Endoscopic treatment of recurrent stones

Patients who are poor risks for re-operation benefit from endoscopic removal of recurrent common bile duct stones. In a large series of 624 patients with recurrent stones,[93] endoscopic clearance was achieved in 88 per cent and long-term stenting was required in 7 per cent. Surgery was carried out in 4 per cent. Recurrent cholangitis was seen in 10 per cent of patients with long-term stents, and this was managed by stent change and antibiotics in all cases. Stones larger than 1.5 cm in diameter are difficult to remove endoscopically, and mechanical lithotripsy may be employed to clear the duct. Chung *et al.*[94] achieved bile duct clearance in 81 per cent of 68 patients with stones measuring 1–4.9 cm in diameter. Pigment stones

Table 10b.5 Lithotripsy for common bile duct stones

Author (reference no.)	Patients	Stones disintegrated	Bile duct clearance	Route
Yoshimoto[87]	31	97%	95%	electrohydraulic (endoscopic)
Siegel[88]	21	?	86%	electrohydraulic (endoscopic)
Sauerbruch[89]	113	91%	86%	extracorporeal shock wave lithotripsy
Wenzel[90]	55	98%	92%	extracorporeal shock wave lithotripsy
Cotton[91]	25	92%	80%	laser (endoscopic)
Ponchon[92]	25	?	88%	laser (endoscopic)
Chung[94]	68	?	81%	mechanical lithotripsy

are easily crushed, while cholesterol stones are often resistant to this method and need surgery.

Re-operation for retained common bile duct stones

In good risk patients (and especially the young), surgery has an edge over endoscopic methods. Re-exploration of the common bile duct can be challenging, but can produce good results in carefully selected cases. Successful surgical clearance of recurrent common bile duct stones was achieved in 69/72 (97 per cent) of cases in one series,[38] with complications arising in six patients (8.3 per cent) and no deaths. Mortality rates of 1.7–4.1 per cent have been recorded for common bile duct re-exploration.[95–98] Most of these deaths occur in older and poor risk patients, and for young (under 60 years) good risk patients, the mortality for re-operation is less than 2 per cent, i.e. comparable to endoscopic sphincterotomy. When the bile duct is wider than 1.5 cm and there is gross choledocholithiasis, or if a stone impacted at the lower end of the common bile duct cannot be removed, a choledochoduodenostomy should be performed. This can be achieved with a mortality of 1.8–2.8 per cent, with cholangitis occurring as a complication in 2.8–5 per cent overall.[99–103] The diameter of the common bile duct is important to the success of this operation. In one series,[100] no patient with a bile duct diameter greater than 1.6 cm developed cholangitis, while 22 per cent of those with ducts smaller than this had post-operative cholangitis. Common bile duct stones lying above a stricture and stones in patients who have had Billroth II partial gastrectomy are usually indications for adoption of a surgical approach.

Conclusions

The success of laparoscopic cholecystectomy in the treatment of symptomatic cholelithiasis has stimulated surgeons to search for a minimally invasive surgical solution to common bile duct stones. Current evidence suggests that surgical methods of bile duct clearance carry a lower morbidity and mortality than endoscopic methods in patients younger than 50 years. The marriage of video-laparoscopic, endoscopic and interventional radiological techniques has led to several innovative methods for the laparoscopic removal of common bile duct stones. At present, transcystic fluoroscopically-guided and choledochoscopic stone removal are the two most popular techniques. The situation is fast changing, and many new methods are being tested. In the hands of the experts, the short-term results of laparoscopic bile duct exploration appear to be as good as those of endoscopic sphincterotomy and open choledocholithotomy. The jury is still out on laparoscopic bile duct exploration, however. It will take till the end of the century for long-term follow-up data to become available on the incidence of recurrent and retained stones. Contrary to the case of laparoscopic cholecystectomy,[104] randomized controlled trials of laparoscopic versus other methods of bile duct clearance should be undertaken, and small numbers may dictate a multi-centre study. In the meantime, careful prospective audit of results will define the role played by laparoscopic methods in the management of bile duct stones.

References

1. Brodish RJ, Fink AS. ERCP, cholangiography and laparoscopic cholecystectomy. *Surg Endosc* 1993; **7**: 3–8.
2. Cotton PB. ERCP and laparoscopic cholecystectomy. *Am J Surg* 1993; **165**: 474–478.
3. Leitman IM, Fisher ML, McKinley MJ, Rothman R, Ward RJ, Reiner DS, Tortolani AJ. The evaluation and management of known or suspected stones of the common bile duct in the era of minimal access surgery. *Surg Gynaecol Obst* 1993; **176**: 527–533.
4. Perissat J, Huibregtse K, Keane FBV, Russell RCG, Neoptolemos JP. Management of bile duct stones in the era of laparoscopic cholecystectomy. *Br J Surg* 1994; **81**: 799–810.
5. Nair RG, Whiteley GSW, McCloy RF. Laparoscopic cholecystectomy in the UK two years on – results and implications for the management of common bile duct stones. *Proc R Coll Physicians Edinb* 1993; **23**: 474–483.
6. Uzer M, Hawes RH. ERCP and laparoscopic cholecystectomy: stones, stents and sphincterotomy. In: Hunter JG (ed.), Laparoscopic Surgery, *Ballière's Clinical Gastroenterology* 1993; **7**(4): 921–940.
7. Scott-Coombes D, Thompson JN. Bile duct stones and laparoscopic cholecystectomy. *Br Med J* 1991; **303**: 1281–1282.
8. Hunter JG. Laparoscopic cholecystectomy and the common bile duct. *Surg Endosc* 1994; **8**: 285–286.
9. Fink AS. Current dilemmas in management of common duct stones. *Surg Endosc* 1993; **7**: 285–291.
10. Cuschieri A, Dubois F, Mouiel J, Mouret P, Becker H *et al*. The European experience with laparoscopic cholecystectomy. *Am J Surg* 1991; **161**: 385–390.
11. Petelin JB. Laparoscopic approach to common duct pathology. *Am J Surg* 1993; **165**: 487–491.
12. Hunter JG. Laparoscopic trans-cystic

common bile duct exploration. *Am J Surg* 1992; **163**: 53–58.

13. Spaw AT, Reddick EJ, Olsen DO. Laparoscopic laser cholecystectomy: analysis of 500 procedures. *Surg Laparosc Endosc* 1991; **1**: 2–7.

14. Sackier JM, Berci G, Phillips E, Carroll B, Shapiro S, Paz-Partlow M. Routine or selective peroperative cholangiography during laparoscopic cholecystectomy? *Arch Surg* 1991; **126**: 1021–1026.

15. Carroll BJ, Fallas MJ, Phillips EH. Laparoscopic transcystic choledochoscopy. *Surg Endosc* 1994; **8**: 310–314.

16. Smith P, Clayman RV, Soper NJ. Laparoscopic cholecystectomy and choledochoscopy for the treatment of cholelithiasis and choledocholithiasis. *Surgery* 1992; **111**: 230–233.

17. Stoker ME, Leveillee RJ, McCann JC, Maini BS. Laparoscopic common bile duct exploration. *J Laparoendosc Surg* 1991; **1**: 287–293.

18. Swanstrom LL. Laparoscopic approaches to the common bile duct stone. In: Hunter JG (ed.), Laparoscopic Surgery, *Ballière's Clinical Gastroenterology* 1993; **7**: 897–920.

19. Ferzli GS, Massaad A, Kiel T, Worth MH. The utility of laparoscopic common bile duct exploration in the treatment of choledocholithiasis. *Surg Endosc* 1994; **8**: 296–298.

20. Franklin ME, Pharand D, Rosenthal D. Laparoscopic common bile duct exploration. *Surg Laparosc Endosc* 1994; **4**: 119–124.

21. Appel S, Krebs, Fern D. Techniques for laparoscopic cholangiography and removal of common duct stones. *Surg Endosc* 1992; **6**: 134–137.

22. Arregui ME, Davis CJ, Arkush AM, Nagan RF. Laparoscopic cholecystectomy combined with endoscopic sphincterotomy and stone extraction or laparoscopic choledochoscopy and electrohydraulic lithotripsy for management of cholelithiasis with choledocholithiasis. *Surg Endosc* 1992; **6**: 10–15.

23. Carroll BJ, Phillips EH, Chandra M, Fallas M. Laparoscopic transcystic duct balloon dilatation of the sphincter of Oddi. *Surg Endosc* 1993; **7**: 514–517.

24. Girard RM, Legros G. Stones in the common bile duct – surgical approaches. In: Blumgart LH (ed.), *Surgery of the Liver and Biliary Tract*. Churchill Livingstone, London, 1988, pages 577–585.

25. Larson RE, Hodgson JR, Priestley JT. The early and long-term results of 500 consecutive explorations of the common duct. *Surg Gynaecol Obst* 1966; **122**: 744–750.

26. Magee RB, Macduffee RC. One thousand consecutive cholecystectomies. *Arch Surg* 1968; **96**: 858–861.

27. Pappas TN, Slimane TB, Brooks DC. One hundred consecutive explorations of the common bile duct without mortality. *Ann Surg* 1990; **211**: 260–262.

28. Davies MG, O'Broin E, Mannion C, McGinley J, Gupta S *et al*. Audit of open cholecystectomy in a district general hospital. *Br J Surg* 1992; **79**: 314–316.

29. Morgenstern L, Wong L, Berci G. Twelve hundred open cholecystectomies before the laparoscopic era. *Arch Surg* 1992; **127**: 400–403.

30. Kramling H-J, Lange V, Schildberg FW, Heberer G. Surgical interventions for bile duct stones. *Ballière's Clinical Gastroenterology* 1992; **6**(4): 819–831.

31. Rogers AL, Farha GJ, Beamer RL, Chang FC. Incidence and associated mortality of retained common bile duct stones. *Am J Surg* 1985; **150**: 690–693.

32. Finnis D, Rowntree T. Choledochoscopy in exploration of the common bile duct. *Br J Surg* 1977; **64**: 661–664.

33. Nora PF, Berci GB, Dorazio RA *et al*. Operative choledochoscopy: Results of a prospective study in several institutions. *Am J Surg* 1977; **133**: 105–110.

34. Berci G, Shore M, Morgenstern L *et al*. Choledochoscopy and operative fluorocholangiography in the prevention of retained stones. *World J Surg* 1978; **2**: 411–427.

35. Jakimowicz JJ, Carol EJ, Mak B *et al.* An operative choledochoscopy using the flexible choledochoscope. *Surg Gynaecol Obst* 1986; **162**: 215–221.

36. Markowitz I, Kappelman MD, Webb WR. Choledochoscopy in prevention of retained common bile duct stones. *Am Surg* 1987; **53**: 558–561.

Yap PC, Atacador M, Yap AG, Yap RG. Choledochoscopy as a complementary procedure to operative cholangiography in biliary surgery. *Am J Surg* 1980; **140**: 648–652.

38. Girard RM, Legros G. Retained and recurrent bile duct stones – surgical or nonsurgical removal. *Ann Surg* 1981; **193**: 150–154.

39. Burdiles P, Csendes A, Diaz JC, Maluenda F, Avila S, Jorquera P, Aldunate M. Factors affecting mortality in patients over 70 years of age submitted to surgery for gallbladder or common bile duct stones. *Hepatogastroenterology* 1989; **36**: 136–139.

40. Lygidakis NJ. Operative risk factors of cholecystectomy-choledochotomy in the elderly. *Surg Gynaecol Obst* 1983; **157**: 15–19.

41. Houghton PWJ, Jenkinson LR, Donaldson LA. Cholecystectomy in the elderly: a prospective study. *Br J Surg* 1985; **72**: 220–222.

42. Leese T, Neoptolemos JP, Baker AR, Carr-Locke DL. Management of acute cholangitis and the impact of endoscopic sphincterotomy. *Br J Surg* 1986; **73**: 988–992.

43. Seifert E. Endoscopic papillotomy and removal of gallstones. *Am J Gastroenterol* 1978; **69**: 154–159.

44. Geenen GE, Vennes JA, Silvis SE. Resume of a seminar on ERCP and endoscopic sphincterotomy. *Gastrointest Endosc* 1981; **27**: 31–38.

45. Cotton PB, Valon AG. British experience with duodenoscopic sphincterotomy for removal of common bile duct stones. *Br J Surg* 1981; **68**: 373–375.

46. Vaira D, Ainley C, Williams S, Cairns S, Salmon P *et al.* Endoscopic sphincterotomy in 1000 consecutive patients. *Lancet* 1989; **ii**: 431–434.

47. Lambert ME, Betts CD, Hill J, Faragher EB, Martin DF, Tweedle DEF. Endoscopic sphincterotomy: the whole truth. *Br J Surg* 1991; **78**: 473–476.

48. Cotton PB. Endoscopic management of bile duct stones; (apples and oranges). *Gut* 1984; **25**: 587–597.

49. Carr-Locke DL. Stones in the common bile duct-endoscopic approaches. In: Blumgart LH (Ed.), *Surgery of the Liver and Biliary Tract*. Churchill Livingstone, London, 1988, pages 587–601.

50. Hawes RH, Cotton PB, Vallon AG. Follow-up 6 to 11 years after duodenoscopic sphincterotomy for stones in patients with prior cholecystectomy. *Gastroenterol* 1990; **98**: 1008–1012.

51. Gregg JA, DeGirolami P, Carr-Locke DL. Effects of sphincteroplasty and endoscopic sphincterotomy on the bacteriological characteristics of the common bile duct. *Am J Surg* 1985; **149**: 668–671.

52. Classen M. Endoscopic papillotomy. In: Sivak M (Ed.), *Gastroenterologic Endoscopy*. W B Saunders, Philadelphia, 1987, pages 631–651.

53. Seifert E, Gail K, Weismuller J. Langzeitresultate nach endoskopischer sphinkterotomie. *Dtsch Med Wochenschr* 1982; **107**: 610–614.

54. Miller BM, Kozarek RA, Ryan JA, Ball TJ, Traverso LW. Surgical versus endoscopic management of common bile duct stones. *Ann Surg* 1988; **207**: 135–141.

55. Neoptolemos JP, Carr-Locke DL, Fossard DP. Prospective randomised study of preoperative endoscopic sphincterotomy versus surgery alone for common bile duct stones. *Br Med J* 1987; **294**: 470–474.

56. Stiegmann GV, Goff JS, Mansour A, Pearlman N, Reveille RM, Norton L. Precholecystectomy endoscopic cholangiography and stone removal is not superior to cholecystectomy, cholangiography and common bile duct exploration. *Am J Surg* 1992; **163**: 227–230.

57. Voyles CR, Sanders DL, Hogan R. Common bile duct evaluation in the era of

laparoscopic cholecystectomy – 1050 cases later. *Ann Surg* 1994; **219**: 744–752.

58. Deziel D, Millikan KW, Economou SG, Doolas A, Ko S-T, Airan MC. Complications of laparoscopic cholecystectomy: a national survey of 4292 hospitals and an analysis of 77604 cases. *Am J Surg* 1993; **165**: 9–14.
59. Macintyre IMC, Wilson RG. Impact of laparoscopic cholecystectomy in the UK: a survey of consultants. *Br J Surg* 1993; **80**: 346.
60. Woods MS, Traverso LW, Kozarek RA, Tsao J, Rossi RL *et al.* Characteristics of biliary tract complications during laparoscopic cholecystectomy: a multi-institutional study. *Am J Surg* 1994; **167**: 27–34.
61. Rosenthal RJ, Steigerwald SD, Imig R, Bockhorn H. Role of intraoperative cholangiography during endoscopic cholecystectomy. *Surg Laparosc Endosc* 1994; **4**: 171–174.
62. Phillips EH. Routine versus selective intraoperative cholangiography. *Am J Surg* 1993; **165**: 505–507.
63. Sherman S, Gottlieb K, Lehman GA. Therapeutic biliary endoscopy. *Endoscopy* 1994; **26**: 93–112.
64. Deslandres E, Gagner M, Pomp A *et al.* Intraoperative endoscopic sphincterotomy for common bile duct stones during laparoscopic cholecystectomy. *Gastrointest Endosc* 1993; **39**: 54–58.
65. Hunter J, Soper NJ. Laparoscopic management of bile duct stones. *Surg Clin N Am* 1992; **72**: 1077.
66. Ko S, Airan M. Therapeutic laparoscopic suturing techniques. *Surg Endosc* 1992; **6**: 41–46.
67. Neuhaus H, Feussner H, Ungeheuer A *et al.* Prospective evaluation of the use of endoscopic retrograde cholangiopancreatography prior to laparoscopic cholecystectomy. *Endoscopy* 1992; **24**: 745–749.
68. Larson GM, Vitale GC, Casey J *et al.* Laparoscopic cholecystectomy expands the role of biliary endoscopy. *Gastrointest Endosc* 1992; **38**: 255.
69. Berci G. Preoperative ERCP and intraoperative cholangiography in the age of laparoscopic cholecystectomy. *Surg Endosc* 1993; **7**: 2.

70. Stain SC, Cohen H, Tsuishoysha M *et al.* Choledocholithiasis. Endoscopic sphincterotomy or common bile duct exploration. *Ann Surg* 1991; **213**: 627–634.
71. The Southern Surgeons Club: a prospective analysis of 1518 laparoscopic cholecystectomies. *N Engl J Med* 1991; **324**: 1073–1078.
72. Sherman S, Ruffolo T, Hawes RH, Lehman GA. Complications of endoscopic sphincterotomy: a prospective series with emphasis on the increased risk associated with sphincter of Oddi dysfunction and nondilated bile ducts. *Gastroenterology* 1991; **101**: 1068–1075.
73. Wilson MS, Tweedle DEF, Martin DF. Common bile duct diameter and complications of endoscopic sphincterotomy. *Br J Surg* 1992; **79**: 1346–1347.
74. Davidson BR, Neoptolemos JP, Carr-Locke DL. Endoscopic sphincterotomy for common bile duct calculi in patients with gallbladders in situ considered unfit for surgery. *Gut* 1988; **29**: 114–120.
75. Ingolby CJH, El-Saadi J, Hall RI, Denyer ME. Late results of endoscopic sphincterotomy for bile duct stones in elderly patients with gallbladders in situ. *Gut* 1989; **30**: 1129–1131.
76. Cotton PB, Vallon AG. Duodenoscopic sphincterotomy for bile duct stones in patients with gallbladders. *Surgery* 1982; **91**: 628–630.
77. Siegel JH, Safrany L, Ben-Zvi JS, Pullano WE, Cooperman A, Stenzel M, Ramsay WHO. Duodenoscopic sphincterotomy in patients with gallbladders in situ: report of a series of 1272 patients. *Am J Gastroenterol* 1988; **83**: 1255–1258.
78. Hansell DT, Millar MA, Murray WR, Gray GR, Gillespie G. Endoscopic sphincterotomy for bile duct stones in patients with intact gallbladders. *Br J Surg* 1989; **76**: 856–858.
79. Escorrou J, Cordova JA, Lazarthes F. Early and late complications after endo-

scopic sphincterotomy for biliary lithiasis with and without their gallbladder in situ. *Gut* 1984; **25**: 598–602.

80. Tanaka M, Ikeda S, Yoshimoto H, Matsumoto S. The long-term fate of the gallbladder after endoscopic sphincterotomy: complete follow-up study of 122 patients. *Am J Surg* 1987; **154**: 505–509.

81. Hill J, Martin DF, Tweedle DEF. Risks of leaving the gallbladder in situ after endoscopic sphincterotomy for bile duct stones. *Br J Surg* 1991; **78**: 554–557.

82. Solhaug JH, Foskuan O, Rosseland A, Rydberg B. Endoscopic sphincterotomy in patients with gallbladder in situ. *Acta Chir Scand* 1984; **150**: 475–478.

83. Dunn D, Nair R, Fowler S, McCloy R. Laparoscopic cholecystectomy in England and Wales: results of an audit by the Royal College of Surgeons of England. *Ann R Coll Surg Engl* 1994; **76**: 269–275.

84. Burhenne HJ. Percutaneous extraction of retained biliary tract stones: 661 patients. *Am J Roengtenol* 1980; **134**: 889–898.

85. Mazzariello RM. A 14-year experience with nonoperative instrumental extraction of retained bile duct stones. *World J Surg* 1978; **2**: 447–455.

86. Palmer KR, Haffman AF. Intraductal mono-octanoin for the direct dissolution of bile duct stones: experience in 343 patients. *Gut* 1986; **27**: 196–202.

87. Yoshimoto H, Ikeda S, Tanaka M, Matsumoto S, Kuroda Y. Choledochoscopic electrohydraulic lithotripsy and lithotomy for stones in the common bile duct, intrahepatic ducts and gallbladder. *Ann Surg* 1989; **210**: 576–582.

88. Siegel JH, Ben-Zvi JS, Pullano WE. Endoscopic electrohydraulic lithotripsy. *Gastrointest Endosc* 1990; **36**: 134–136.

89. Sauerbruch T, Stern M and the Study group for shock-wave lithotripsy of bile duct stones. Fragmentation of bile duct stones by extracorporeal shock waves. A new approach to biliary calculi after failure of routine endoscopic measures. *Gastroenterology* 1989; **96**: 146–152.

90. Wenzel H, Greiner L, Jakobeit Ch, Lazica M, Thuroff J. Extrakorporale stosswellenlithotripsie von gallengangssteinen. *Deutsche Medizinische Wochenschrift* 1989; **114**: 738–743.

91. Cotton PB, Kozarek RA, Schapiro RH et al. Endoscopic laser lithotripsy of large bile duct stones. *Gastroenterology* 1990; **99**: 1128–1133.

92. Ponchon T, Gagnon P, Valette PJ et al. Pulsed dye laser lithotripsy of bile duct stones. *Gastroenterology* 1991; **100**: 1730–1736.

93. Cairns SR, Dias L, Cotton PB, Salmon PR, Russell RCG. Additional endoscopic procedures instead of urgent surgery for retained common bile duct stones. *Gut* 1989; **30**: 535–540.

94. Chung SCS, Leung JWC, Leong HT, Li AKC. Mechanical lithotripsy of large common bile duct stones using a basket. *Br J Surg* 1991; **78**: 1448–1450.

95. Allen B, Shapiro W, Way LW. Management of recurrent and residual common bile duct stones. *Am J Surg* 1981; **142**: 41–47.

96. DeAlmeida AM, Cruz AG, Aldeia FJ. Side-to-side choledochoduodenostomy in the management of choledocholithiasis and associated disease. Facts and fiction. *Am J Surg* 1984; **147**: 253–259.

97. Lygidakis NJ. Surgical approaches to postcholecystectomy choledocholithiasis. *Arch Surgery* 1982; **117**: 481–484.

98. McSherry CK, Glenn F. The incidence and causes of death following surgery for nonmalignant biliary tract disease. *Surg Gynaecol Obst* 1980; **191**: 271–275.

99. Parrilla P, Ramirez P, Sanchez Bueno F et al. Long-term results of choledochoduodenostomy in the treatment of choledocholithiasis: assessment of 225 cases. *Br J Surg* 1991; **78**: 470–472.

100. Kraus MA, Wilson SD. Choledochoduodenostomy. Importance of common duct size and occurrence of cholangitis. *Arch Surg* 1980; **115**: 1212–1213.

101. Berlatsky Y, Freund H. Choledocho-duodenostomy in the treatment of benign biliary tract disease. *Am J Surg* 1981; **141**: 90–93.
102. Huguier M, Houry S, Pascal G. Chole-dochoduodenostomy for calculous biliary disease. *Arch Surg* 1985; **120**: 241–242.
103. Gaskill HV, Levine BA, Sirinek KR, Aust JB. Frequency and indication for choledochoduodenostomy in benign biliary tract disease. *Am J Surg* 1982; **144**: 682–684.
104. Neugebauer E, Troidl H, Spangenberger W, Dietrich A, Lefering R, and the cholecystectomy study group. Conventional versus laparoscopic cholecystectomy and the randomised controlled trial. *Br J Surg* 1991; **78**: 150–154.

11a

The upper gastrointestinal tract: thoracoscopic dissection of the oesophagus

O.J. McAnena

Introduction

Patients with carcinoma of the oesophagus pose major problems for the clinician. Fifty per cent of patients present too late to be candidates for surgical resection.[1] The majority are elderly and frequently suffer from concomitant medical conditions.[2, 3] While various approaches have been made combining chemotherapy and radiotherapy, either prior to or after surgical resection, removal of the tumour is the mainstay of potentially curative treatment for carcinoma of the oesophagus.

The difficulties encountered with surgery for oesophageal carcinoma derive from its relative inaccessibility. Lying in the posterior mediastinum, it is intimately associated with the posterior wall of the trachea anteriorly in its upper third, the pulmonary vessels, aorta, and heart in its middle third, and the descending aorta in its lower third. Historically, there have been three different approaches to the oesophagus: the three-stage (thoracic, abdominal, cervical)[4] the trans-hiatal (abdomino-cervical)[5], and the thoraco-abdominal.[6] Each approach has serious drawbacks. The blunt or trans-hiatal approach appears to decrease the risk of post-operative pulmonary dysfunction.[1] However, because it is a blind procedure, there is a risk of serious haemorrhage either from the intercostal or aortic arterial branches that give the oesophagus its blood supply, or perhaps more importantly from the azygos vein. There is also a risk of chylous leak from thoracic duct injury which is potentially fatal.[7] In addition, the incidences of tumour rupture and damage to the membranous part of the bronchus, particularly in middle-third carcinomas, are significantly increased.[8] Many would argue that the inability to perform nodal dissection decreases the chances of long-term survival.[9]

Three-stage or thoraco-abdominal approaches to dissect the oesophagus also have disadvantages.[10] While nodal dissection under direct vision is possible by these approaches, the risk of post-operative pulmonary complications is increased. In addition, serious morbidity can occur from thoracic wound pain. This multicavity approach prolongs the operating time and magnifies the physiological insult.

Access to intra-abdominal and intra-thoracic disease has been improved by laparoscopy and thoracoscopy. Mobilization of the oesophagus under direct vision at thoracoscopy should decrease the risk of haemorrhage and thoracic duct injury associated with blunt dissection, whilst enabling the surgeon to dissect the mediastinal lymph nodes. Video-assisted thoracic surgery in the treatment of emphysematous bullae, particularly in the young patient, has proven an effective form of treatment and decreases the post-operative morbidity and hospital stay. The concept of applying video-assisted thoracic surgery to the dissection of the intra-thoracic part of the oesophagus carries much appeal. The perceived insult of a thoracic incision and exposure of the thoracic cavity is avoided through this video thoracoscopic approach.[11]

Another minimally invasive approach to the oesophagus has been described by Professor Buess in Germany: the mediastinum is dissected under direct vision using a special endoscopic dissector.[12] Our own technique has utilized the standard telescope through the right chest and it is this which is described herein.[13]

Pre-operative preparation ───────────

Thoracoscopic-assisted oesophagectomy is a new procedure. The surgeon submitting a patient to this approach must have extensive experience in complex minimally invasive surgical techniques. He or she must also have prior experience in the open thoracic approach to the oesophagus. Ideally, the surgeon should first pursue a preceptorship, under the guidance of a surgeon already experienced in this approach.

The patients must be selected carefully. The procedure is most ideally suited to the approach of benign conditions of the oesophagus such as lye strictures, etc. Unfortunately, almost invariably the indication for oesophagectomy in the Western hemisphere is for malignant disease. Therefore, it is preferable to select those with early lower third oesophageal carcinomas or tumours of the oesphago-gastric junction.

Pre-operative evaluation is essentially the same as that for open surgery of the oesophagus. Endoscopy and biopsy, barium swallow and meal, liver ultrasound, bronchoscopy for middle and upper third tumours, and computerized tomographic scanning of the thorax and upper abdomen are essential to provide adequate information prior to surgery. Evaluation of pulmonary function by spirometry and arterial blood gases are essential. Intravenous digoxin may be considered in the peri-operative period to decrease the risk of post-operative arrhythmias, although there are no data to support this practice. The co-operation of an anaesthetist experienced in thoracic surgery is essential. Physiotherapy is as essential before this operation as it is before the open procedure. High quality videoscopic equipment and a 30° telescope are vital.

The standard surgical procedure

Epidural anaesthesia is useful in controlling post-operative abdominal pain. Following double-lumen anaesthesia, right internal jugular CVP and left radial artery line placements, pulse oximetry measurement and bladder catheterization, a gastroscope is placed in the oesophagus and the patient draped. The patient is turned from a supine to a standard right thoracotomy position (Fig. 11a.1). A major problem in the use of video-endoscopic equipment is the lack of space in the area around the operating table.

At the sites of port placement we routinely utilize pre-emptive analgesia, using 0.5 per cent Bupivicaine. The first 10 mm trocar is sited in the fifth interspace in the anterior axillary line. Once the telescope is advanced into the chest cavity, the remaining ports are placed as far away from each other as possible, while at the same time the instruments can be moved in all directions as freely as possible. The trocars must allow repositioning of the telescope wherever they are placed and it is therefore preferable to utilize 10 mm ports. The further the trocars are sited away from each other, the less likelihood is there of 'crossing swords' during the operative procedure. One must be careful not to go too far anteriorly as there is a risk to mediastinal structures; equally, by going too far posteriorly, movement within the chest cavity is limited by the thoracic spine.

Despite the use of double-lumen anaesthesia and collapse of the right lung, it may be necessary to use carbon dioxide insufflation for the first twenty minutes of the procedure. The automatic insufflator should be set at no more than 5 mm Hg pressure. If it is delivered at the conventional laparoscopic pressure (approximately 15 mm Hg), there is a real risk of a tension pneumothorax. It may be necessary to use up to one litre of carbon dioxide insufflation, which will aid in

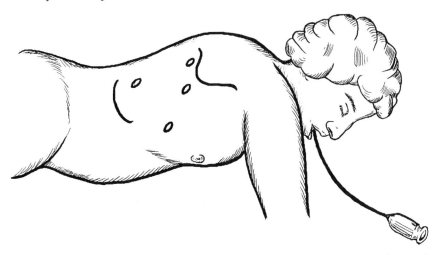

Fig. 11a.1   The patient is placed in a right thoracotomy position. The endoscope is introduced prior to draping.

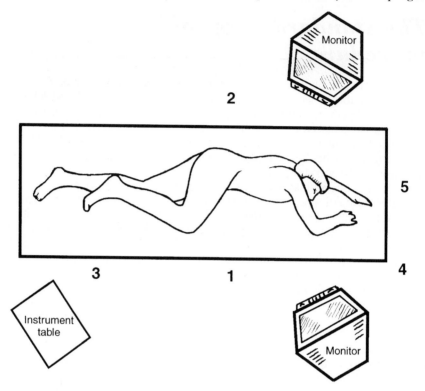

Fig. 11a.2   Position of surgeon and assistants: 1 surgeon; 2 first assistant; 3 scrub
nurse; 4 endoscopist; 5 anaesthetist.

compressing the right lung if residual air is present in the lung. Positioning the
patient in a more prone position may reduce post-operative respiratory complications.

Initially, the operating surgeon stands on the patient's left-hand side and the
operating monitor is placed opposite, to the left of the operating assistant's
shoulder. The assistant's monitor is placed to the right of the operation surgeon
(Fig. 11a.2). The nurse stands to the left of the operating surgeon. A second
assistant, who is experienced in gastroscopy is placed sitting beside the anaesthetist at the head of the table in a manner that does not interfere with anaesthetic
intervention.

From time to time the dissection will require the operating surgeon to transfer
to the opposite side of the table. On the patient's right-hand side, dissection of the
upper third of the oesophagus is facilitated. The gastroscope is used to provide
additional light within the mediastinum. It also confirms the exact position and
enables distraction of the oesophagus in the posterior mediastinum. The tumour
is inspected to detect any invasion of the adjacent structures that may have been
missed on pre-operative imaging. The thoracic cavity is examined to identify the
presence of any unforeseen pleural metastatic deposits. Once the lesion has been

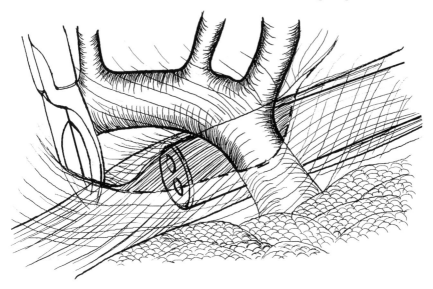

Fig. 11a.3   Dissection is initiated at the pleura over the azygos vein. Note the endoscope illuminates the oesophagus in the mediastinum.

confirmed to be resectable, dissection is started, preferably at a site where the oesophagus is not involved with tumour. The initial steps are designed to encircle the oesophagus (Fig. 11a.3). The parietal pleura overlying the oesophagus is divided by sharp dissection. The author uses an ultrasonic coagulating device (Harmonic® scalpel, Ultracision, Providence, Rhode Island, USA) rather than monopolar diathermy for dissection. Ultrasonic coagulation works by denaturing protein. This reduces the risk of adjacent organ damage because not only do the tissue temperatures remain relatively low, but there is also no risk of arcing or capacitance coupling. This is especially important at the middle third of the oesophagus where its anterior wall is in intimate association with the thin posterior membranous lower trachea at the level of the carina. An adequate suction-irrigation system is mandatory because even small amounts of blood in the operating field will absorb light and significantly diminish the picture quality.

Dissection for lower third tumours begins just below the azygos vein, and preferably proceeds caudally towards the inferior pulmonary ligament. Control of the azygos vein is an integral part of encircling the oesophagus. The pleura overlying the azygos is therefore carefully mobilized and divided cephalad to the thoracic inlet. Careful scissors dissection close to the under surface of the azygos vein is the key to its mobilization. It is important to avoid the small vascular tributaries that occasionally enter its under surface and are best controlled with clips. The azygos vein is then divided using the vascular Endo GIA®, (US Surgical Corp, CT), which applies three rows of staples to each side of the divided vein (Fig. 11a.4). The oesophagus is then mobilized over a distance of 3–4 cms by a combination of distraction of the oesophageal wall utilizing the gastroscope within it and sharp dissection outside. Numerous vessels from the anterior wall

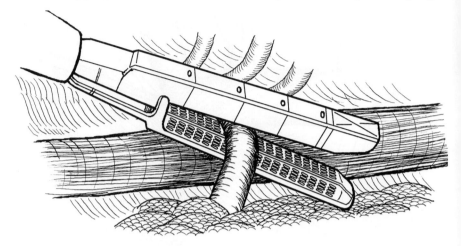

Fig. 11a.4   Division of the azygos vein using an Endo-GIA® 30 mm stapler. This facilitates oesophageal encirclement.

of the thoracic aorta and from the intercostal arteries, which are the mainstay of the blood supply to the oesophagus, can be clearly identified at thoracoscopy. These are clipped and divided. It will take some time before the posterior and left walls of the oesophagus are sufficiently free to permit the passage of a shaped memory instrument (Roticulating Endograsp®, Autosuture, Ascot, UK), under the oesophagus. Once it encircles the oesophagus it can be used to provide traction and angulation in each direction to facilitate further the oesophageal dissection on the surface opposite the telescope (Fig. 11a.5). It is preferable to perform dissection between the oesophagus and the trachea by scissors dissection rather than diathermy. The author has preferred to use the Harmonic scalpel dissector in this instance. Because the membranous trachea is so thin in its lower part, heat injury by diathermy may result in perforation.

Formal dissection of the mediastinal nodes requires experience: it is difficult and time consuming. The potential benefits of radical lymph node dissection must be weighed against the prolonged operative time and potential post-operative complications.

The dissection can continue headwards to behind the thyroid gland and distally to the diaphragmatic hiatus and indeed into the abdominal cavity if necessary. The larger the tumour, the more hazardous and difficult the dissection.

In some instances resection of the contra-lateral mediastinal pleura may be necessary. Frequent irrigation of the mediastinal bed to clear any blood clots is imperative to provide adequate visualization. Once haemostasis has been achieved, an angulated 32 French thoracostomy tube is advanced through the most inferior and anterior port before the lung is inflated under direct vision. It may be necessary to close the thoracoscopy wounds using a J needle with 'O' Vicryl (Ethicon®, UK) prior to closing the skin.

The patient is then placed in the supine position. The remainder of the operation is performed as if one was doing a trans-hiatal oesophagectomy. Using a

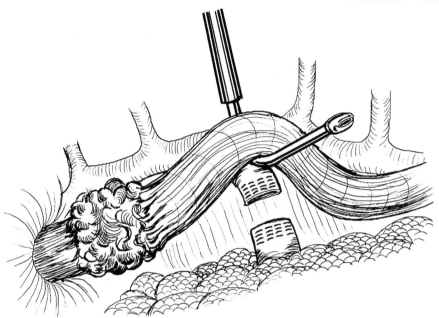

Fig. 11a.5   A Roticulating Endo Grasp® is placed under the oesophagus. Traction and angulation helps in completion of dissection.

bilateral sub-costal (Chevron) incision, gastric mobilization is performed on the right gastro-epiploic artery. The usual attention must be given to ligating carefully the short gastric vessels without injury to the spleen. A greater curvature gastric tube is constructed and positioned in the posterior mediastinal tunnel. The neck dissection is usually performed on the left side. The left recurrent laryngeal nerve must be identified and preserved. Then the stomach tube is pulled up to the neck, and the thoracic oesophagus is excised. An oesophago-gastrostomy is then performed in the neck using 3.0 Maxon® (Davis and Geck, UK). We routinely utilize jejunostomy feeding post-operatively. This is initiated within 36 hours of surgery. Patients are transferred to the Intensive Care Unit post-operatively. We prefer, where possible, to extubate the patient sooner rather than later.

Discussion

The thoracoscopic approach to oesophageal mobilization for cancer has the theoretical appeal that dissection of the oesophagus and haemostasis can be acheived under direct vision while avoiding the need for an open thoracotomy.[13] In the initial stages it was hoped that this would overcome the adverse problems of open thoracotomy, as seen in the three-stage or Ivor–Lewis oesophagectomy, and of the blunt nature of oesophageal trans-hiatal dissection.

The literature on thoracoscopic-assisted oesophagectomy is limited. In our own series the mean time for oesophageal mobilization ranged from 100–160 minutes. The mean operating time ranged from 250–360 minutes. We feel that prolonged right lung collapse increases the risk of post-operative pulmonary complications. All patients who have such prolonged collapse will, after re-expansion of the lung, have evidence of persistent segmental collapse on immediate post-operative chest X-ray. This has usually resulted in significant pulmonary problems. Thus, in our own experience, the expected potential for improved post-operative pulmonary function and diminished pulmonary complications has not yet been realized.

Cuschieri has reported that placing the patient in the prone position on the table tends to reduce post-operative complications. In particular, the number of reported incidences of post-operative pneumonia was 3 out of 26 procedures.[14] In our own experience the single most significant complication has been pulmonary.

Buess and Manncke have described the technique of trans-mediastinal endoscopic oesophageal dissection.[15] This approach avoids thoracotomy. Using a mediastinoscope, video endoscopy and dedicated instruments, the oesophagus is dissected out through the mediastinum. The major structures within the mediastinum are identified. In their experience, simultaneous mediastinal dissection can be performed with the abdominal approach. This shortens the operative procedure. Intra-mediastinal nodes can be identified.

In their series, the major operative complications were rare (5.3 per cent). Only one patient required thoracotomy. This group of workers have suggested that their technique results in a low rate of post-operative pulmonary complications and recurrent laryngeal nerve palsy. Although this is an improvement it does not solve the problem of limited dissection associated with trans-hiatal oesophagectomy. The exact technique would require a period of instruction from one of the surgeons who have learned this technique before embarking upon it.

Other experimental technologies have been addressed. Bessel *et al.*[16] have described a combined thoracoscopic and laparoscopic approach with oesophago-gastric reconstruction in the chest. The operation is performed in three stages. Firstly, the thoracoscopic oesophageal dissection, followed by laparoscopic gastric mobilization and finally a thoracoscopic oesophago-gastric anastomosis is performed, using a circular endoluminal stapler. Buess *et al.* have utilized a similar approach with an intra-thoracic stapled anastomosis. Using firstly a trans-oral approach, the stapler is inserted from above. The anvil, which is connected to a wire, is drawn into the abdomen together with the distal oesophagus. Retracting the wire pulls both the anvil and the stomach up into the thorax after the insertion of the anvil. Secondly, the trans-hiatal approach requires a special attachment to introduce the anvil into the thorax and then into the oesophageal stump. The gastric tube is pushed into the thorax by the stapler gun which is inserted into the stomach through a gastrostomy. The insertion of the anvil into the oesophageal stump is also achieved with the support of a flexible endoscope, including a polyp snare.

All of these approaches are modifications of the traditional Ivor–Lewis operation. Many surgeons are concerned about the risk of breakdown of an intra-thoracic anastomosis leading to mediastinitis.[17] Undoubtedly however, the final choice of approach is an individual surgical preference based on experience.

Conclusion ————————————————

The management of oesophageal carcinoma remains a perplexing problem for the surgical oncologist. Because so many patients present at a late stage with treatment limited to palliation, many therapies have evolved. These include the treatment of the symptoms themselves by dilatation, laser therapy, electro-coagulation and intubation, or by various forms of surgery.[18]

Undoubtedly, resection when performed with curative intent gives the best relief of dysphagia and remains the only hope of cure. The conventional options for surgery carry certain advantages and disadvantages. The school of surgeons who promulgate trans-hiatal oesophagectomy believe that there is a lower incidence of post-operative pulmonary complications compared to either the three-stage or thoraco-abdominal approaches. Trans-hiatal oesophagectomy, however, is a blind procedure. There is a small but definite risk of haemorrhage from bleeding oesophageal vessels or from the azygos vein or its tributaries. Bronchial rupture may occur, particularly with middle third carcinomas, and the incidence of thoracic duct injury seems higher than in open surgery. The school of surgeons who promote open thoracotomy rightly state that lymph node dissection is not an option with trans-hiatal resection. There is evidence that extensive lymph node dissection may improve survival in some cases.[19] Thoracotomy incisions facilitate dissection under direct vision and allow for lymph node dissection. It would appear that the risks of chylothorax rupture into a bronchus or rupture of the tumour itself and haemorrhage are diminished. Long-term discomfort may result from thoracotomy incisions. Either way the present conventional surgical approaches to oesophageal resecton involve significant post-operative morbidity, particularly undesirable in patients with a poor long-term outlook.

The right thoracoscopic-assisted oesophagectomy appeals in that it appears to marry the advantages of the open traditional approach with those of the closed trans-hiatal dissection, without having the drawbacks of either. A thoracotomy incision is avoided and dissection and haemostasis are performed under direct vision. Formal mediastinal lymph node dissection has not been performed by us, although we believe it feasible through this approach with increasing experience. It is in this respect superior to the mediastinascopic approach developed by Buess *et al.* Because the mediastinascope is straight, the olive at its end impinges on the aorta when the lower third of the thoracic oesophagus is reached, rendering this part of the dissection difficult unless the instrument is held in the correct alignment by the abdominal surgeon. However, the mediastinoscopic technique has the advantage that the entire operation can be performed without changing the position of the patient on the operating table.

If one decides to embark on the thoracoscopic-assisted operation, then patients must be selected who have small, mobile tumours. With larger tumours there is a risk of injury to mediastinal structures because of a loss of the surgical planes and the difficulty in separating the tumour from the surrounding structures in the face of a limited two-dimensional image. It might perhaps be more appropriate to attempt this type of surgery initially on patients with benign conditions of the oesophagus.

The technique of thoracoscopically-assisted mobilization of the oesophagus has some potential for future management of oesophageal problems. Undoubtedly, surgeons who undertake this form of surgery must have the training to enable them to proceed immediately to standard open thoracotomy if necessary. The canine model in the laboratory is useful but the author finds the bovine model not particularly helpful in learning thorascopic oesophageal dissection techniques.

The present available data suggest that hospital stay is not shortened. Therefore, as it presently stands it would appear that the morbidity is equivalent to that following trans-hiatal dissection. It is technically a demanding and difficult procedure and the expected benefits have not yet materialized. Until better results are demonstrated from specialist centres, the technique cannot be universally recommended.

References

1. Muller JM, Erasmi H, Stelzner M and Zieren H *et al.* Surgical therapy of oesophageal carcinoma. *Br J Surg* 1990; **77**: 45–57.
2. Mitchell RL. Abdominal and right thoracotomy approach as standard procedure for oesophago-gastrectomy with low morbidity. *J Thorac Cardiovasc Surg* 1987; **93**: 205–211.
3. Lam K, Cheung HC, Wong J, Ong GB. The present state of surgical treatment of carcinoma of the oesophagus. *J R Coll Surg Edinb* 1982; **27**: 315–326.
4. McKeown KC. The surgical treatment of carcinoma of the oesophagus. A review of the results in 478 cases, *J R Coll Surg Edinb* 1985; **30**: 1–14.
5. Orringer MB. Trans-thoracic versus trans-hiatal oesophagectomy: what difference does it make? *Ann Thorac Surg* 1987; **44**: 116–118.
6. Tanner NC. The present position of carcinoma of the oesophagus. *Postgrad Med J* 1947; **23**: 109–139.
7. Bolger C, Walsh TN, Tanner WA, Keeling P, Hennessy TPJ. Chylothorax after oesophagectomy. *Br J Surg* 1991; **78**: 587–589.
8. Fok M, Siu KF, Wong J. A comparison of transhiatal and transthoracic resection for carcinoma of the thoracic oesophagus. *Am J Surg* 1989; **158**: 414–419.
9. Khoury GA. Oesophageal surgery under Akiyama. *Lancet* 1989; **i**: 91–92.
10. Gotley DC, Beard J, Kruper MJ *et al.* Abdomino-cervical transhiatal oesophagectomy in the management of oesophageal carcinoma *Br J Surg* 1990; **77**: 815–819.
11. Cuschieri A, Shimi S, Banting S. Endoscopic oesophagectomy through a right thoracoscopic approach. *J R Coll Surg Edinb* 1992; **27**: 7–11.
12. Buess G. Kipfmuller K, Nahrun M, Melzer A. Endoskopischemikrochirurgische dissektion des osophagus. In: Buess G, (ed.) *Endoskopie.* Arzte-Verlag, Koln, 1990, pages 338–375.
13. McAnena OJ, Rogers J, Williams NS. Right thoracoscopically assisted oesophagectomy for cancer. *Br J Surg* 1994; **81**: 236–238.
14. Cuschieri A. Thoracoscopic subtotal oesophagectomy. *Endosc Surg Allied Technol* 1994; **2**: 21–25.
15. Manncke K, Raestrup H, Walter D *et al.* Technique of endoscopic mediastinal dissection of the oesophagus. *Endosc Surg Allied Technol* 1994; **1**: 10–15.
16. Bessell JR, Maddern GJ, Manncke K, Ludbrook G, Jameson GG. Combined thoracoscopic and laparoscopic oesophagectomy and oesophago-gastric reconstruction. *Endosc Surg Allied Technol* 1994; **1**: 32–36.
17. Lund O, Kimose HH, Aagaard MT *et al.* Risk stratification and long term results after surgical treatment of carcinomas

of the thoracic oesophagus and cardia. *J Thorac Cardiovasc Surg* 1990; **99**: 200–290.

18. Watson AA. A study of the quality and duration of survival following resection, endoscopic intubation and surgical intubation in oesophageal carcinoma. *Br J Surg* 1982; **69**: 585–588.

19. Akiyama H, Tsurumaru M, Kawamura T, Ono Y. Principles of surgical treatment for carcinoma of the oesophagus. *Ann Surg* 1981; **194**: 438–446.

11b

The upper gastrointestinal tract: the laparoscopic management of gastro-oesophageal reflux disease and peptic ulceration

T.V. Taylor

Introduction

There have been radical changes in the mangement of acid related disorders in recent years. Some 15 years ago, neither peptic ulcer nor gastro-oesophageal reflux disease (GORD) were amenable to effective healing therapy and all that was available to relieve persistent painful symptoms was conventional antacid medication. Surgery, however, offered the potential of 'cure' of these disorders via either an acid reducing or an anti-reflux procedure, but at the price of open operation and often disabling side effects of which many have been incurable. In recent years, there have been major advances in the medical treatment of both conditions which need to be weighed against the feasibility, efficacy, safety and cost of surgery in the laparoscopic era.

The presence of acid is essential for both disorders. The disorders in other ways, however, differ fundamentally. GORD results from the exposure of the oesophagus to acid, in either sufficient concentration or duration to damage the stratified squamous epithelium. It is rarely a life-threatening condition but may be very disabling. Peptic ulceration remains a potential killer as a result of the complications of bleeding and perforation, both of which still carry a mortality of at least 10 per cent. Perhaps, ironically, this mortality is increasing in most Western countries, particularly in the elderly female.

Gastro-oesophageal reflux disease

Pathogenesis

Gastro-oesophageal reflux disease, the commonest cause of dyspepsia, varies from a mildly symptomatic entity to a complicated aggressive disorder that can lead to stricture formation, pulmonary complications and possibly Barrett's oesophagus. It has been established that approximately 10 per cent of the US population have heartburn daily and more than one third have intermittent symptoms. Furthermore, in up to 50 per cent of patients with non-cardiac chest pain, 78 per cent of patients with chronic hoarseness, and 82 per cent of patients with asthma, an association with reflux disease may be noted.[1-4]

The causes of failure of the anti-reflux mechanism may lie in inadequacies of the oesophageal pump or the lower oesophageal sphincter, or else in abnormalities in the gastric reservoir. The lower oesophageal sphincter (LES) may fail for reasons of lack of strength, duration of contraction and relaxation, length and position. Subtle changes in vagal function may alter these variables and may be the leading factor in the pathogenesis of the condition in the absence of hiatal hernia. It is now recognized that transient relaxation of the lower oesophageal sphincter, not resting pressure level, is the most important determinant of reflux.[5] Episodes of transient relaxation are more common after a meal and are stimulated by fat in the duodenum, which also slows gastric emptying. Although pathological reflux can occur in the absence of hiatal hernia, herniation leads to loss of the positive pressure effect on the intra-abdominal oesophagus; loss of the oesophago-gastric angle; impairment of the 'mucosal rosette' phenomenon; and sometimes impaired gastric emptying. Duration of contact of acid/pepsin on the mucosa is affected by both frequency of reflux and oesophageal peristalsis.

Clinical evaluation

In evaluating the patient, the history is important, and the therapeutic effect of empiric antacids may contribute to making the diagnosis. Thereafter endoscopy is the first line and most cost-effective investigation. It is valuable for grading and stratifying the extent of the reflux disease. Several biopsies of the diseased area should be taken to rule out Barrett's oesophagus or a potential malignancy; in immune-compromised patients these biopsies should be cultured. A barium swallow examination may be a useful adjunct to endoscopy, particularly when a stricture is suspected, under which circumstances it should precede endoscopy. The Bernstein test of mucosal sensitivity to acid is fairly reliable for confirming that symptoms are acid related, though there is likely to be a lack of positivity in patients with Barrett's oesophagus.

Unfortunately, the data obtained by 24-hour ambulatory lower oesophageal pH and manometry, though demonstrating reasonable specificity and sensitivity, do not always correlate well with symptom severity score or with severity of oesophagitis as graded endoscopically. Accepted limits of normality also vary, and herein lies a dilemma.[6] The clinician is after all treating symptoms in gastroesophageal disease, though other considerations are also pertinent, such as the development of Barrett's oesophagus with its underlying potential for malignancy. The major role of ambulatory pH and manometry in this situation is to evaluate those patients with atypical reflux symptoms, non-cardiac chest pain, unexplained pulmonary symptoms or hoarseness. Manometry is helpful in positioning the oesophageal probe, and a high percentage of abnormal oesophageal contractions or the presence of a hypotensive lower oesophageal sphincter supports a diagnosis of a severe type of GORD.

Clinical management

Medical

Lifestyle modifications are to be recommended, such as elevation of the head of the bed, avoidance of fat, reduction of alcohol intake, cessation of smoking and avoidance of eating prior to sleeping. Weight reduction is often the key to achieving improvement of symptoms and relatively minor weight reduction may alleviate even severe symptoms. Conventional over-the-counter antacids and alginates are more beneficial than placebo. Variable and often unimpressive results have been associated with the use of H2-receptor antagonist therapy, in conventional dosage, in this disorder. Standard doses produce symptomatic relief in 32 to 82 per cent of patients and resolution of endoscopically confirmed oesophagitis was demonstrated in 0 to 82 per cent (mean 48 per cent). Most effective control is achieved with high dose regimes given four times daily.[7] The proton pump inhibitors omeprazole and lansoprazole are effective in a high proportion of patients with erosive oesophagitis which is resistant to even high dose H2-receptor blockade. The usual dosage of omeprazole is 20 mg daily, some will require 40 mg daily, and a number can be maintained on 20 mg taken on alternate days. There is a limited place for using prokinetic drugs such as cisapride as an adjunct to H2-receptor antagonists.

   Maintenance therapy after healing is the crucial problem underlying medical therapy. Early relapse of symptoms most frequently follows cessation of medication. Omeprazole is most effective in prevention and the dose may be reduced, but there are some anxieties, probably totally unfounded, about its long term use and the issue of genotoxicity.

Surgical management

Over the past half century, the surgical management of GORD has evolved from anatomical correction of the hiatal defect to the development of many anti-reflux procedures most of which involve some degree of fundoplication, partial or complete. Correction of the hiatal hernia and restoration of the lower oesophageal sphincter to the abdominal cavity do not achieve adequate control of reflux. Nissen's fundoplication may produce overkill by inducing dysphagia and 'gas bloat'. Partial wraps in the form of anterior or posterior fundoplications or 270° fundic wraps have been associated with good results, at least in the short term and warrant further scrutiny. Perhaps the surgical profession's concern, scepticism and perhaps disillusion with conventional anti-reflux surgery was best epitomized by the enthusiasm with which Angelchik's silicone-collar anti-reflux device was adopted. The device has largely been abandoned in the laparoscopic era. Nissen's fundoplication however, despite its short-term complications and not infrequent long-term failure, remains the 'gold standard' against which all other anti-reflux procedures should be compared.

Laparoscopic anti-reflux surgery

In 1991, Dallamagne from Belgium[8] performed the first laparoscopic Nissen fundoplication. Since then, surgeons in increasing numbers have been using the laparoscopic approach for the treatment of gastro-oesophageal reflux. A number of different techniques have been described for the performance of this procedure but the essentials of the operation are (a) establishment of the pneumoperitoneum and placement of ports; (b) exposure of the proximal stomach and abdominal oesophagus; (c) dissection of the abdominal oesophagus; (d) identification of the anterior and posterior vagus nerves; (e) identification of the diaphragmatic crura; (f) establishment of a window, behind the oesophagus, for the wrap; (g) approximation of the crura; (h) mobilization of the upper 255 mm of gastric greater curvature; and (i) the fundoplication technique.[9]

Under general anesthetic, the patient is placed supine or in the lithotomy position; the former is certainly adequate. The table should be tilted into the

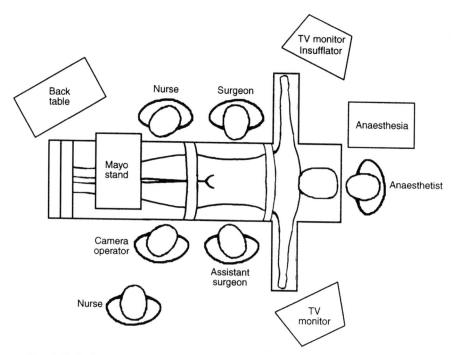

Fig. 11b.1   Layout of operating room for laparoscopic Nissen fundoplication.

anti-Trendelenburg position, while the arms are placed out on boards (Fig. 11b.1). Two television monitors are placed at 45° to the head of the operating table. The surgeon and the nurse stand on the right side of the table, the assistant and video-camera operator stand on the left. A pneumoperitoneum is established at the site of the umbilicus using a disposable Verres needle inserted in the sagittal plane angled down to the pelvis. About four to five litres of carbon dioxide are insufflated until the intra-abdominal pressure is approximately 15 mm of mercury. A 10–11 mm trocar is then inserted, again in the sagittal plane aimed down into the pelvis. Five to six 10–11 mm trocars are used in all (Fig. 11b.2). The second is placed just below the xiphoid process and slightly to the left of the falciform ligament. The third is placed between the xiphoid and the umbilicus slightly to the left of the falciform ligament. The fourth trocar is placed in the right anterior axillary line below the level of the liver; this is used for liver retraction. The fifth trocar is placed under the subcostal area on the left anterior axillary line. A sixth trocar is optional, and may be inserted about 50 mm below and medial to the fifth trocar. A 30° to 40° reverse Trendelenburg position with 20° to 30° rotation of the patient to the right will allow optimal exposure of the hiatus. Both a 0° and a 30° forward viewing scope should be used at various stages of the procedure, through the umbilical port.

A fan-like expandable liver retractor is used to retract the left lobe of the liver.

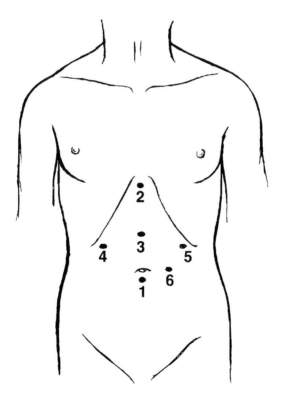

Fig. 11b.2 Positioning of ports, all are 10–11 mm.

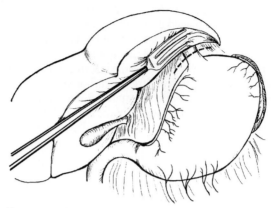

Fig. 11b.3 Exposure of distal oesophagus.

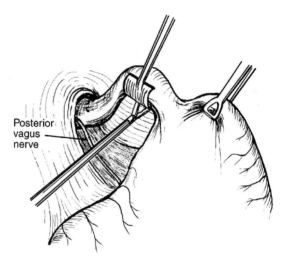

Posterior
vagus
nerve

Fig. 11b.4 Mobilization of the distal oesophagus.

The surgeon uses the upper midline and left subcostal ports in a two-handed approach to the hiatus. The assistants retract the liver and oesophagus, the latter via the left lateral port.

The gastro-hepatic omentum is divided above the hepatic branches of the anterior vagus and the peritoneum over the distal oesophagus is divided (Fig. 11b.3). Fatty and areolar tissue is dissected off the distal oesophagus which is exposed; electrocautery may be used. The right crus is identified. The oesophagus is retracted to the left and the posterior vagus nerve is identified and dissected off the oesophagus (Fig. 11b.4). Further division of soft tissues then exposes the left crus. To ensure that the crural defect is not made too small a size 58 or 60 F Maloney bougie is placed within the oesophagus. A soft rubber sling is placed around the distal oesophagus which is retracted so that the crura can be sutured

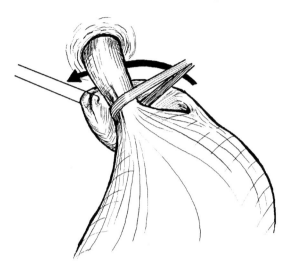

Fig. 11b.5 The posterior fundic wrap.

using the Auto suture needle holder (endostitch) with a short (< 1 cm) transverse needle which is transferable from one limb of the needle holder to the other. Depending upon the size of the defect, about three sutures are placed through the crura.

The short gastric vessels are next divided between surgical clips, by using the linear stapler/cutter or alternatively the harmonic scalpel and about 10 to 15 cm of gastric fundus is mobilized. The posterior fundus of the stomach is grasped behind the oesophagus and brought through to lie on the right side of the structure (Fig. 11b.5). A second grasper is placed on the anterior gastric wall which is pulled around to create a loose wrap. Pulling the posterior fundus around the back of the oesophagus may be facilitated by the use of a roticulator endo-dissector (Auto suture 174213) which is easily manipulated into the space behind the oesophagus. The apices of the fundic wrap are approximated and sutured in position by picking up the seromuscular layers of the stomach and the muscular wall of the oesophagus. About three sutures are inserted with the endostitch needle holder and short double-ended transverse needle (Auto suture) described above (Fig. 11b.6). The wrap should be short and 'floppy'. The fundoplication may finally be anchored to the under surface of the diaphragm. Knot tying can be done intracorporeally or extracorporeally. A nasogastric tube is left in place over night and fluids are begun the following day. The average hospital stay is two days.

Vertical gastric plication

Another surgical option for the treatment of GORD which could be carried out laparoscopically is the technique of vertical gastric plication. Described by the author,[10] this procedure, rather like an undivided Collis gastroplasty, effectively lengthens the 'intra-abdominal oesophagus', sharpens the angle of entry into the stomach and reinforces the lower oesophageal sphincter (Fig. 11b.7).

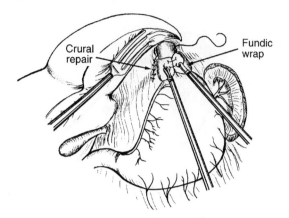

Fig. 11b.6   The crural repair and the sutured fundoplication.

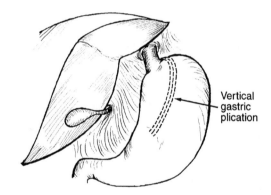

Fig. 11b.7   Vertical gastric plication.

Partial wraps

Partial fundoplication carried out by forming an anterior or posterior wrap are equally feasible to the Nissen procedure. The Toupet partial fundoplication, in addition, is a modification of the complete wrap aimed at reducing the side effects of the Nissen fundoplication. In this procedure, a 270° gastric wrap of the oesophagus with the gastric fundus on either side of the wrap is anchored to the crus of the diaphragm. On the whole, the short gastric vessels are not divided with the Toupet technique.

The Angelchik prosthesis

In performing this procedure the lower oesophagus is mobilized and a C-shaped silicone collar or cuff is placed around the distal oesophagus and clips are put

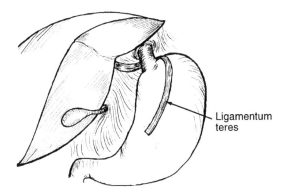

Fig. 11b.8 Ligamentum teres gastropexy.

across the silicone ties, which emanate from the cuff, to hold it in position. The collar lies, like a horse's halter, loosely around the lower oesophagus.

Laparoscopic ligamentum teres cardiopexy

Nathanson[11] described laparoscopic gastropexy with a ligamentum teres wrap in patients with intractable gastro-oesophageal reflux disease. The mechanism is thought to be one of lengthening the intra-abdominal oesophagus and accentuating the angle of His. Good results were claimed in five patients (Fig. 11b.8).

Endoscopic techniques

Endoscopic injection of the gastro-oesophageal junction with scar-inducing agents has been investigated and shown to enhance the gastro-oesophageal barrier function, at least in the short term. Donahue and his colleagues[12] injected 4 ml of 5 per cent sodium morrhuate solution into the submucosa of the gastric cardia of an experimental canine reflux model at 6 injection sites arranged in a horseshoe pattern 1 to 2 cm below the gastro-oesophageal junction. These injections were performed four times in each dog at 3 to 4 week intervals. Endoscopic sclerosis was effective in preventing reflux induced by high-dose atropine. It was thought that reflux prevention was probably related to enhancement of the gastric component of the reflux barrier. McGowan and Galloway[13] attempted to increase yield pressure endoscopically in the dog by using the N2-YAG laser to produce a deep fibrous scar at the cardia in the approximate line of the gastric sling fibres. One of the ten dogs developed a gastric perforation.

Discussion

When Dallemagne introduced laparoscopic Nissen fundoplication, his preliminary report in 1991 was based on 12 patients. Post-operative results based on endoscopy, manometry and barium contrast studies were reported as excellent.[8]

One of the patients underwent conversion to an open procedure because of a tear in the greater curvature at the site of the short gastric vessels. The only complication was pneumonia which occurred in one patient. Post-operative pain was minimal and the hospital stay was reduced to three days. After six months, all 6 patients reviewed were well.

In 1992 Bagnato reported on 16 patients treated with Nissen fundoplication, 14 with persistent gastro-oesophageal reflux and 2 with achalasia.[9] Two required open conversion because of difficulties in defining the anatomy of the posterior oesophagus. Three or four sutures were used in achieving a complete 360° wrap. The patients with achalasia also underwent a laparoscopic trans-abdominal Heller's myotomy. All 16 patients reported complete relief of symptoms over a mean follow-up period of nine months. Hinder and Filipi in 1992 reported encouraging results in 40 laparoscopic Nissen fundoplication procedures performed over a one-year period between 1991 and 1992.[11] Cuschieri, Shimi and Nathanson claimed that total fundoplication and crural repair was feasible in 8 elderly patients, aged between 60 and 76 years, who had large hiatal hernias, either sliding or mixed.[15] The average operating time was three hours and the only complications were a single pneumothorax and surgical emphysema put down to migration of CO_2 through the mediastinum. These authors emphasize the importance of using a 30° forward viewing telescope which allows much better visualization of the region of the gastro-oesophageal junction. Geagea in 1991 reported on 10 cases of laparoscopic Nissen fundoplication without morbidity or mortality.[16] Dallemagne went on in 1993 to report the results of Nissen fundoplication in 132 patients in whom the indication for laparoscopic intervention was symptomatic reflux disease not responding to medical treatment.[17] There was no operative related mortality. The overall morbidity was 7.5 per cent. Ninety-eight patients were seen three months after surgery and evaluated for control of reflux symptoms; however, endoscopic examination revealed no evidence of recurrent oesophagitis. Three complained of occasional dysphagia, and two of mild dysphagia. One patient required re-operation for persistent severe dysphagia.

In a series of 35 patients Bittner and colleagues, 1993, reported a higher morbidity rate of 25.7 per cent.[18] Five required conversion to an open procedure as a result, in three patients, of haemodynamic instability secondary to presumed pneumothorax and colotomy and a distal oesophageal perforation in two patients. Ten per cent had significant dysphagia. The clinical outcome was regarded as good or excellent in 87 per cent and unsatisfactory in 13 per cent.

In a recent study reported from Bordeaux and Brussels 758 patients underwent a laparoscopic procedure for reflux disease, while during the same period 38 underwent an elective laparotomy. In the laparoscopic group there were 294 Nissen, 334 Nissen–Rossetti placements, 106 Toupet procedures, and 24 Angelchik prosthesis placements.[19] The conversion rate was only 4.2 per cent (32 cases). In 7 cases the conversion was due to an intra-operative complication, whereas in 25 cases the conversion was done because of technical difficulties. Thirty post-operative complications occurred (4 per cent), leading to a re-operation in 12 cases. The major complications were haemorrhage in 4; gastric perforation in 2; oesophageal perforation in 2; and colonic perforation in 1. This is an important and large study which goes some way to answering the question of whether laparoscopic access is associated with a higher mortality or morbidity rate and whether the advantages of laparoscopic access are not reduced by a possibly higher surgical risk. The results reported in this study suggest that laparoscopic treatment, when performed by an experienced laparoscopic surgeon, is as safe as open surgery. There was no mortality, and morbidity compared favourably; hence laparoscopic treatment would seem to have more advantages than disadvantages. There are two important caveats to this conclusion. One is that no long-term results of laparoscopic anti-reflux surgery exist; though there is no reason to believe that they should be materially worse than those following a short-term effective open operative procedure. The second and most important concern is that the results described in this combined Belgian and French study are based on cases done by experienced laparoscopic surgeons, even though they include their own particular learning curve for this procedure. This is not to say that equally good results could be obtained 'across the board' for this difficult operation. The inexperienced and less technically skilled surgeon may find himself in trouble with oesophageal, gastric or even colonic perforations leading, in the case of the former, to possible corrective oesophageal resection with ensuing septic complications and possible multiple organ failure.

The surgeon has an escape clause – conversion to the time-honoured open procedure. Conversion may be necessary in two types of circumstance. The first of these is technical operative difficulty. Obesity, adhesions, enlarged left hepatic lobe, or annoying oozing of blood are the most common reasons for conversion, and account for about 80 per cent of cases. If the procedure is not progressing satisfactorily after about one hour of dissection then it would seem wise to convert it. Secondly, conversion may be necessary because of an intra-operative complication that cannot be managed laparoscopically. The most serious complication, perforation of the posterior aspect of the oesophagus has already been mentioned. Recognition is of fundamental importance, so as to allow expeditious and life-saving correction of the problem. The repair should be done immediately by converting to open laparotomy and correction of the defect by primary surgical repair. If the injury is not appreciated immediately and repair is delayed, oesophageal resection with its attendant high morbidity and mortality may be required. Careful dissection of the oesophagus should prevent this complication. The dissection involves the hiatal orifice rather than the oesophagus itself. Mobilization begins on the right crus, having divided the upper part of the gastrohepatic ligament, and continues until the junction with the left crus is reached and the left subdiaphragmatic space is entered. A large retro-oesophageal window should be created so as to facilitate an unrestricted loose and floppy fundic wrap. Staying close to the hiatal orifice prevents pleural laceration and possible pneumothorax. Suturing a gastric perforation is more feasible laparoscopically, and less likely to give rise to the problems which may be encountered with an oesophageal tear. The Babcock forceps should be used very cautiously; it is capable, particularly when placed under tension, of tearing the stomach. Another cause of gastric perforation is acute gastric dilatation which may occur in a vulnerable patient following too early withdrawal of the nasogastric tube. Gross gastric dilatation leads to ischaemia, particularly of the devascularized area of the greater curvature. Splenic laceration is another potential problem but seems to occur rarely. The incidence of respiratory complications, most notably atelectasis and pleural effusion, is probably lower than that associated with the open operation.

In the large study of Collet and Cadiere (1995)[19] 24 patients underwent laparoscopic placement of an Angelchik prosthesis; the morbidity was 12.5 per cent compared with 2.3 per cent after the Nissen fundoplication. Angelchik and his coworkers evaluated the prothesis in 10 pigs in 1991, concluding that the antireflux prosthesis can be safely and effectively placed using laparoscopic methods.[20] The higher morbidity in the Belgian/French large study and the potential which the prosthesis has shown in previous studies to migrate would provide sufficient evidence, in the author's opinion, that the device should not be used. The current controversy surrounding the systemic effects associated with breast implants would further suggest that silicone prostheses should not be inserted into body cavities where alternative satisfactory methods of treatment exist.

In conclusion, laparoscopic treatment for GORD can be safe and effective in the hands of accomplished laparoscopic surgeons. Laparoscopy obviates the disadvantages of laparotomy and enables exactly the same operative procedure to be performed as at open operation. The surgery should only be performed by experienced laparoscopic surgeons, probably those who have done at least one hundred cholecystectomies laparoscopically and have attended at least one course on advanced laparoscopic surgery which provides hands-on experience of the Nissen fundoplication in the pig or dog. These courses are run in several centres in the USA. Obviously, long-term studies are required, but as the intraperitoneal procedures in the open and laparoscopic operations are the same then one would expect to achieve similar results to those obtained by traditional surgery.

Peptic ulcer disease

Aetiology and pathogenesis

For most of this century, peptic ulceration has been regarded as being due, predominantly, to the erosive effects of acid and pepsin upon a vulnerable or weakened gastric or duodenal mucosal barrier. Acid is essential for ulceration and the aphorism of Schwartz, 'No acid – no ulcer' remains true today. Until recently, chronic peptic ulcer disease was curable only by acid-reducing surgery. The introduction of the H2-receptor antagonists in 1977 provided efficacious antisecretory medication resulting in the short-term healing of the vast majority of ulcers. With one month's medication 65 per cent of ulcers, both gastric and duodenal, healed; a two-month course resulted in the healing of some 85 per cent.[21] Cessation of treatment, however, rapidly led to a return of secretion to pretreatment levels with, in consequence, a high incidence of recurrent ulceration, some 90 per cent at two years.[22] None the less the number of patients undergoing elective ulcer surgery began to decline dramatically in the early 1980s.

The mid-1980s brought about the discovery of the micro-organism. *Helicobacter pylori*, with subsequent ever increasing evidence of its implication in the aetiology of peptic ulcer disease.[23,24] Many, if not most, now assign causative roles to *Helicobacter* infection in duodenal and the vast majority of gastric ulcers. They list as proof that successful eradication of *H pylori*, unlike the H2 receptor antagonists, not only heals the ulcer but achieves long-term eradication and possible cure.[25]

Helicobacter pylori infection must be added to the ulcer equation which becomes: acid/pepsin +/− *H pylori* infection versus the mucosal resistance.[25,26] Furthermore, particularly in the elderly, NSAID use is a factor and probably a dominant variable. *H pylori* infection should now be investigated in patients with ulcer disease undergoing endoscopy. It has been suggested that *H pylori* infection is the most common cause of peptic ulceration and that NSAID use is the second major cause.[27] Acid is, however, still important in the pathogenesis of ulcer disease as evidenced in the rare Zollinger–Ellison syndrome, and by the good results of surgical vagotomy. In terms of pathogenesis the ulcer crater is not the result of *H pylori* activity alone; *H pylori* merely compromises protective mechanisms, breaching the gastric mucosal barrier and leaving the mucosa of the stomach and duodenum vulnerable to acid and peptic damage.[28] There would appear, therefore to be two main types of peptic ulcer, the *H pylori* related and the non-*H pylori* related. In the latter category the major aetiological factor would appear to be the taking of NSAIDs and aspirin. Alcohol and smoking also influence ulceration but are not causative.

A thesis implicating *H pylori* infection as the major cause of peptic ulceration has further reduced the amount of elective surgery being carried out for peptic ulcer and soon surgical trainees will gain little or no experience of gastric surgery. Surgical therapy for ulcer disease, however, is effective in achieving the long-term or permanent healing of the vast majority of ulcers so treated.[29–31] In consequence these patients no longer run the risk of developing the potentially fatal side effects of bleeding and perforation, both of which carry a mortality of at least 10 per cent. Furthermore, the mortality associated with peptic ulcer disease in the United Kingdom and in Finland is increasing despite the advances in medical therapy which have occurred over the past 17 years.[32,33]

The 1994 United States National Institutes of Health Consensus Conference guidelines recommend that all patients with a new or recurrent peptic ulcer should be tested for *H pylori* infection.[34] Recurrence rates of ulceration are certainly much lower after eradication of the organism than after successful healing with H2-receptor antagonist therapy and currently quoted reinfection rates are low.[35] A number of combinations of antimicrobial agents have been shown to be effective against the organism in a high proportion of cases.[36] If medication fails and the patient develops recurrent ulceration I would try one further two-week course of antimicrobial therapy.[37] The success rate of triple therapy in eradicating the organism is of the order of 80 per cent. Recurrent rates of infection are, in the short term, low. It remains crucial to this strategy to know long-term ulcer recurrence rates. Currently these are running at low levels after one year. We do not yet know whether eradication of *H pylori* reduces the subsequent risk of gastric cancer in these patients. In *H pylori*-associated ulcers, in the absence of NSAID use, I would not use prolonged courses of H2-receptor therapy. These drugs are helpful in initial therapy in combination with antimicrobials, because they help to achieve more rapid symptomatic relief. The other main use of H2-receptor antagonist drugs in peptic ulcer disease is, I believe, in the management of patients with NSAID-induced ulcers, both to establish short-term healing and where it is necessary for the patient to continue to take NSAIDs as adjunctive long-term prophylaxis.[38]

Patients who repeatedly develop recurrent ulceration, either due to failed eradication of the organism or for other reasons, should be considered for elective surgery, particularly if they have reached the age of 50 years, after which they run a much increased chance of developing potentially fatal complications. Clearly the number of such patients has dramatically declined in recent years and now probably too few patients are being offered the option of the surgical method of permanent cure of their ulcer. In these patients the Zollinger–Ellison syndrome should be ruled out by serum gastrin estimations. The elective operation of choice is either a standard highly selective vagotomy or a lesser curve seromyotomy with posterior truncal vagotomy. The surgeon may elect to do the procedure of his choice, either of the above, laparoscopically.[39–41] There are inherent advantages in this approach provided that the procedure is performed in a technically adequate manner.[42]

Complicated ulcer

Haemorrhage from peptic ulcer remains a common problem. The mortality associated with major upper gastrointestinal tract haemorrhage remains, as it has been for most of this century, 10 per cent. Endoscopic intervention with adrenaline injection or the use of a heater probe or similar modality has reduced the number of open operations performed, though this has not, as yet, been convincingly associated with a reduction in mortality. Furthermore, patients who have had one or more episodes of bleeding from a peptic ulcer are at a greatly increased risk of having further potentially lethal haemorrhage. Where stigmata suggesting continued or repeated bleeding are present, such as the presence of a visible vessel in the ulcer crater, or where bleeding continues, surgery should be carried out expeditiously. It is of fundamental importance that the ulcer crater should be oversewn with non-absorbable suture material. This is feasible through a duodenotomy, while preserving the pyloric sphincter. In addition a highly selective vagotomy or a lesser curve seromyotomy with posterior truncal vagotomy should be carried out and also the patient should be assessed, at this time, for *H pylori* status. In the elderly frail, unstable patient, truncal vagotomy and pyloroplasty may be expedient and life saving.

Because of side effects I would not routinely advocate truncal vagotomy and antrectomy but if there is marked scarring with a very large ulcer crater then antrectomy with a Billroth II reconstruction may be most appropriate. Should the patient develop a recurrent ulcer after the pylorus preserving vagotomy, this should be treated by eradication of *H pylori* if the organism was found to be present.[43] There is no evidence that antisecretory medication with intravenous H2-receptor antagonists is of any value in the treatment of the acutely bleeding ulcer. Intravenous omeprazole has not been shown to be efficacious in this situation and concerns have been expressed as to its safety in view of ophthalmological complications which have been reported in Germany.[44]

The NSAID-induced bleeding peptic ulcer is more likely to require surgery, particularly in the elderly patient who has coexisting cardiovascular and respiratory pathology. The high mortality inherent in this group of patients relates more to their associated medical problems than to uncontrolled haemorrhage per se, but having become haemodynamically unstable there is a tendency to lapse into the acute respiratory distress syndrome and multiple organ failure.

Surgery remains the choice of treatment for perforated peptic ulcer. Simple oversewing of the perforation with an omental patch has been the standard treatment for many years. It may be argued, however, that any patient who has an ulcer diathesis which is aggressive enough to perforate on one occasion may do so again; therefore it would be logical to perform an acid reducing vagotomy at the time of oversew. Some surgeons reserve acid-reducing surgery for those whose perforation occurs after a long history of a symptomatic ulcer diathesis, while performing a simple oversew in those patients who acutely perforate without prodromal symptoms. If acid-reducing surgery is carried out it should take the form of a pylorus-preserving vagotomy as described above. It is possible to close the perforation and even add a seromyotomy or HSV laparoscopically. In addition it is well worthwhile assessing the *H pylori* status on patients with ulcer perforation.[45]

While to the present day little has been written on the association between *H pylori* infection and perforation, eradication of the organism would seem warranted. For those who perforate an ulcer while taking NSAIDs and who need to continue with the latter, acid-reducing surgery should accompany oversewing the perforation. It is important that data should be obtained on long-term follow-up of perforation in patients who have been treated by simple over-sewing of their ulcers and *H pylori* eradication. Closure of perforation may be performed laparoscopically and recently a simple technique of injecting the perforation with fibrin gel has been developed.

In the presence of a major degree of tight pyloric stenosis the treatment of choice is either HSV or seromyotomy with posterior truncal vagotomy and either pyloroplasty or gastroenterostomy. Mild degrees of pyloric stenosis may respond to endoscopic dilatation, which may be carried out at the time of diagnostic endoscopy; *H pylori* status should be assessed concurrently.

In these days of more effective medical management of peptic ulceration there is little place in elective management for truncal vagotomy with either a drainage procedure or an antrectomy. The side effects of severe diarrhoea, dumping or bilious vomiting may be prolonged, disabling and incurable; therefore the risks of encountering these should not be run.[46] There is an insignificant risk of developing severe diarrhoea or dumping with either of the pylorus-preserving procedures mentioned.

Laparoscopic vagotomy

Four procedures have been performed laparoscopically for the treatment of chronic duodenal ulcer: truncal vagotomy and pyloric dilatation; anterior lesser curve seromyotomy with posterior truncal vagotomy; highly selective vagotomy; linear gastrectomy and posterior truncal vagotomy.

Truncal vagotomy

In exposing the distal oesophagus, truncal vagotomy is feasible; the technique is similar to the early steps of the Nissen fundoplication procedure described above. The posterior vagus is divided and a segment of nerve is removed. The anterior nerve requires mobilization from the anterior wall of the oesophagus to which it is adherent. The lower end of the nerve trunk is spatulate in shape at the level of the oesophago-gastric junction, a feature which helps in identification. On occasions there may be more than two main trunks; the additional trunks must be divided in order to achieve a total truncal vagotomy. The pylorus should be dilated endoscopically with a 30 mm balloon inflated to 45 psi for 10 minutes.

Anterior lesser curve seromyotomy with posterior truncal vagotomy[47–51]

The patient is positioned either in the supine position or in a full lithotomy position.[52] The surgeon may stand on the patient's right side or between the legs. The first assistant is on the patient's left and the second assistant on the right. The television monitors are placed each at 45° to the table at the level of the patient's head. The peritoneal cavity is insufflated through the umbilicus. The first 10–11 mm trocar is placed in the midline about two inches above the umbilicus; the video-laparoscope is placed through this. The second, sub-xiphoid 10 mm trocar is inserted just to the left of the falciform ligament. Third and fourth 5 mm trocars are placed in the right and left subcostal regions and a final 10–11 mm trocar is placed to the left of the midline. An expandable liver retractor is inserted through the subxiphoid port to retract the left lobe of the liver and achieve better exposure of the gastro-oesophageal area.

The peritoneum overlying the upper aspect of the lesser curve of the stomach and the peritoneal reflection from the under surface of the diaphragm are divided. Areolar and fatty tissues are dissected free to expose the right crus of the diaphragm. As the oesophagus is displaced anteriorly and to the left, the posterior vagus nerve trunk is recognized and dissected free. The nerve is then transected between clips and about one inch (25 mm) of its length is removed.

The anterior seromyotomy is next performed by stretching the anterior surface of the stomach with the grasping forceps. The line of dissection is placed between 1 and 1.5 cm from the lesser curvature, extending from a point approximately 6 cm proximal to the pylorus at the crow's foot to the gastro-oesophageal junction. Two inferior branches of the crow's foot are preserved. The seromuscular incision is performed with the electric hook coagulator using a blended monopolar current. Two grasping forceps are used to stretch the circular muscle fibres while the hook coagulator is used to divide these. When the muscular layer is divided the submucosa can be seen to protrude and there is wide separation of the divided muscle. Above the crow's foot, as the dissection is performed exactly parallel to the lesser curvature about three to five short vessels are encountered; these are clipped and divided (Fig. 11b.9). The branches of the nerve of Latarjet cross the stomach in a plane superficial to the serosa so that when the seromuscular layer has been incised all of the vagal branches passing across the myotomy to the

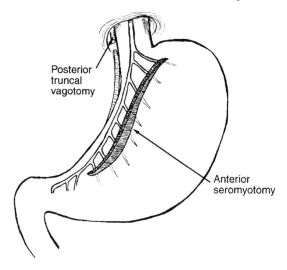

Fig. 11b.9   Anterior lesser curve seromyotomy with posterior truncal vagotomy.

parietal cell mass are divided. The stomach should be inflated with air at the end
of the procedure to check that the mucosa has not been breached.

Highly selective vagotomy

Conventional highly selective vagotomy was modified for use by the laparoscope
by Dallemagne.[53] The dissection is begun at a point 6 cm proximal to the pylorus
at the crow's foot in a plane between the nerve of Latarjet and the lesser
curvature. Small leashes of tissue with blood vessels are isolated, clipped and
divided as the lesser curvature is denuded to a point 3 cm above the oesophago-
gastric junction. Great care must be taken not to damage the nerves of Latarjet or
even the main vagal trunks. The operation is somewhat tedious and time consuming to perform. Recurrence rates, due largely to incomplete vagotomy when
the operation is performed by open surgery, are often high and there is no reason
to believe that they should be any lower when the procedure is carried out
laparoscopically (Fig. 11b.10).

Linear gastrectomy: anterior highly selective with posterior truncal vagotomy

For technical expediency to overcome the difficult and sometimes tedious dissection involved in conventional highly selective vagotomy, Hannon and his colleа-
gues[54] developed a technique of denervating the anterior parietal cell area using
an endoscopic stapling device, the Endo-GIA.

In this procedure the ports are placed as for the previous operations described
herein but a 12 mm port is in addition inserted in the right mid- to lower abdomen

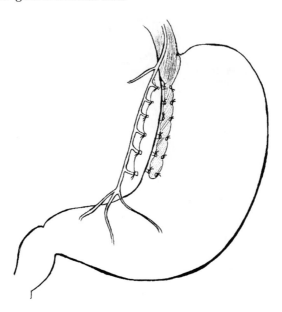

Fig. 11b.10   Highly selective vagotomy.

for the Endo-GIA stapler. The posterior vagus nerve is divided. Starting 6–7 cm proximal to the pylorus a fold of the anterior gastric wall is pulled between the jaws of the stapler which is placed so as to divide and reanastomose the full thickness of the gastric wall removing a linear strip of stomach from the starting point, parallel to and 1 cm from the lesser curvature, up to the gastro-oesophageal junction. The procedure is facilitated by the use of a 46 French bougie which is passed into the proximal stomach. On completion of the linear stapling the stomach is inflated with air to check the integrity of the anastomosis.

Thoracoscopic vagotomy

A report exists of a patient who developed a stomal ulcer following a Polya gastrectomy and underwent thoracoscopic vagotomy.[55] The inferior pulmonary ligament was freed, and the lung was retracted cephalad. The space behind the pericardiophrenic junction medial to the aorta was opened and the oesophagus was identified. The vagal trunks were clipped and divided. Endoscopy three months after the procedure showed that the ulcer had healed.

Laparoscopic treatment of perforated peptic ulcer

Perforated duodenal and gastric ulcer can be treated laparoscopically. The perforation is usually easily identified and can be closed by suture or with a fibrin sealant and an omental patch can be placed over the defect. Large gastric perforations may be converted into a gastrostomy by inserting a Foley Catheter through the perforation. Patients should be treated with antibiotics and either omeprazole or an H2-blocker. They should then undergo investigation of *Helicobacter* status and if present, the organism should be eradicated.[56]

Discussion

That laparoscopic vagotomy is feasible and, in experienced hands, safe, is beyond question. As with antireflux surgery, the same intra-abdominal procedure can be performed laparoscopically as at open surgery. One would expect therefore that potentially the same long-term results could be achieved with laparoscopic as with open vagotomy. Because of the side effects associated with truncal vagotomy and drainage, elective ulcer surgery today should be confined to the pylorus-preserving procedures. Highly selective vagotomy, however, has been associated with a high incidence of ulcer recurrence, even amounting to as many as 30 per cent of cases, at long-term follow-up, 14–18 years.[57] The major cause of this recurrence has been incomplete vagotomy due to an inadequate technical procedure having been performed at open operation: laparoscopic surgery undoubtedly adds another dimension of difficulty to any procedure and it might be assumed, not unreasonably, that the adequacy of highly selective vagotomy may be more limited when performed laparoscopically. Anterior lesser curve seromyotomy with posterior truncal vagotomy, however, permits a greater degree of vagal denervation, the whole posterior gastric wall, than does highly selective vagotomy and it is technically feasible through the laparoscope. Recurrence rates have been lower with this procedure than with highly selective vagotomy, probably as a result of a greater degree of gastric denervation. The seromyotomy procedure is also better suited to the obese patient as there is no fat on the gastric wall at the site of the seromyotomy, though the fat on the lesser curvature can be an encumbrance in the performance of highly selective vagotomy. It is probably down to a question of personal preference as to which procedure is favoured by the particular surgeon but several highly experienced laparoscopists such as Cuschieri of Dundee[58,59] and Dubois of Paris have abandoned highly selective vagotomy in favour of lesser curve seromyotomy with posterior truncal vagotomy. The author found that this operation gave results superior to those of truncal vagotomy and drainage because of a reduction in the incidence of diarrhoea and dumping.[48]

Katkouda and Mouiel have reported the largest series of laparoscopic anterior lesser curve seromyotomy with posterior truncal vagotomy in over 80 patients.[60] Their initial detailed study of 10 patients had a mean operative duration of sixty minutes. Acid inhibition was in keeping with that which would be expected from an operation producing total vagotomy of the parietal cell area of the stomach with an 80 per cent reduction in basal and an 83 per cent reduction in stimulated acid output. These workers have reported a very low complication rate. Clearly, this operation has much to commend it but very few patients are now referred for elective peptic ulcer surgery. Only time will tell whether the attractions of laparoscopic vagotomy with short hospital stay, minimal morbidity, long-term healing and possibly relatively low cost are sufficient to sway some clinicians back to at least a selective policy of elective surgery for uncomplicated peptic ulcer. Hannon's procedure of linear gastrectomy offers an alternative technical approach to performing an anterior lesser curve seromyotomy with posterior truncal vagotomy.

As stated, thoracoscopic vagotomy is also feasible; it has all the problems of truncal vagotomy associated with it and may only be of very occasional value in the case of a recurrent stomal ulcer after previous gastric resection or gastro-jejunostomy.[52]

Bleeding peptic ulcers are now best treated initially by injection of adrenaline or a sclerosing agent into the ulcer crater. Alternative endoscopic techniques utilize monopolar or bipolar electrodes or a heater probe; laser coagulation is expensive and of little value. When these methods fail, open operation is indicated and the ulcer is oversewn. Perforated peptic ulcer, on the other hand, lends itself to treatment by laparoscopy where simple oversew with reinforcement by an omental patch is the treatment of choice. The injection into the ulcer crater perforation of fibrin glue needs further evaluation. Thereafter the patient's *Helicobacter* status should be assessed and, if positive, the organism should be eradicated.

Both peptic ulceration and GORD are common disorders; some patients have both conditions. Although many fewer patients are now candidates for elective ulcer surgery than a decade ago, there is a need for major academic centres with an interest in gastroenterology to develop and train surgeons to perform laparo-scopic pylorus-preserving vagotomy.

References

1. Nebel OT, Fornes MF, Castell DO. Symptomatic gastroesophageal reflux: incidence and precipitating factors. *Am J Dig Dis* 1976; **21**: 953–956.
2. Hewson EG, Sinclair JW, Dalton CB, Richter JE. Twenty-four hour esophageal pH monitoring: the most useful test for evaluating non-cardiac chest pain. *Am J Med* 1991; **90**: 576–583.
3. Wiener GJ, Koufman JA, Wu WC, Cooper JB, Richter JE, Castell DO. Chronic hoarseness secondary to gastroesophageal reflux disease: documentation with 24 hour ambulatory pH monitoring. *Am J Gastro* 1989; **84**: 1503–1508.
4. Sontag SJ, O'Connell S, Khandelwal S, Miller T, Nemchausky B, Schnell TG.

Most asthmatics have gastroesophageal reflux with or without bronchodilator therapy. *Gastroenterol* 1990; **99**: 613–620.
5. Dodds WJ, Dent J, Hogan WJ. Mechanics of gastroesophageal reflux in patients with reflux esophagitis. *New Eng J Med* 1982; **307**: 1574–1582.
6. Schlesinger PK, Donohue PE, Schmid B, Layden TJ. Limitations of 24 hour intra-esophageal pH recording in the hospital setting. *Gastroenterol* 1985; **89**: 797–804.
7. Johnson NJ, Boyd EJ, Mills JG, Wood JR. Acute treatment of reflux esophagitis: A multicenter trial to compare 150 mg ranitidine b.d. with 300 mg q.d.s. *Aliment Pharm Therapeut* 1989; **3**: 259–266.

8. Dallemagne B, Weerts JM, Jeheas C, Markiewiez S, Lombard R. Laparoscopic Nissen fundoplication: Preliminary report. *Surg Laparosc Endosc* 1991; **1**: 138–143.

9. Bagnato VJ. Laparoscopic Nissen fundoplication. *Surg Laparosc Endosc* 1992; **2**: 188–190.

10. Taylor TV, Knox RA, Dullan BR. Vertical gastric plication: An operation for gastro-oesophageal reflux. *Ann R Col Surg Engl* 1989; **71**: 31–36.

11. Nathanson LK, Shimi S, Cuschieri A. Laparoscopic ligamentum teres cardiopexy. *Br J Surg* 1991; **78**: 947.

12. Donohue PE, Carvalho JPC, Davis PE, Shen YJE, Miidla I, Bombeck T, Nylms L. Endoscopic sclerosis of the gastric cardia for prevention of experimental gastro-oesophageal reflux, *Gastrointest Endosc* 1990; **36**: 253–256.

13. McGowan RCM, Galloway JM. A laser induced scar at the cardia increases the yield pressure of the lower esophageal sphincter. *Gastrointest Endosc* 1990; **36**: 439–443.

14. Hinder RA, Filipi CJ. The technique of laparoscopic Nissen fundoplication. *Surg Laparosc Endosc* 1992; **2**: 265–272.

15. Cuschieri A, Shimi S, Nathanson LK. Laparoscopic reduction, crural repair, and fundoplication of large hiatal hernia. *Am J Surg* 1992; **163**: 425–430.

16. Geagea T. Laparoscopic Nissen's fundal plication is feasible. *Can J Surg* 1991; **34**: 313.

17. Weerts JM, Dallemagne B, Hamoir E, DeMarche M, Markiewitz S, Jehaes C. Laparoscopic Nissen fundoplication, detailed analysis of 132 patients. *Surg Laparosc Endosc* 1993; **3**: 359–364.

18. Bittner H, Meyers WC, Brazer SR, Pappas TN. Laparoscopic Nissen fundoplication: Operative results and short-term follow-up. *Am J Surg* 1994; **167**: 193–196.

19. Collet D, Cadiere GB. Conversions and complications of laparoscopic treatment of gastro-esophageal reflux disease. *Am J Surg* 1995; **169**: 622–626.

20. Berguer R, Stiegmann GV, Mamamoto M, Kim J, Mansour A, Denton J, Norton LW, Angelchik JP. Minimal access surgery for gastro-esophageal reflux: laparoscopic placement of the Angelchik prosthesis in pigs. *Surg Endosc* 1991; **5**: 123–126.

21. Penston JG, Wormsley KG. Review article: maintenance treatment with H2-receptor antagonists for peptic ulcer disease. *Aliment Pharmacol Ther* 1992; **6**: 3–29.

22. Van Deventer GM, Elashoff JD, Reedy TJ, Schneidman D, Walsh JH. A randomized study of maintenance therapy with ranitidine to prevent the recurrence of duodenal ulcer. *N Engl J Med* 1989; **320**: 1113–1119.

23. Graham DY. Helicobacter pylori: its epidemiology and its role in duodenal ulcer disease. *J Gastroenterol Hepatol* 1991; **6**: 105–113.

24. Dixon MF. *Helicobacter pylori* and peptic ulceration: histopathological aspects. *J Gastroenterol Hepatol* 1991; **6**: 125–130.

25. Graham DY, Go MF. Helicobacter pylori: current status. *Gastroeneterol* 1993; **105**: 279–282.

26. Taylor TV. Current indications for elective peptic ulcer surgery. *Br J Surg* 1989; **76**: 427–428.

27. Soll AH. Pathogenesis of peptic ulcer and implications for therapy. *N Engl J Med* 1990; **322**: 909–916.

28. Dixon MF. Pathophysiology of Helicobacter pylori infection. *Scand J Gastroenterol* 1994; **29**: (Suppl 201): 7–10.

29. Herrington JL Jr, Davidson J, Shumway SJ. Proximal gastric vagotomy: follow-up of 109 patients for 6–13 years. *Am Surg* 1986; **204**: 108–113.

30. Goligher JC, Hill GL, Kenny JE, Nutter E. Proximal gastric vagotomy without drainage for duodenal ulcer: results after 5–8 years. *Br J Surg* 1978; **65**: 145–148.

31. Taylor TV, Thomas PE, Lythgoe PJ, MacFarland JB. Anterior lesser curve seromyotomy and posterior truncal vagotomy versus vagotomy and pyloroplasty in the treatment of duodenal ulcer – results of a prospective con-

trolled trial. *Brit J Surg* 1990; **77**: 1007–1009.

32. Mortality Statistics (General). *Review of Registrar General on Deaths in England and Wales 1990.* Series DH1 number 24, page 32, HMSO, London.

33. Taylor TV. Deaths from peptic ulcer. *Brit Med J* 1985; **291**: 653–655.

34. Peura DA. Recognition and eradication of *Helicobacter Pylori. Federal Practitioner* 1994; **10**: 83–87.

35. Marshall BJ, Goodwin CS, Warren JR *et al.* Prospective double-blind trial of duodenal ulcer relapse after eradication of Campylobacter pylori. *Lancet* 1988; **2**: 1437–1442.

36. Hentschel E, Brandstatter G, Dragosics B *et al.* Effect of ranitidine and amoxicillin plus metronidazole on the eradication of *Helicobacter pylori* and the recurrence of duodenal ulcer. *N Engl J Med* 1993; **328**: 308–312.

37. Graham DY. Treatment of peptic ulcers caused by *Helocobacter pylori. N Engl J Med* 1993; **328**: 349–350.

38. Rubin R. Medical treatment of peptic ulcer disease. *Med Clin N Amer* 1991; **75**: 981–988.

39. Shapiro S, Gordon L, Daznovsky L, Grundfest W, Chandra M. Development of laparoscopic anterior seromyotomy and right posterior truncal vagotomy for ulcer prophylaxis. *J Laparosc Endosc* 1991; **1**: 277–286.

40. Voeller GR, Pridgen WL, Mangaint EC. Laparoscopic posterior truncal and anterior seromyotomy: A pig model. *J Laparo Endosc Surg* 1991; **1**: 357–359.

41. Hunter JG, Becker JM, Lee RG, Christien PE, Doxon JA. Anterior lesser curve seromyotomy with posterior truncal vagotomy: a potential treatment for peptic ulcer disease. *Brit J Surg* 1989; **76**: 949–952.

42. Katkhouda N, Moueil J. A new surgical technique of treatment of chronic duodenal ulcer without laparotomy by videocoelioscopy. *Am J Surg* 1991; **161**: 361–364.

43. Graham DY, Hepps KS, Ramirez FC, Lew GM, Saeed ZA. Treatment of *H pylori* reduces the rate of rebleeding in peptic ulcer disease. *Scand J Gastroenterol* 1994; **28**: 939–942.

44. der Arzneimittezdommission der Deutschen Apotteker Wichtige Mitteilungen. *MSD Muenchen* 1994; **134**: 18–19.

45. Roth SH, Bennett RE. Nonsteroidal antiinflammatory drug gastropathy – recognition and response. *Arch Int Med* 1987; **147**: 2093–2100.

46. Taylor TV. The post vagotomy and cholecystectomy syndrome. *Ann Surg* 1981; **194**: 625–629.

47. Taylor TV, Macleod DAD, Gunn AA, Maclennan I. Anterior lesser curve seromyotomy and posterior truncal vagotomy in the treatment of chronic duodenal ulcer. *Lancet* 1982; **2**: 846–848.

48. Oostvogel HJM, Van Vroonhoven TJMV. Anterior lesser curve seromyotomy with posterior truncal vagotomy versus proximal gastric vagotomy. *Br J Surg* 1988; **75**: 121–124.

49. Taylor TV, Gunn AA, Macleod DAD *et al.* Morbidity and mortality after anterior lesser curve seromyotomy and posterior truncal vagotomy for duodenal ulcer. *Br J Surg* 1985; **72**: 950–951.

50. Taylor TV, Holt S, Heading RC. Gastric emptying after anterior lesser curve seromyotomy and posterior truncal vagotomy. *Br J Surg* 1987; **72**: 620–622.

51. Taylor TV, Lythgoe JP, McFarland JP, Gilmore IT, Thomas PE, Ferguson GH. Anterior lesser curve seromyotomy and posterior truncal vagotomy versus truncal vagotomy and pyloroplasty in the treatment of chronic duodenal ulcer. *Br J Surg* 1990; **77**: 1007–1009.

52. Katkhouda N, Mouiel J. A new technique of surgical treatment of chronic duodenal ulcer without laparotomy by videocoelioscopy. *Am J Surg* 1991; **161**: 361–364.

53. Dallemagne B, Weerts JM, Jeheas C, Markiewiez S, Lombard R. Laparoscopic highly selective vagotomy. *Br J Surg* 1994; **81**: 554–556.

54. Hannon JK, Snow LL, Weinstein LS. Linear gastrectomy: an endoscopic staple assisted anterior highly selective

vagotomy combined with posterior truncal vagotomy for treatment of peptic ulcer disease. *Surg Laparosc Endosc*, 1992; **2**: 254–257.

55. Chisholm EM, Chung SCS, Sunderland GT, Leong HT, Li AKC. Thoracoscopic vagotomy: a new use for the laparoscope. *Br J Surg* 1992; **79**: 254.

56. Mouset P, Franciois, Vignal J, Barth X, Lambard Platet R. Laparoscopic treatment of perforated peptic ulcer. *Br J Surg* 1990; **77**: 1006.

57. Hoffman J, Olsen A, Jensen HE. Prospective 14 to 18 year follow-up study after parietal cell vagotomy. *Br J Surg* 1987; **74**: 1056–1059.

58. Cuschieri A. Laparoscopic vagotomy: gimmick or reality? *Surg Clin N Am* 1992; **72**: 357–367.

59. Collett D, Cadiere GB. Conversions and complications of laparoscopic treatment of gastroesophageal reflux disease. *Am J Surg* 1995; **169**: 622–626.

60. Moueil J, Katkhouda N. Laparoscopic vagotomy for chronic duodenal ulcer disease. *World J Surg* 1993; **17**: 34–39.

12

Laparoscopic appendicectomy

H. Gajraj, G.S. Carr-White, A. Loh and R.S. Taylor

Introduction

The first appendicectomy was performed by Claudius Amyand at St George's Hospital, London in 1735; an 11-year-old boy had injured his appendix (which lay in a scrotal hernia) with a pin.[1] Over 150 years elapsed before the first appendicectomy for appendicitis was performed.[2,3] Appendicitis is now the commonest condition requiring emergency surgery,[4–7] and the operative treatment has changed little in the last 100 years.

However, the morbidity and mortality of this condition have decreased significantly over the last century, mainly due to advances in anaesthesia, peri-operative care and the use of prophylactic antibiotics.[5] The high prevalence of appendicitis and the relative technical simplicity of appendicectomy have led to complacency.[5] Although the overall mortality of appendicectomy is low (about 1 per cent),[8–12] complications are common, occurring in approximately 20 per cent of patients.[10,12] Perforation is the most important factor influencing morbidity and mortality. With perforation the mortality rate rises to approximately 8.5 per cent[8] and the complication rate rises to just under 50 per cent.[10]

Laparoscopy is the most exciting innovation in both the diagnosis and treatment of appendicitis. It offers the prospect of earlier diagnosis and, therefore, reductions in both morbidity and mortality as well as accurate diagnosis of conditions mimicking appendicitis. Laparoscopic appendicectomy is associated with fewer complications, less pain, shorter hospital stay and earlier resumption of normal activities. Long-term studies may show that laparoscopic appendicectomy is associated with a reduction in other complications such as adhesions, infertility in females and right inguinal herniation. In this chapter we present data on the use of laparoscopy in the diagnosis of appendicitis and data on laparoscopic appendicectomy from case series and trials. We also describe in detail how we perform laparoscopic appendicectomy.

Diagnosis

The diagnosis of appendicitis may be difficult. This is reflected in the frequency with which patients, thought clinically to have appendicitis, undergo appendicectomy and subsequently no abnormality of the appendix is found (negative appendicectomy). The negative appendicectomy rate varies between 25 per cent and 40 per cent overall.[4,6,7,13] For women of child-bearing age it is consistently higher;[4,7,13–15] as many as half undergo a negative appendicectomy. In the past, this has been regarded as the price paid for early diagnosis and treatment. The length of the history appears to be a major determinant of the risk of perforation.[10,16,17] In one large series, perforation was nearly three times more likely if symptoms had been present for more than 24 hours.[10] Although surgical delay has not been consistently implicated in the risk of perforation,[11,17] one study suggested that perforation was twice as likely if the operation was performed more than 24 hours after admission.[10] A large multicentre study on the use of computer-aided diagnosis noted that earlier diagnosis of appendicitis halved the perforation rate (23.7 per cent versus 11.5 per cent).[18] It is often regarded as acceptable to remove a number of normal appendices rather than miss a case of appendicitis that would subsequently proceed to perforation with its associated increased morbidity and mortality. However, 15 per cent of patients who undergo negative appendicectomy suffer significant morbidity.[4,19] A high negative appendicectomy rate and its associated morbidity are now no longer acceptable.[20] Adjunctive tests to improve diagnostic accuracy include serial white cell counts, ultrasonography, barium enema, computerized tomography, peritoneal cytology and clinical scores.[20–22] However, although these do improve diagnostic accuracy, none has gained general acceptance.[20,23]

Involvement of general surgeons in laparoscopic cholecystectomy and the widespread availability of video-laparoscopy have renewed interest in the use of laparoscopy in the diagnosis of appendicitis. A number of studies support the use of laparoscopy in the management of patients with acute abdominal pain. In patients with a clinical diagnosis of appendicitis, it allows direct visualization of the appendix, confirms pathology of other organs that may mimic appendicitis and allows a prompt and confident diagnosis of non-specific abdominal pain (NSAP). Laparoscopy in the diagnosis of appendicitis in women of child-bearing age is supported by a number of studies.[14,24–33] In this group, a clinical diagnosis of appendicitis is twice as likely to be incorrect than in men.[7,19] Compared to the muscle splitting right iliac fossa incision, it allows a more complete examination of the pelvic organs and its use can more confidently establish a diagnosis of pelvic inflammatory disease (PID). This is an important condition that mimics appendicitis and its incidence is increasing.[34] At laparoscopy fluid can be taken from the pelvis for microbiological examination and appropriate antibiotic therapy can be instituted. NSAP is now the commonest reason for emergency surgical admission.[6,7,35] This diagnosis is more frequently made in women and it may be that many cases of PID are being misdiagnosed as NSAP.[35] Widespread use of laparoscopy in the diagnosis of the acute abdomen has been associated with a reduction in the frequency with which NSAP is diagnosed.[36] Patients with NSAP have numerous investigations to exclude other conditions[6] and in one large study, remained in hospital for a mean of four days.[18] Laparoscopy may allow early discharge of these patients.

Laparoscopy is no substitute for a careful clinical assessment. However, for those patients thought to have appendicitis there are strong data supporting the use of laparoscopy to establish the diagnosis (Table 12.1).[24,25,27,28–33,37–44] The complication rate of a negative laparoscopy is much lower than that of a negative appendicectomy.[27,30] In addition, laparoscopy allows a complete inspection of other intra-abdominal organs.

Treatment

The first laparoscopic appendicectomy for a non-inflamed appendix was described by Semm in 1983.[45] In 1985, Fleming first described the technique of laparoscopically directed appendicectomy.[46] Laparoscopic appendicectomy for appendicitis was first described in 1987 by Schreiber.[47] Considerable data from case series (Table 12.2),[26,46,48–57] comparisons based on historical controls, non-randomized trials and randomized prospective trials support laparoscopic appendicectomy as the treatment of choice for acute appendicitis (Table 12.3).[58–69] A number of studies have shown that laparoscopic appendicectomy is associated with less post-operative pain,[59,63,65,67–69] a shorter hospital stay,[58,60,63,64–67,69] fewer complications,[58,62–65,68] and earlier return to full activity.[58–60,62,65]

Controversy surrounds the subject of appendicectomy for patients whose appendix appears normal. Our own practice for those patients with a clinical diagnosis of appendicitis and whose laparoscopy shows no abnormality (i.e. for patients with NSAP) is to perform laparoscopic appendicectomy. This practice is supported by the discrepancy between the macroscopic appearance of the appendix at operation and the results of histological examination.[70,71] In young patients, the life-long risk of developing appendicitis is quite high.[72] In our opinion, the low morbidity associated with laparoscopic appendicectomy supports this practice of 'incidental' appendicectomy. When laparoscopy shows a definite cause for the patient's symptoms (other than appendicitis) our current practice is not to perform appendicectomy. Others have strongly argued that in young patients laparoscopic appendicectomy is still justified.[72,73] However, the appendix has a number of uses in reconstructive surgery and for this reason we take a more conservative approach.[74]

Technique

Once laparoscopy has confirmed the diagnosis, the laparoscope may be used to direct the siting of a small incision over the appendix. The appendix is then delivered through the abdominal wall on to its surface where an otherwise conventional appendicectomy is performed.[46,48,49,57]

This technique (often described as 'laparoscopically-guided') has been criticized as failing to reduce septic wound complications which are the main source of morbidity associated with open appendicectomy. Other techniques involve intra-

Table 12.1 Diagnostic laparoscopy

First author	Year	No. of pts	Type of pts	Comments
Anteby[25]	1974	223	Women with acute lower abdominal pain	Agreement between clinical and laparoscopic diagnosis in only 57 patients (26 per cent). Of 35 patients thought to have appendicitis only 8 confirmed by laparoscopy (23 per cent).
Sugarbaker[44]	1975	56	Acute abdominal pain	29 underwent a preliminary laparotomy and 18 (62 per cent) did not require laparotomy.
Leape[40]	1980	32	Questionable appendicitis	Appendicitis confirmed in 17 (53 per cent); 12 (38 per cent) did not require laparotomy.
Anderson[24]	1981	27	Acute lower abdominal pain: 19 had clinical diagnosis of appendicitis	Laparoscopy confirmed appendicitis in 9 patients 15 patients required no further exploration.
Deutsch[27]	1982	36	Women of child-bearing age (18–45 yrs) with a diagnosis of appendicitis	12 (33 per cent) had a gynaecological condition not requiring surgery.
Reiertsen[43]	1985	81	Acute abdominal pain	Of 40 patients with a clinical diagnosis of appendicitis, 17 (43 per cent) were excluded by laparoscopy.
Clarke[37]	1986	46	Clinical diagnosis of appendicitis	Diagnosis revised in 10 (22 per cent).
Spirtos[32]	1987	87	Women of child-bearing age with a diagnosis of appendicitis	22 (26 per cent) did not require laparotomy. In non-pregnant women PID was the most common alternative diagnosis.

Author	Year	n	Inclusion criteria	Comments
Paterson-Brown[30]	1988	90	Clinical diagnosis of appendicitis	Reduced the negative appendicectomy rate, especially in women.
Whitworth[33]	1988	51	Women (19–48 yrs) with clinical diagnosis of appendicitis	Laparoscopy improved diagnostic accuracy of conditions affecting diagnosis of reproductive organs. Negative appendicectomy rate not affected.
Graham[28]	1991	79	Clinical diagnosis of appendicitis	27 (34 per cent) required appendicectomy. 2.2 per cent negative appendicectomy rate.
Kuster[39]	1992	38	Undiagnosed right iliac fossa pain	Appendicitis confirmed in only 10 (26 per cent); PID the most common alternative diagnosis. Performed under local anaesthesia.
Kum[38]	1993	102	Clinical diagnosis of appendicitis. 28 patients had equivocal signs after 8–12 hours	Of the 28, only 18 (64 per cent) had appendicitis.
Olsen[29]	1993	60	Women aged 15–56 years	Group of 30 who were randomized to laparoscopy had 2 negative appendicectomies compared to 11 in control group.
Scott[31]	1993	77	Acute abdominal pain	Altered clinical diagnosis in 19 per cent and management in 13 per cent.

Table 12.2 Laparoscopic appendicectomy

First author	Year	No. of pts	Comments
Fleming[46]	1985	15	Guided siting of stab incision; appendix delivered onto abdominal wall surface. Mean post-operative stay 3 days.
Gangal[51]	1987	73	Application of bands. Technique described; no follow-up data.
Schreiber[47]	1987	70	Women aged 15–65 yrs; 3 pregnant. Endoloops used. Mean hospital stay 8.1 days. 3 conversions; 1 laparotomy for electrocautery damage to caecum.
Gotz[52]	1990	388	12 converted to open procedure; endoloops used. No wound infections; no prophylactic antibiotics given. Mean operating time 20 mins.
Cristalli[50]	1991	31	20 laparoscopic appendicectomies; clips applied to appendix. Mean operating time 36.5 mins. No complications.
Nowzaradan[54]	1991	43	2 converted to open procedure; endoloops used. No wound infections.
Pier[55]	1991	625	14 converted out of 639 laparoscopic appendicectomies; endoloops used. 2 intra-abdominal abscesses; 14 wound infections.
Saye[56]	1991	109	Endoloops used. Mean post-operative stay 23 hrs. Mean operating time 20 mins. Only 10 per cent of appendices were inflamed. Appendicectomy performed 'incidentally' in most cases as part of another procedure.
Valla[57]	1991	465	Children under 16 yrs. Endoloops and clips used for truly laparoscopic technique; laparoscopically guided technique with appendix delivered onto abdominal surface also used. 3 intra-abdominal abscesses; 2 hernias; no wound infections.
Byrne[48]	1992	25	6 converted to open procedure; appendix delivered onto abdominal surface. Median time to discharge 2 days; 14 days to normal activity. Mean operating time 62 mins.
Choy[49]	1993	23	2 converted to open procedure; appendix delivered onto abdominal surface. Median time to discharge 3 days. Median operating time 55 mins. 2 wound infections.
Cox[26]	1993	81	7 converted; endoloops used. Median post-operative stay 2 days. 8 days to normal activity. Median operating time 55 mins. 1 wound infection.
Ludwig[53]	1993	29	2 converted to open procedure; endoloops, clips and staples used. Median post-operative stay 2 days; 7 days to normal activity.

Table 12.3 Laparoscopic versus open appendicectomy

First author	Year	No. of pts	Design	Comments
Hill[61]	1991	23	Non-randomized prospective	No differences.
Attwood[58]	1992	62	Randomized prospective	Reduced hospital stay, fewer complications, more rapid return to activity, no difference in operating time.
Gilchrist[60]	1992	64	Non-randomized prospective	Reduced hospital stay, more rapid return to full activity. No difference in operating time.
McAnena[63]	1992	65	Non-randomized prospective	Reduced hospital stay, less pain, fewer wound complications. No difference in operating time.
Kum[62]	1993	137	Randomized prospective; normal or perforated appendices excluded	No wound infections in laparoscopic group (vs 9 in open), earlier return to normal or full activity, less pain. No difference in operating time.
Nowzaradan[65]	1993	200	Retrospective; historical controls for open group	Reduced hospital stay, less pain, more rapid return to normal activity and fewer complications.
Schirmer[66]	1993	122	Retrospective	No difference.
Schroder[67]	1993	200	Non-randomized prospective	Reduced hospital stay, less post-operative pain. No difference in complications; operating time prolonged.
Tate[68]	1993	155	Non-randomized prospective	Less post-operative pain, fewer wound infections.
Vallina[69]	1993	35	Retrospective; historical controls for open group	Reduced hospital stay, less post-operative pain. No difference in time to full activity. Operating time prolonged.
Mompean[64]	1994	200	Non-randomized prospective	Reduced hospital stay, fewer wound infections. No difference in operating time.
Frazee[59]	1994	75	Randomized prospective	No difference in hospital stay or complications. Less pain, more rapid return to full activity. Longer operating time.

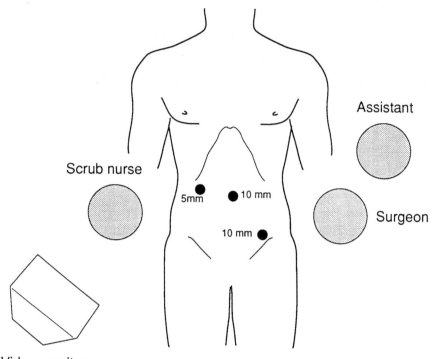

Assistant

Scrub nurse

5mm   ● 10 mm

10 mm ●

Surgeon

Video monitor

Fig. 12.1   Diagram showing position of port sites, surgical staff and video monitor.

corporeal suturing and knot tying,[75] the use of clips[50,57,76] or staples[53] or the use of pre-tied loops.[26,47,52–57,77] These techniques are *truly* laparoscopic: after intra-abdominal appendicectomy, the appendix is delivered via the port and does not come into contact with the abdominal wall. Our technique at St George's Hospital is based on two years' experience of over 100 appendicectomies and will be described in detail (Figs 12.1 and 12.2).

The operation is performed under general anaesthesia. A bladder catheter and naso-gastric intubation are not routinely used. The patient empties his bladder just prior to transfer to the operating theatre. Male patients are placed supine. Female patients are placed in the lithotomy position with the hips flexed to 35° and widely abducted. This allows vaginal examination and uterine sounds to be placed. The uterus can be manipulated to provide better visualization of the female reproductive organs. The operating table is positioned head down. The surgeon stands on the patient's left and his assistant stands to his right. The scrub nurse stands on the patient's right. The monitor is placed near the patient's right foot (Fig. 12.1). Peritoneal insufflation is through a Verres needle sited at the umbilicus and a 10 mm port is placed through an incision just below the umbilicus. A laparoscopic examination of the appendix and other intra-abdominal organs is performed. The operating table may be tilted left-side down to allow better visualization of the appendix. For the retrocaecal appendix, retraction of

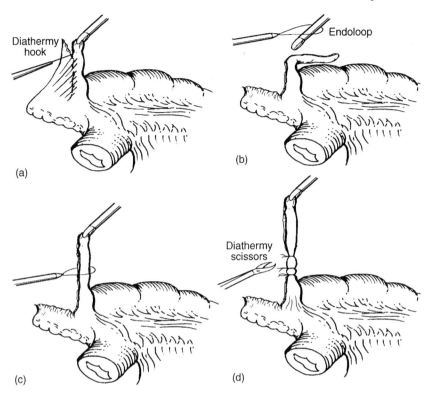

Fig. 12.2   Steps in laparoscopic appendicectomy. (a) division of the mesoappendix
with diathermy hook; (b) grasping forceps through endoloop; (c) appendix
pulled through endoloop; (d) division of appendix between endoloops.

the caecum medially will aid exposure. After establishing a diagnosis of appendicitis or NSAP laparoscopic appendicectomy is performed (Fig. 12.2). A 10 mm
port is placed low in the left lower quadrant of the abdomen under direct vision. A
5 mm port is placed in the right upper quadrant of the abdomen under direct
vision. The appendix is grasped with forceps, introduced through the right upper
quadrant port and is lifted cephalad. With a diathermy hook introduced through
the left lower quadrant port, the mesoappendix is divided close to the appendix.
Catgut endoloops (Endoloop, Ethicon Ltd, UK) are then introduced through this
10 mm port; two endoloops are applied to the base of the appendix 5 mm apart
and one more distally. Diathermy scissors are then introduced through the 10 mm
port and the appendix is divided. Diathermy is used sparingly to avoid injury to
the appendix stump. When small enough, the appendix is withdrawn through the
10 mm port, otherwise it is manipulated into a retrieval bag and this is withdrawn
through the incision in the left lower quadrant after the port has been removed. In
cases of difficulty, an additional 5 mm port may be placed low down in the right
lower quadrant. Scissors introduced via this port can be used to divide the lateral
peritoneal reflection of the caecum, which can then be mobilized medially and

cephalad. An inflamed retrocaecal appendix may then be excised in the way just described. After the appendix has been removed, pus is carefully aspirated from all intra-abdominal compartments and the area of the inflamed appendix is carefully irrigated with saline. We do not invaginate the appendix as this has been shown to be unnecessary.[78] Under direct vision, the instrument ports are removed and the pneumoperitoneum is released. Then, the laparoscopic port is removed. The port sites are examined digitally to confirm that bowel has not been 'sucked up' and the skin is closed with a fine absorbable subcuticular stitch. With these precautions, we believe that a deep myofascial suture is not necessary and may indeed risk catching the bowel.

The need for prophylactic antibiotics in laparoscopic appendicectomy is not established. A large series of 388 laparoscopic appendicectomies has been performed without prophylactic antibiotics and there were no wound infections.[52] Our own practice is to give patients 1 g metronidazole rectally once a clinical diagnosis of appendicitis is made. Further antibiotic therapy is given only if the appendix is perforated or there is generalized peritonitis.

Laparoscopic appendicectomy can be performed using a number of port configurations. We use our combination for a number of reasons:

1. The two instrument ports are widely separated, preventing 'crowding' of the instruments and 'knitting needle' movements.
2. The laparoscope views the operation from a central position between the two instruments, allowing a good view and easy orientation.
3. The surgeon can stand comfortably, facing the monitor and working in the direction of the appendix.

Occasionally, we site the 5 mm port in the right lower quadrant so that the resulting scar is hidden by underwear. However, with this configuration, the surgeon and the laparoscope are 'working' in different directions which can make orientation difficult.

When we have encountered difficulty with this configuration, we place the laparoscope through the 10 mm lower left quadrant port and use the umbilical port for instrumentation. However, in our experience, instrument crowding may be a problem. We believe the 5 mm right upper quadrant incision to be cosmetically acceptable and we would recommend this configuration to beginners.

The results of our own prospective study comparing laparoscopic and open appendicectomy have been extremely encouraging (data to be published). Hospital stay has been shortened and there has been an earlier return to normal activities. In agreement with many other studies we have noted a marked reduction in wound complications. Currently, our conversion rate to open appendicectomy is less than 5 per cent.

The future

Laparoscopic diagnosis of appendicitis and laparoscopic appendicectomy have established themselves in current surgical practice.[79,80] Until now these procedures have been performed by senior surgeons who hitherto would have delegated apendicectomy to more junior staff. Many of these senior surgeons have already had experience with laparoscopic cholecystectomy. The main challenge for the future is to train young surgeons to be proficient with the laparoscope and to perform laparoscopic appendicectomy.[81] In many respects laparoscopic appendicectomy is technically easier than laparoscopic cholecystectomy and trainees should in the future gain experience of laparoscopic appendicectomy early in their training.[55,82,83]

References

1. Creese PG. The first appendectomy. *Surg Gynecol Obstet* 1953; **97**: 643–652.
2. Morton TG. The diagnosis of pericaecal abscess, and its radical treatment by removal of the appendix vermiformis. *JAMA* 1888; **10**: 733–739.
3. McBurney C. Experience with early operative interference in cases of disease of the vermiform appendix. *NY Med J* 1889; **50**: 676–684.
4. Chang FC, Hogle HH, Welling DR. The fate of the negative appendix. *Am J Surg* 1973; **126**: 752–754.
5. Cooperman, M. Complications of appendectomy. *Surg Clin N Am* 1983; **63**: 1233–1247.
6. Hawthorne IE. Abdominal pain as a cause of acute admission to hospital. *J R Coll Surg Edinb* 1992; **37**(6): 389–393.
7. Irvin TT. Abdominal pain: a surgical audit of 1190 emergency admissions. *Br J Surg* 1989; **76**: 1121–1125.
8. Hauswald KR, Bivins BA, Meeker WR, Griffen WO. Analysis of the causes of mortality from appendicitis. *Am Surg* 1976; **42**: 761–766.
9. Peltokallio P, Tykka H. Evolution of the age distribution and mortality of acute appendicitis. *Arch Surg* 1981; **116**: 153–156.
10. Scher KS, Coil JA. The continuing challenge of perforating appendicitis. *Surg Gynecol Obstet* 1980; **150**: 535–538.
11. Silberman VA. Appendectomy in a large metropolitan hospital: retrospective analysis of 1013 cases. *Am J Surg* 1981; **142**: 615–618.
12. Sussman EJ, Kastanis JN, Feigin W, Rosen HM. Surgical outcome for resi-

dent and attending surgeons. *Am J Surg* 1982; **144**: 250–253.
13. Baigrie RJ, Scott-Coombes D, Saidan Z, Vipond MN, Paterson-Brown S, Thompson JN. The selective use of fine catheter peritoneal cytology and laparoscopy reduces the unnecessary appendicectomy rate. *Br J Clin Pract* 1992; **46**(3): 173–176.
14. Foster HMcA. Which patients should undergo laparoscopy? *Br Med J* 1988; **297**: 489.
15. Lewis FR, Holcroft JW, Boey J, Dunphy E. Appendicitis: a critical review of diagnosis and treatment in 1000 cases. *Arch Surg* 1975; **110**: 677–683.
16. Hunter IC, Paterson JG, Davidson AI. Deaths from acute appendicitis: a review of twenty-one cases in Scotland from 1974–1979. *J R Coll Surg Edinb* 1986; **31**: 161–163.
17. Koepsell TD, Inui TS, Farewell VT. Factors affecting perforation in acute appendicitis. *Surg Gynecol Obstet* 1981; **153**: 508–510.
18. Adams ID, Chan M, Clifford PC *et al.* Computer aided diagnosis of acute abdominal pain: a multicentre study. *Br Med J* 1986; **293**: 800–804.
19. Deutsch AA, Shani N, Reiss R. Are some appendicectomies unnecessary? *J R Coll Surg Edinb* 1983; **28**: 35–40.
20. Hoffmann J, Rasmussen OO. Aids in the diagnosis of acute appendicitis. *Br J Surg* 1989; **76**: 774–779.
21. Ooms HWA, Koumans RJK, Ho Kang You PJ, Puylaert JBCM. Ultrasonography in the diagnosis of acute

appendicitis. *Br J Surg* 1991; **78**: 315–318.

22. Thompson MM, Underwood MJ, Dookeran KA, Lloyd DM, Bell PRF. Role of sequential leucocyte counts and C-reactive protein measurements in acute appendicitis. *Br J Surg* 1992; **79**(8): 822–824.

23. Sarfati MR, Hunter GC, Witzke DB, Bebb GG, Smythe SH, Boyan S, Rappaport WD. Impact on adjunctive testing on the diagnosis and clinical course of patients with acute appendicitis. *Am J Surg* 1993; **166**: 660–664.

24. Anderson JL, Bridgewater FHG. Laparoscopy in the diagnosis of acute lower abdominal pain. *Aust NZ J Surg* 1981; **51**: 462–464.

25. Anteby SO, Schenker JG, Polishuk WZ. The value of laparoscopy in acute pelvic pain. *Ann Surg* 1975: **181**: 484–486.

26. Cox MR, McCall JL, Wilson TG, Padbury RTA, Jeans PL, Toouli J. Laparoscopic appendicectomy: a prospective analysis. *Aust NZ J Surg* 1993; **63**(11): 840–847.

27. Deutsch AA, Zelikovsky A, Reiss R. Laparoscopy in the prevention of unnecessary appendicectomies: a prospective study. *Br J Surg* 1982; **69**: 336–337.

28. Graham A, Henley C, Mobley J. Laparoscopic evaluation of acute abdominal pain. *J Laparoendosc Surg* 1991; **1**(3): 165–168.

29. Olsen JB, Myren CH, Haahr PE. Randomized study of the value of laparoscopy before appendicectomy. *Br J Surg* 1993; **80**: 922–923.

30. Paterson-Brown S, Thompson JN, Eckersley JRT, Ponting GA, Dudley HAF. Which patient with suspected appendicitis should undergo laparoscopy? *Br Med J* 1988; **296**: 1363–1364.

31. Scott JH, Rosin RD. The influence of diagnostic and therapeutic laparoscopy on patients presenting with an acute abdomen. *J R Soc Med* 1993; **86**(12): 699–701.

32. Spirtos NM, Eisenkop SM, Spirtos TW, Poliakin RI, Hibbard LT. Laparascopy – a diagnostic aid in cases of suspected appendicitis. Its use in women of reproductive age. *Am J Obstet Gynecol* 1987; **156**: 90–94.

33. Whitworth CM, Whitworth PW, Sanfillipo J, Polk HC. Value of diagnostic laparoscopy in young women with possible appendicitis. *Surg Gynecol Obstet* 1988; **167**: 187–190.

34. Pearce JM. Pelvic inflammatory disease: a sexually transmitted disease with potentially serious sequels that is often treated poorly. *Br Med J* 1990; **300**: 1090–1091.

35. Gray DWR, Collin J. Non-specific abdominal pain as a cause of acute admission to hospital. *Br J Surg* 1987; **74**: 239–242.

36. Paterson-Brown S. The acute abdomen – the role of laparoscopy. *Baillières Clinical Gastroenterology* 1991; **5**(3 pt 1): 691–703.

37. Clarke PJ, Hands LJ, Gough MH, Kettlewell MG. The use of laparoscopy in the management of right iliac fossa pain. *Ann R Coll Surg Engl* 1986; **68**: 68–69.

38. Kum CK, Sim EKW, Goh PMY, Ngoi SS, Rauff A. Diagnostic laparoscopy: reducing the number of normal appendicectomies. *Dis Colon Rectum* 1993; **36**: 763–766.

39. Kuster GGR, Gilroy SBC. The role of laparoscopy in the diagnosis of acute appendicitis. *Am Surg* 1992; **58**(10): 627–629.

40. Leape LL, Ramenofsky ML. Laparoscopy for questionable appendicitis – can it reduce the negative appendicectomy rate? *Ann Surg* 1980; **191**: 410–413.

41. Paterson-Brown S, Olufunwa SA, Galazka N, Simmons SC. Visualisation of the normal appendix at laparoscopy. *J R Coll Surg Edinb* 1986; **31**: 106–107.

42. Paterson-Brown S, Eckersley JRT, Sim AJW, Dudley HAF. Laparoscopy as an adjunct to decision-making in the 'acute abdomen'. *Br J Surg* 1986; **73**: 1022–1024.

43. Reiertsen O, Rosseland AR, Hoivik B, Solheim K. Laparoscopy in patients admitted for acute abdominal pain. *Acta Chir Scand* 1985; **151**: 521–524.

44. Sugarbaker PH, Bloom BS, Sanders JH, Wilson RE. Preoperative laparoscopy in diagnosis of acute abdominal pain. *Lancet* 1975; **1**: 442–445.
45. Semm K. Endoscopic appendectomy. *Endosc* 1983; **15**: 59–64.
46. Fleming JS. Laparoscopically directed appendicectomy. *Aust NZ J Obstet Gynaecol* 1985; **25**: 238–240.
47. Schreiber JH. Early experience with laparoscopic appendicectomy in women. *Surg Endosc* 1987; **1**: 211–216.
48. Byrne DS, Bell G, Morrice JJ, Orr G. Technique for laparoscopic appendicectomy. *Br J Surg* 1992; **79**: 574–575.
49. Choy A, McGuinness C, Gajraj H, Bett NJ, Chilvers AS. Low cost laparoscopic appendicectomy. *Min Invas Ther* 1993; **2**: 15–17.
50. Cristalli BG, Izard V, Jacob D, Levardon M. Laparoscopic appendectomy using a clip applier. *Surg Endosc* 1991; **5**(4): 176–178.
51. Gangal HT, Gangal MH. Laparoscopic appendicectomy. *Endosc* 1987; **19**: 127–129.
52. Gotz F, Pier A, Bacher C. Modified laparoscopic appendectomy in surgery: a report of 388 operations. *Surg Endosc* 1990; **4**: 6–9.
53. Ludwig KA, Cattey RP, Henry LG. Initial experience with laparoscopic appendectomy. *Dis Col and Rect* 1993; **36**(5): 463–467.
54. Nowzaradan Y, Westmoreland J, McCarver CT, Harris RJ. Laparoscopic appendectomy for acute appendicitis: indications and current use. *J Laparoendosc Surg* 1991; **1**(5): 247–257.
55. Pier A, Gotz F, Bacher C. Laparoscopic appendectomy in 625 cases: from innovation to routine. *Surg Laparosc Endosc* 1991; **1**: 8–13.
56. Saye WB, Rives DA, Cochran EB. Laparoscopic appendectomy: three years' experience. *Surg Laparosc Endosc* 1991; **1**: 109–115.
57. Valla JS, Limonne B, Valla V, *et al.* Laparoscopic appendectomy in children: report of 465 cases. *Surg Laparosc Endosc* 1991; **1**: 166–172.
58. Attwood SEA, Hill ADK, Murphy PG, Thornton J, Stephens RB. A prospective randomized trial of laparoscopic versus open appendectomy. *Surg* 1992; **112**(3): 497–501.
59. Frazee RC, Roberts JW, Symmonds RE, *et al.* A prospective randomized trial comparing open versus laparoscopic appendectomy. *Ann Surg* 1994; **219**: 725–731.
60. Gilchrist BR, Lobe TE, Schropp KP, *et al.* Is there a role for laparoscopic appendectomy in pediatric surgery? *J Paed Surg* 1992; **27**(2): 209–212.
61. Hill ADK, Attwood SEA, Stephens RB. Laparoscopic appendicectomy is feasible and safe in acute appendicitis. *Ir J Med Sci* 1991; **160**(9): 268–270.
62. Kum CK, Ngoi SS, Goh PMY, Tekant Y, Isaac JR. Randomized controlled trial comparing laparoscopic and open appendicectomy. *Br J Surg* 1993; **80**: 1599–1600.
63. McAnena OJ, Austin O, O'Connell PR, Hederman WP, Gorey TF, Fitzpatrick J. Laparoscopic versus open appendicectomy: a prospective evaluation. *Br J Surg* 1992; **79**: 818–820.
64. Mompean JAL, Campos RR, Paricio PP, Aledo VS, Ayllon JG. Laparoscopic versus open appendicectomy: a prospective assessment. *Br J Surg* 1994; **81**: 133–135.
65. Nowzaradan Y, Barnes JP, Westmoreland J, Hojabri M. Laparoscopic appendectomy: treatment of choice for suspected appendicitis. *Surg Laparosc Endosc* 1993; **3**(5): 411–416.
66. Schrimer BD, Schmieg RE, Dix J, Edge SB, Hanks JB. Laparoscopic versus traditional appendectomy for suspected appendicitis. *Am J Surg* 1993; **165**(6): 670–675.
67. Schroder DM, Lathrop JC, Lloyd LR, Boccaccio JE, Hawasli A. Laparoscopic appendectomy for acute appendicitis: is there really any benefit? *Am Surg* 1993; **59**(8): 541–547.
68. Tate JJT, Chung SC, Dawson J, Leong HT, Chan A, Lau WY, Li AKC. Conventional versus laparoscopic surgery for acute appendicitis. *Br J Surg* 1993; **80**: 761–764.

69. Vallina VL, Velasco JM, McCulloch CS. Laparoscopic versus conventional appendectomy. *Ann Surg* 1993; **218**(5): 685–692.

70. Grunewald B, Keating J. Should the 'normal' appendix be removed at operation for appendicitis? *J R Coll Surg Edinb* 1993; **38**(3): 158–160.

71. Lau WY, Fan ST, Yin TF, Chu KW, Suen HC, Wong KK. The clinical significance of routine histopathological study of the resected appendix and safety of appendiceal inversion. *Surg Gynecol Obstet* 1986; **162**: 256–258.

72. Welch NT, Hinder RA, Fitzgibbons RJ. Laparoscopic incidental appendectomy. *Surg Laparosc Endosc* 1991; **1**(2): 116–118.

73. Seow-Choen F. Randomized study of the value of laparoscopy before appendectomy. *Br J Surg* 1994; **81**: 146.

74. Wheeler RA, Malone PS. Use of the appendix in reconstructive surgery: a case against incidental appendicectomy. *Br J Surg* 1991; **78**: 1283–1285.

75. Semm K, Freys I. Endoscopic appendectomy: technical operative steps. *Min Invas Ther* 1991; **1**: 41–50.

76. Leahy PF. Technique of laparoscopic appendicectomy. *Br J Surg* 1989; **76**: 616.

77. Tate JJT, Chung SCS, Li AKC. Laparoscopic appendicectomy: a two-handed technique. *Br J Surg* 1993; **80**: 764.

78. Engstrom L, Fenyo G. Appendicectomy: assessment of stump invagination versus simple ligation – a prospective, randomized trial. *Br J Surg* 1985; **72**: 971–972.

79. MacFayden BV, Wolfe BM, McKernan JB. Laparoscopic management of the acute abdomen, appendix and small and large bowel. *Surg Clin N Am* 1992; **72**(5): 1169–1183.

80. Paterson-Brown S. Emergency laparoscopic surgery. *Br J Surg* 1993; **80**: 279–283.

81. Banerjee AK. Laparoscopic appendicectomy. *Lancet* 1991; **338**: 893.

82. Loh A, Taylor RS. Laparoscopic appendicectomy. *Br J Surg* 1992; **79**: 289–290.

83. Scott-Conner CE, Hall TJ, Anglin BL, Muakkassa FF. Laparoscopic appendectomy. Initial experience in a teaching program. *Ann Surg* 1992; **215**(6): 660–667.

13a

The lower gastrointestinal tract: colorectal cancer

J.E. Hartley and J.R.T. Monson

Introduction

Basic familiarity with diagnostic and therapeutic laparoscopy has rapidly become a requirement for the abdominal surgeon within Western society. This enthusiasm for minimally invasive techniques stems from the widespread success of laparoscopic cholecystectomy which has rapidly become the treatment of choice for the symptomatic gallbladder.[1] The laparoscopic approach has since been adapted to a wide range of general surgical procedures including herniorrhaphy[2] appendicectomy,[3] Nissen fundoplication[4] and oesophagectomy.[5]

The application of laparoscopic techniques to coloproctology was therefore inevitable with the first reports of laparoscopic approaches to colorectal resection appearing in 1991;[6-9] Cooperman and co-workers describing the laparoscopic assisted removal of a villous adenoma of the ascending colon,[6] followed by Fowler and White's report of the use of a laparoscopic linear stapler to divide the large bowel and mesentery during resection of the sigmoid colon.[8] However, although large numbers of laparoscopic colorectal procedures have been performed worldwide, this application has not developed at the same rate as other areas. Reasons for this include the high degree of laparoscopic skills required, expensive instrumentation and inevitably protracted operating times, but, most significantly, the uncertain oncological safety of this technology.

The relatively uncontrolled introduction of these techniques has occurred in the face of well publicized dissent from the colorectal community. However, large series have been accrued with apparent clinical benefit – particularly in the United States. Thus, although minimally invasive surgical techniques have undoubtedly benefited many patients around the world thanks to smaller incisions and reduced surgical trauma, the case for their use should be considered unproven.[10]

The purpose of this communication is to review the current state of laparoscopic surgery for colorectal cancer in terms of the indications and contra-indications for the approach, the operative principles and technical pitfalls, and the results achieved to date. As is often the case in clinical surgery much of what follows cannot withstand critical scientific appraisal since no randomized controlled trial of this technology has been performed, and indeed it seems to us increasingly unlikely that such a study will ever be completed. However, this chapter is a synthesis of our own experience and the published experience of others which we hope goes some way towards representing a balanced view of this increasingly important field.

Indications and contraindications

In the six years since the inception of minimally invasive colorectal surgery the laparoscopic approach has rapidly been adapted to the whole range of recognized colorectal resections for both benign and malignant disease. However, it is the benign conditions such as diverticular disease and inflammatory bowel disease and non-curative resections for malignancy which have provided the most widely accepted indication for the laparoscopic approach.[11]

Laparoscopy for potentially curable colorectal cancer has yet to be whole-heartedly embraced, and in both the United States and Europe it is widely held that such surgery should not be performed outside of properly controlled clinical studies. However, even if one takes the view that laparoscopy is justifiable under such circumstances, the question remains as to which lesions are suitable. While the occasional colorectal laparoscopist may report favourable experiences with laparoscopic right colonic resections, correspondingly fewer feel that rectal carcinoma ought to be approached in this fashion. There can be little doubt that the low anterior resection for carcinoma represents perhaps the most technically demanding procedure in colorectal surgery, as evidenced by the wide extremes of outcome illustrated in a range of studies.[12,13] One could therefore present an excellent case for the avoidance of laparoscopic rectal cancer surgery until the case for the approach *per se* is conclusively proven. We, however, would suggest that the magnified views obtained deep within the pelvis, may allow for a more accurate pelvic dissection and excision of the intact mesorectum as advocated by Heald and co-workers.[14,15] Given the current body of evidence this constitutes largely a matter of personal preference, and ongoing randomized trials of this intervention for colorectal cancer have remained essentially pragmatic in their recruitment of patients with carcinomas below the pelvic brim.

Laparoscopic resection for cancer is in the early stages of its clinical evaluation so that, other than faecal peritonitis or obstructing carcinoma, specific contra-indications to the approach have not been uniformly accepted. The size of the lesion and inflammatory or neoplastic involvement of adjacent structures in our view represent relative contra-indications to laparoscopic resection. Our philosophy in approaching this form of resection is that principles established at open surgery should not be contravened at laparoscopy. Thus we see little objection in approaching such lesions laparoscopically albeit with a low threshold for conversion in the face of anatomical uncertainty or difficulty in determining the correct plane of dissection. Attempts at pre-operative staging are, nonetheless, appropriate. The choice of imaging modalities depends to a large extent on the facilities available but include pelvic CT,[16] MRI[17] and endoanal USS.[18] The extent to which the use of such imaging pre-operatively influences subsequent conversion rates to formal laparotomy has yet to be determined.

In addition to tumour-related factors and increasing awareness of the pathophysiology, laparoscopy allows some general observations pertinent to case selection. Firstly, a protracted pneumo-peritoneum, with its attendant cardiovascular and respiratory effects, is required. In such patients the decrease in venous return consequent upon the pneumo-peritoneum may lead to a significant reduction in cardiac output.[19] In addition, significant absorption of carbon dioxide is the inevitable consequence of a protracted pneumo-peritoneum and is normally readily dealt with by appropriate increases in the respiratory minute volume, guided by end tidal carbon dioxide measurements.[20] In patients in whom the pulmonary reserve is limited such compensation may not be possible. Under such circumstances accumulation of carbon dioxide may lead to the development of a respiratory acidosis which may in turn provoke cardiac arrhythmias.[19] At present, therefore, avoidance of the laparoscopic approach in those patients with significant cardiorespiratory compromise would appear to be a reasonable precaution. A variety of avenues by which such difficulties might be avoided have been explored; these include gasless laparoscopy incorporating abdominal wall lifting devices which obviate the requirement for a pneumo-peritoneum,[21] and alternative gases, including helium, which avoid the potential acid-base problems associated with carbon dioxide.[22] However, at present there is insufficient evidence to support the widespread usage of these alternatives.

Finally, the technical problems associated with laparoscopy in the grossly obese or those with previous abdominal surgery justifiably influence decision-making and both represent at least relative contraindications to laparoscopy.

Technical considerations ⎯⎯⎯⎯⎯⎯

There are a number of detailed accounts of the individual laparoscopic colorectal resections to which the interested reader is commended.[23–27] The following narrative is therefore limited to discussion of the general principles governing successful laparoscopic surgery.

Pre-operative preparation

The preparation of patients for laparoscopic colorectal resection is in essence identical to that of patients undergoing conventional surgery, with pre-operative bowel preparation, antibiotic and thromboembolic prophylaxis all being undertaken according to those regimens established for open colorectal surgery.

We would add one important proviso; which is that all patients who are to undergo laparoscopic resection should have a pre-operative contrast examination of the colon. This is because colonoscopy may be inaccurate with regard to the

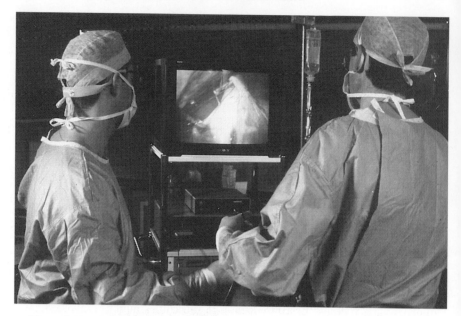

Fig. 13a.1   Full video-laparoscopy facilities are requisite for safe laparoscopic colorectal resection.

anatomical position of lesions within the colon, with for example, the hepatic flexure being frequently mistaken for the caecum.[28] In the absence of serosal involvement the site of the lesion may not be obvious at laparoscopy, so that if undue reliance is placed on the colonoscopy report the wrong segment of colon may be removed,[29] or synchronous lesions may be missed.[30] Indian ink, injected at the base of the lesion at colonoscopy, can clearly be seen at subsequent laparoscopy and may help avoid the former pitfall.

Instrumentation

Full video-laparoscopy facilities are required (Fig. 13a.1), along with a selection of laparoscopic instruments, of which the most important are: Babcock-type bowel grasping instruments, curved disposable endoscopic scissors, and an endoscopic linear stapling device (Fig. 13a.2), used to divide the bowel and mesenteric vessels. In addition laparoscopic ultrasound transducers, while not essential, are used increasingly for assessment of the liver during colorectal surgery (Fig. 13a.3).

Operative principles

The fundamental components of a laparoscopic operation for colorectal cancer are identical to those employed in open colorectal surgery. Under general anaesthesia the patient is placed in a modified Lloyd–Davies position in which the legs are held almost straight (this prevents the legs impinging upon the movements of the

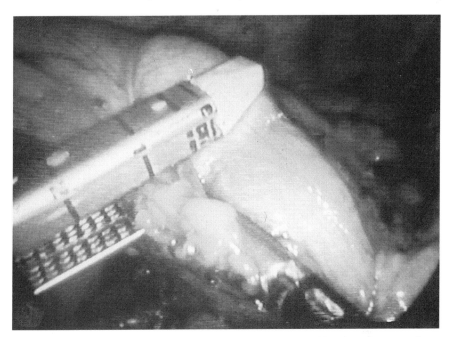

Fig. 13a.2 Endoscopic linear staplers are used to divide either bowel or vascular pedicles.

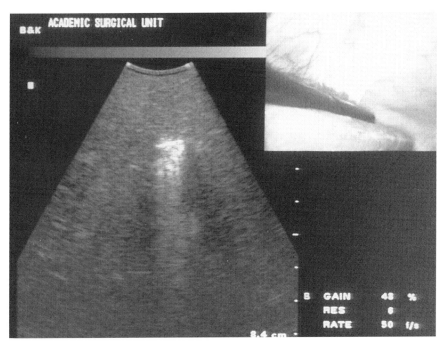

Fig. 13a.3 Laparoscopic ultrasound transducers have been used increasingly for assessment of the liver during minimally colorectal procedures.

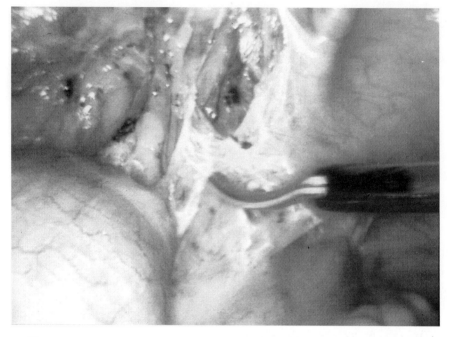

Fig. 13a.4   The colon is progressively mobilized by division of its peritoneal attachments using electrocautery scissors.

long-handled laparoscopic instruments). A urinary catheter and nasogastric tube are mandatory and help guard against trocar injury to the viscera. Carbon dioxide pneumo-peritoneum is achieved in the standard fashion using either a Verres needle or some modification of the Hassan 'open' technique. Most colorectal procedures use 4 or 5 laparoscopy ports, with the camera used via the subumbilical port and further ports in each of the four quadrants of the abdomen.

The principle steps of laparoscopic colorectal resection are identical to those of the corresponding open procedure and comprise: mobilization of the bowel, interruption of its vascular supply, resection of the appropriate segment, and finally restoration of intestinal continuity or formation of a stoma.[27]

The colon is mobilized by a combination of Babcock retraction and division of the peritoneal attachments with electrocautery scissors (Fig. 13a.4). With care and meticulous attention to haemostasis the whole of the colon and rectum can, if necessary, be mobilized in this fashion. Probably the most difficult region to approach in this way is the transverse colon, since the middle colic artery, stomach, and duodenum are all at risk of injury during mobilization of the greater omentum off the colon. The rectum can, if desired, be mobilized with intact mesorectum down to the level of the pelvic floor during either anterior resection or abdominoperineal excision. Indeed, the magnified views obtained at laparoscopy deep within the pelvis (Fig. 13a.5) appear to us to facilitate accurate sharp dissection of the mesorectum as advocated by Heald and co-workers.[15]

The technical difficulty of the procedure is greatly influenced by the bodily

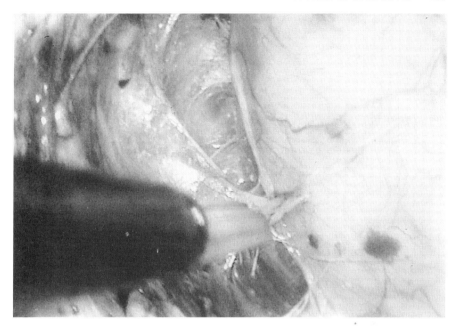

Fig. 13a.5 The magnified views obtained at laparoscopy deep within the pelvis may facilitate sharp dissection of the intact mesorectum.

habitus of the patient, with obesity presenting particular difficulties. In addition the surgeon's orientation at laparoscopy is often particularly influenced by the presence of colonic adhesions, whether congenital or inflammatory. However, perhaps the major factor with which the laparoscopic colonic surgeon must come to terms is the near total reliance on gravity as a means of retraction. Such differences may be particularly acute when dealing with the small bowel since the laparoscopist has no facility to pack away and protect the intestine during extensive dissection. Instead, however, there is a critical angle of Trendelenburg tilt beyond which the small bowel will fall away out of the pelvis and operative field. Any adhesions of small bowel to pelvic structures must therefore be divided at an early stage in the procedure. If the small bowel is not afforded some protection by these means there is the danger of inadvert diathermy injury or enterotomy.

A further major difference consequent upon the laparoscopic approach is the surgeon's reliance on endoscopic instruments. Instrument trauma is a very real concern. At open surgery the surgeon can readily use a hand or swab in order to distract the colon. At laparoscopy Babcock-type instruments must be used. In contrast to a hand or swab these are relatively traumatic and ineffective. In general the more effective the laparoscopic instrument the more traumatic it is likely to be. Since the retracting instruments are out of camera view for protracted periods of time any injury may go unnoticed, with disastrous consequences. It is also clearly important to avoid undue manipulation of the tumour since seeding via instruments to the laparoscopic trocars is one of the putative mechanisms for the phenomenon of port-site metastasis as discussed below. The risks of diathermy injury are also clear[31] and at present the best policy by which such injuries may be avoided lies in constant awareness of the danger. During colorectal surgery the structure at greatest risk from thermal injury is the ureter, particularly on the left side, and excessive diathermy must be avoided until this structure has been identified.

Having mobilized the appropriate segment of colon the vascular supply to the bowel is thereafter best divided intracorporeally using a linear stapler (Fig. 13a.6). The subsequent small incision required for specimen delivery (governed largely by the size of the specimen) can then be sited over the tumour, or the intended site of anastomosis, without consideration for the relative ease or difficulty with which the vascular pedicle may be divided via such access. The mobilized bowel is then delivered (Fig. 13a.7) and resected (Fig. 13a.8). The incision must be of sufficient size to avoid squeezing the tumour, with the risk of spillage of cells, during specimen delivery (Fig. 13a.9). Some authors have advocated the use of specimen bags in order to minimize this risk, but these have not gained widespread favour.

An extracorporeal anastomosis is then performed by either a suture or stapled technique. Intracorporeal anastomosis, by sutured or stapled techniques is technically possible as part of a 'totally-laparoscopic' operation, which obviates the requirement for a significant abdominal incision. However, we remain to be convinced that the extra time and effort required for such an anastomosis is worthwhile. In addition such an approach creates problems with regard to mode of specimen delivery. Although resected specimens can be removed transanally, this requires unphysiological dilatation of the sphincters and, for malignant lesions, there is a theoretical risk of tumour seeding.

Laparoscopic abdominoperineal excision represents the only 'totally-laparoscopic' resection in common practice, since having mobilized the rectum laparoscopically to the pelvic floor the perineal surgeon completes the excision and extracts the specimen via the perineum. The proximal colon is then brought out through the left iliac fossa port site as an end stoma.

Results

The uptake of laparoscopic colorectal surgery, although not nearly as dramatic as that of laparoscopic cholecystectomy, has nevertheless been substantial with over 1000 cases having been reported in over 50 publications, approximately two thirds of these having been for malignant disease. These publications mainly take the form of case series, or of prospective studies in which the results of laparoscopy are compared with those of historical control groups of patients undergoing open surgery. Unfortunately only a handful of these reports concern themselves exclusively with malignant disease,[32] so that useful comment on the value of these techniques in colorectal cancer surgery is difficult. In addition, a voluntary audit of this form of surgery for benign and malignant disease from the United States – the Laparoscopic Bowel Surgery Registry sponsored by the

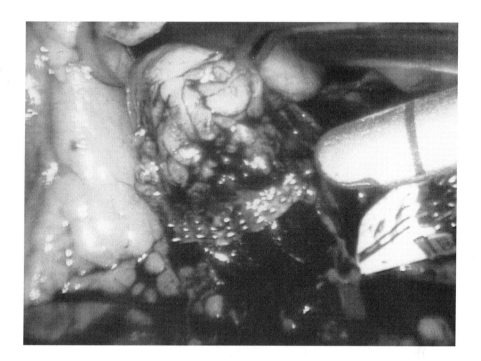

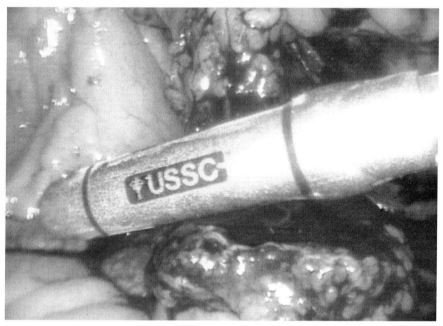

Fig. 13a.6 High ligation of the inferior mesenteric artery during laparoscopic anterior resection using an endoscopic linear stapler (a) about to fire and (b) division completed between rows of staples. These figures are also reproduced in colour between pages 276 and 277.

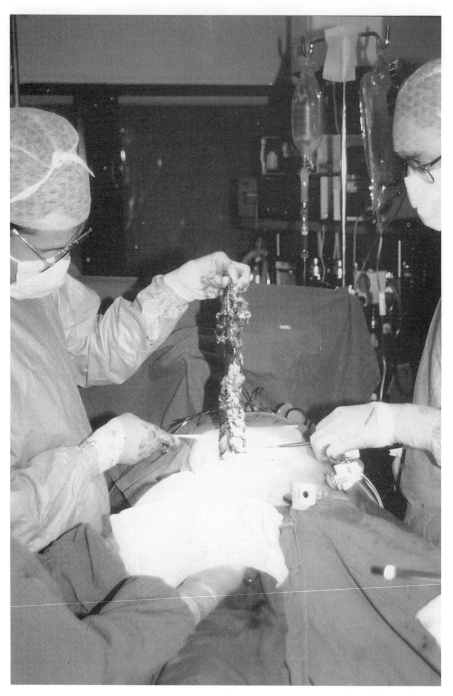

Fig. 13a.7 Specimen delivery during laparoscopic-assisted right hemicolectomy.

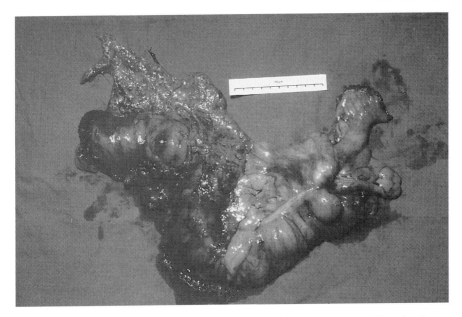

Fig. 13a.8 Comparable specimens can be obtained using laparoscopic-assisted techniques, in this case after right hemicolectomy.

American Society of Colon and Rectal Surgeons, the Society of American Gastrointestinal Endoscopic Surgeons, and the American College of Surgeons Commission on Cancer – has provided useful preliminary data.[33] However, in the absence of data from randomized controlled studies, careful appraisal of the published data, at present, allows only the following general observations to be made regarding this new technology.

Firstly, it is clear that not all patients are suitable for a laparoscopic approach to colonic resection, with the reported rates of conversion to formal laparotomy ranging from 0 to 48 per cent.[11,34,35] Clearly this rate is a reflection of multiple factors including the expertise of the operating team, equipment reliability, and the pressure of time available to complete the list, in addition to those patient-related variables such as obesity and previous surgery, and site, size and extent of tumour. Unfortunately, few studies detail the criteria upon which the decision to undertake laparoscopy was based, or the factors which led to conversion to formal laparotomy. Within our own unit approximately 20 per cent of patients undergoing laparoscopy for colorectal cancer require conversion to formal laparotomy usually because of technical difficulties created by gross obesity, adhesions, or tumour adherence or fixity.[36] As might be anticipated, this requirement for conversion does appear to be reduced as experience with laparoscopy is accrued.

Secondly, laparoscopic colorectal procedures almost invariably take longer than the corresponding open operation. Again this difference does decrease with experience. The increased times are a feature not only of the operation, which in our hands takes approximately one hour longer than the corresponding open

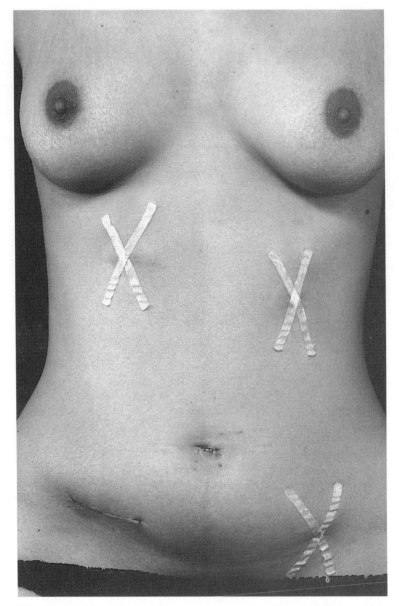

Fig. 13a.9   The abdomen following laparoscopic-assisted right hemicolectomy.

procedure, but also in the setting up, and dismantling, of the requisite equipment. Time factors are clearly an issue which varies in significance with the service commitment of the individual unit. For the busy surgeon the simple factor of limited operating theatre time may mitigate against a laparoscopic approach to colorectal cancer.

Reported figures, from the major series and registry data, for operative morbidity and mortality are comparable to those expected in open surgery.[25,33-35,37-39] However, anecdotal and largely unpublished reports would suggest that major haemorrhage, small bowel enterotomy, ureteral transection, iliac arteriotomy, epigastric vessel lacerations, and pancreatic injury have all occurred.[40] We would strongly contend that most major intra-operative complications are the result of the laparoscopist's persistence in the face of difficulties such that he or she tries to do what they would not attempt during open surgery. Conversely, we feel justified in offering most patients with colorectal cancer a laparoscopic approach with the proviso that early conversion is the response to major difficulties, particularly in definition of the ureter or in mobilization of the tumour. It is far better to admit defeat at laparoscopy than to leave one's patient with positive margins of excision.

On a more positive note, patients undergoing laparoscopic colorectal resection do appear to gain advantage in the post-operative period by virtue of smaller wounds and reduced overall trauma. Reduced pain scores and analgesia requirements, earlier resolution of post-operative ileus, lower rates of wound and chest morbidity, earlier mobilization, reduction in length of hospital stay, and quicker return to normal activity, have been relatively consistent observations.[11,25,33-35] However, such findings have not been entirely uniform, with a smaller number of groups, including our own, specifically reporting no significant difference in post-operative outcome following laparoscopic-assisted colorectal surgery.[36,41] This failure to demonstrate major advantages for laparoscopic-assisted surgery may, in part, be explained by the requirement for an abdominal incision, albeit a smaller one, in order to deliver the resected specimen.

Finally, any procedure resulting in decreased hospital stay and an earlier return to useful activity carries the potential for cost savings. For laparoscopic colorectal surgery these savings must be balanced against increased costs of instrumentation and longer operating times. Studies addressing these issues for laparoscopic colorectal surgery have demonstrated equivalent or reduced total hospital costs for laparoscopic surgery as compared with conventional operations, with savings being attributed to a decrease in the requirement for hospital care.[42]

Safety in malignancy

Colorectal cancer is the only commonly curable visceral malignancy, so that at present approximately 50 per cent of patients presenting with the disease can be treated with the reasonable expectation of cure, of whom 50 per cent again can be expected to be alive 5 years later.[12, 43] Clearly, any new treatment modality in such patients cannot be countenanced unless it is seen at least to match such a survival profile. In the case of the laparoscopic approach to the resection of colorectal cancer we are clearly some years from being able reliably to provide such data, and for the present there are a number of points of controversy which require clarification.

The adequacy of surgical excision at laparoscopy

The perceived wisdom in colorectal cancer surgery has long been that the widest possible excision of the tumour and associated lymphatic tissues should be undertaken. However, there are few conclusive data to support such a policy; for instance no survival advantage can be demonstrated for those patients undergoing a 'high' (and hence wider lymphatic clearance) rather than 'low' ligation of the inferior mesenteric pedicle during anterior resection.[44] For rectal cancer it is apparent that the widest possible radial tumour clearance should be undertaken, since the presence of histologically positive circumferential resection margins is associated with rates of local recurrence in excess of 80 per cent.[45] There are fewer data concerning the relevance of radial tumour clearance for colon as distinct from rectal cancer, though it seems reasonable to anticipate similar recurrence rates.

So how should the adequacy of surgical excision be measured? To date, most reports of laparoscopic and laparoscopic-assisted resections for colorectal cancer have emphasized the equivalent mesenteric and longitudinal margins of excision accomplished at laparoscopy compared, either prospectively or retrospectively, with the same parameters measured following use of conventional surgical techniques.[32,34,35,36,37,46–49]

There are few data reporting radial margins of excision achieved at laparoscopy. However, our own preliminary experiences of the laparoscopic approach to the resection of rectal cancer with total mesorectal excision have suggested that comparable resections are possible, although local recurrence data are awaited.[50] The lymph node yield has also been put forward as a measure of the adequacy of tumour clearance, and again most studies have reported comparable lymph node harvests at laparoscopy and conventional surgery.[32,34,35,36,37,46–49] While such data are reassuring no study has ever shown the absolute number of lymph nodes resected with the specimen to have any influence on disease recurrence and survival. In addition such figures must be interpreted with the utmost caution since widespread variation in lymph node yields has been demonstrated both within and between institutions;[51] the techniques of pathological examination also has a bearing, with the use of fat clearance techniques significantly increasing the likelihood of patients being ascribed to a Dukes C staging.

Rectal cancer surgery

We have already alluded to the reservations expressed by perhaps the majority of colorectal surgeons with regard to the suitability of rectal carcinoma to laparoscopic resection. In addition to concerns about the ability of the laparoscopist to undertake an excision of the intact mesorectum as advocated by Heald and co-workers,[15] other specialist observers have pointed to the relatively high proportion of patients undergoing laparoscopic surgery for rectal cancer who in fact proceeded to abdominoperineal resection.[52] This observation may simply be the result of case-mix factors, but it has led to fears that avoidable sphincter sacrifice may be a consequence of laparoscopic surgery for rectal cancer, where ordinarily in the best hands one would anticipate an abdominoperineal resection rate in the region of 5–10 per cent.

In our view the decision as to whether to submit the patient to laparoscopic abdominoperineal resection or to a sphincter saving procedure must be made pre-operatively. Abdominoperineal resection must be reserved for those patients presenting with lesions less than 4–5 cm from the anal verge. During conventional open surgery it is common practice to make the final decision after a trial pelvic dissection, and to counsel the patient pre-operatively. There is no such facility at laparoscopic abdominoperineal resection where in the vast majority of cases, if these strict selection criteria are applied, the abdominal surgeon will not visualize the tumour. Both surgeon and patient must therefore be certain of the intended resection pre-operatively. We would certainly contend that laparoscopic abdomi-noperineal excision in our own hands constitutes a worthwhile minimally inva-sive procedure since there is no requirement for a significant abdominal incision.[53]

Staging issues

The ability of the surgeon to stage colorectal cancer accurately at laparoscopy has also been questioned. Clearly, much tactile information is lost at laparoscopy and this may create difficulties in the assessment of lymphatic involvement and tumour adherence to, or invasion of, adjacent structures. In addition, and by the same reasoning, liver involvement might feasibly be underestimated at laparo-scopy in the absence of obvious surface metastases. Understaging may result in patients being denied appropriate additional treatment, and also cause problems in clinical trials of adjuvant therapy since such understaged patients would receive adjuvant therapy inappropriately. Modern pre-operative imaging such as CT, MRI and extracorporeal and transrectal ultrasound certainly has a role to play in the assessment of patients prior to laparoscopic colorectal surgery. Such imaging modalities may be of use in assessing the suitability of individual patients for a laparoscopic approach – a role which is currently under investiga-tion in a number of centres. Thus patients with locally advanced disease which may not be detected clinically could be spared a lengthy, and ultimately doomed, preliminary laparoscopy or, if appropriate, be referred for pre-operative radio-therapy or combination therapy.

Alternatively one can envisage a scenario in which all patients would undergo laparoscopy as a staging procedure which would utilize laparoscopic ultrasono-graphy to assess the primary lesion, to search for synchronous colonic pathology, and assess the liver for metastatic disease. The latter indication would seem to us to be the logical extension of advances in laparoscopic and ultrasound technology, given the widespread use of conventional ultrasound for the detection of hepatic metastases during conventional colorectal resection.[54] Recent work within our own unit has shown laparoscopic ultrasound to be as effective as MRI for this indication, although further follow-up is needed to determine the 'false negative' rate of the two modalities.[55]

Port site and wound recurrence

The appearance of isolated reports of abdominal wall recurrence following laparoscopy for cancer has led to speculation that the pattern of disease recurrence may be altered by laparoscopy since wound recurrence after open surgery has long been held to be uncommon, with an incidence of less than 1 per cent.[56] Although these reports are alarming the true extent of this problem remains unclear since few of the major series appear to acknowledge such complications. A recent report from the American Society of Colon and Rectal Surgeons National Register documented only four cases of port site recurrence in some 200 laparoscopic colorectal procedures for neoplasia. All such events were associated with widespread recurrent disease in patients with advanced primary lesions.[57] Nevertheless, over 30 cases of port site recurrence following laparoscopic resection of colorectal cancer have appeared in the world literature,[58,59] with a smaller number occurring after removal of Dukes A lesions.[60,61] The mechanism of this phenomenon is at present unclear, though a number of mechanisms specific to laparoscopy have been postulated. Firstly, repeated passes of laparoscopic instruments through the port may bring exfoliated cancer cells into contact with the trocar wound. The adherence of tumour cells to surgical instrumentation has been well documented,[62] as has the detection of circulating and intraperitoneal malignant cells during colorectal cancer surgery,[63,64] and it has been suggested that an element of local ischaemia at the trocar site may facilitate tumour cell implantation under these circumstances. Secondly, inappropriate manipulation of the tumour – which would not be countenanced at open surgery – may be a feature of laparoscopic resections thanks to the inevitable loss of tactile information, and result in increased shedding of tumour cells. Finally, a high pressure pneumoperitoneum may in some way enhance dissemination and survival of malignant cells. Recent work has identified clumps of whole cells in electrocoagulation smoke produced at laparoscopy,[65] and as gas escapes under high pressure it is possible that such cells may be seeded into the wound. Thus far, however, none of these suggested mechanisms has been substantiated.

Tantalizing clues as to the mechanism of wound recurrence following laparoscopic surgery have recently emerged. A number of animal studies have demonstrated preservation of the systemic immune response after laparoscopy in comparison with laparotomy.[66–68] Such studies have been extended to illustrate a permissive effect on tumour growth following laparotomy when compared to laparoscopy, with this being ascribed to the relatively increased immunosuppression which follows the former intervention.[69–71] Recent studies have also demonstrated that the intraperitoneal as well as the systemic cytokine response to surgery is differentially preserved after laparoscopy compared with laparotomy,[72] and that neutrophil function is also relatively spared.[68] Despite this evidence which would suggest that the laparoscopy may confer benefits in preservation of the immune response, similar models have also suggested increases in wound implantation of tumour cells following laparoscopy.[73,74]

Further work is clearly required, both to determine the true significance of this problem and also to elucidate the mechanism. In the meantime, however, measures designed to reduce the likelihood of tumour cell implantation at the abdominal wall would seem prudent. Such measures include avoidance of manipulation of the tumour with relatively traumatic endoscopic instruments since malignant cells may be dislodged, dispersed and thereafter perhaps implanted at the abdominal wall. The specimen extraction site should also be large enough to deliver the resected colon without undue force and a plastic shield to protect the extraction site may be of value.

Disease recurrence and survival

The true assessment of the safety of laparoscopic techniques in neoplasia will only come from long-term follow-up of patients operated upon using such techniques. Thus far, few data on this issue have been published. The Norfolk surgical group have presented the only 24-month follow-up data thus far published in which of 39 patients the cancer specific mortality at 24 months was 6 per cent, with an overall recurrence of 9 per cent. Importantly, no wound or port-site metastases were detected. The actuarial 3-year survival for this same group of patients was 92 per cent for node negative, and 79 per cent for node positive patients.[75] Although the number of patients presented was small, such survival and recurrence profiles are similar to those which would be anticipated following open surgery, with no unusual pattern of loco-regional recurrence being identified.

Conclusions

For the last five years the colon and rectum have provided an exciting field for innovations in laparoscopic surgery. Laparoscopic colorectal procedures are technically demanding and require expensive instrumentation and protracted operating times. These factors alone may conspire to ensure that such procedures remain beyond the remit of most practising coloproctologists for the foreseeable future. However, in skilled hands, and in carefully selected patients, there seems little doubt that these procedures can be performed safely and with the potential for clinical advantage for the post-operative patient. It is also apparent that in the best hands, colorectal cancer can be reliably excised in a fashion that seems, in the absence of long-term survival data, comparable to that which can be achieved at open surgery. Taken in its broadest context, however, minimally invasive colorectal surgery must be considered an experimental technology whose indications, efficacy, and oncological safety remain unproven.

The real test of the safety of laparoscopic surgery in neoplasia will lie in reliable comparison of local recurrence and survival through properly controlled randomized comparisons with open resection. It is incumbent upon the colorectal community to be clear on these issues before proceeding with the development of these techniques. A number of prospective randomized trials of laparoscopic colorectal cancer surgery are currently underway around the world. However, it remains to be seen whether the surgical profession will demonstrate the collective will to see these trials through to completion. Lessons from the past in this respect bear little encouragement since, as is frequently acknowledged, no major surgical advance has ever been proven in this manner. Nevertheless, until these ongoing studies have reported, or until good prospective follow-up data on survival are

210   *The lower gastrointestinal tract: colorectal cancer*

available, the widespread use of laparoscopic techniques for colorectal malignancy cannot be endorsed.

References

1. Dubois F. Laparoscopic cholecystectomy: historical perspective and personal experience. *Surg Laparosc Endosc* 1991; **1**: 52–57.
2. Nyhus LM. Laparoscopic hernia repair: a point of view. *Arch Surg* 1992; **127**: 137.
3. Attwood S, Hill A, Murphy P, Thornton J, Stephens R. A prospective randomised trial of laparoscopic versus open appendicectomy. *Surg* 1992; **112**: 497–501.
4. Cuschieri A, Shimi S, Nathanson LK. Laparoscopic reduction, crural repair, and fundoplication of large hiatal-hernia. *Am J Surg* 1992; **163**: 425–430.
5. Hill ADK, Darzi A, Monson JRT. Thoracoscopic esophagectomy: Minimally invasive direct-vision esophageal mobilisation for cancer. In: Steichen FM, Welter R (eds) *Minimally Invasive Surgery and New Technology*. Quality Medical Publishing, St Louis, Missouri, 1994; 547–549.
6. Cooperman AM, Katz V, Zimmon D, Botero G. Laparoscopic colon resection: a case report. *J Laparoendosc Surg* 1991; **1**: 221–224.
7. Saclarides TJ, Ko ST, Airan M, Dillon C, Franklin J. Laparoscopic removal of a large colonic lipoma. Report of a case. *Dis Colon Rectum* 1991; **34**: 1027–1029.
8. Fowler DL, White SA. Laparoscopy-assisted sigmoid resection. *Surg Laparosc Endosc* 1991; **1**: 183–188.
9. Schlinkert RT. Laparoscopic-assisted right hemicolectomy. *Dis Colon Rectum* 1991; **34**: 1030–1031.
10. American Society of Colon and Rectal Surgeons. Policy Statement on Laparoscopic Colectomy. *Dis Colon Rectum* 1994; **37**(6).
11. Monson JRT, Hill ADK, Darzi A. Laparoscopic colonic surgery. *Br J Surg* 1995; **82**: 150–157.
12. Phillips R, Hittinger R, Blesovsky L, Fry J, Fielding L. Local recurrence following 'curative' surgery for large bowel cancer: I. The overall picture. *Br J Surg* 1984; **71**: 12–16.
13. Phillips RKS, Hittinger R, Blesovsky L, Fry JS, Fielding LP. Local recurrence following curative surgery for large bowel cancer: II. The rectum and sigmoid. *Br J Surg* 1984; **71**: 17–20.
14. Heald RJ, Husband EM, Ryall RDH. The mesorectum in rectal cancer surgery – the clue to pelvic recurrence? *Br J Surg* 1982; **69**: 613–616.
15. Heald RJ, Ryall RDH. Recurrence and survival after total mesorectal excision for rectal cancer. *Lancet* 1986; **i**: 1479–1482.
16. Freeny PC, Marks WM, Ryan JA, Bolen JW. Colorectal carcinoma evaluation with CT: preoperative staging and detection of postoperative recurrence. *Radiology* 1986; **158**: 347–353.
17. Balzarini L, Ceglia E, D'Ippolito G, Petrillo R, Tess JD, Musuneci R. Local recurrence of rectosigmoid cancer: what about the choice of MRI for diagnosis? *Gastrointest Radiol* 1990; **15**: 338–342.
18. Beynon J, Mortensen NJMcC, Foy DM, Channer JL, Rigby H, Virjee J. The detection and evaluation of locally recurrent rectal cancer with rectal endosonography. *Dis Colon Rectum* 1989; **32**: 509–517.
19. Safran DB, Orlando R. Physiologic effects of pneumoperitoneum. *Am J Surg* 1994; **167**: 281–286.
20. McMahon AJ, Baxter JN, Kenny G, O'Dwyer PJ. Ventilatory and blood gas changes during laparoscopic and open cholecystectomy. *Br J Surg* 1993; **80**: 1252–1254.
21. Tsoi EKM, Smith RS, Fry WR, Henderson VJ, Organ CH. Laparoscopic sur-

gery without pneumoperitoneum: a preliminary report. *Surg Endosc* 1994; **8**: 382–383.

22. McMahon AJ, Baxter JN, Murray W, Imrie CW, Kenny G, O'Dwyer PJ. Helium pneumoperitoneum for laparoscopic cholecystectomy: ventilatory and blood gas changes. *Br J Surg* 1994; **81**: 1033–1036.

23. Darzi A, Hill ADK, Henry MM, Guillou PJ, Monson JRT. Laparoscopic assisted surgery of the colon. Operative technique. *End Surg* 1993; **1**: 13–15.

24. Jager RM. Laparoscopic right hemicolectomy in left lateral decubitus position. *Surg Laparosc Endosc* 1994; **4**: 348–352.

25. Phillips E, Franklin M, Carroll B, Fallas M, Ramos R, Rosenthal D. Laparoscopic colectomy. *Ann Surg* 1992; **216**: 703–707.

26. Elftmann TD, Nelson H, Ota DM, Pemberton JH, Beart RW. Laparoscopic-assisted segmental colectomy: Surgical techniques. *Mayo Clin Proc* 1994; **69**: 825–833.

27. Monson JRT, Darzi A. *Laparoscopic colorectal surgery*. Isis Medical Media, Oxford, 1995.

28. Cotton PB, Williams CB. *Practical Gastrointestinal Endoscopy*. Blackwell Scientific Publications, Oxford, 1990.

29. Hill ADK, Banwell PB, Darzi A. Laparoscopic colonic surgery: the unseen lesion. *Minim Invas Ther* 1993; **1**. 13–15.

30. McDermott JP, Devereaux DA, Caushaj PF. Pitfall of laparoscopic colectomy. *Dis Colon Rectum* 1994; **37**: 602–603.

31. McMahon AJ, Baxter JN, O'Dwyer PJ. Preventing complications of laparoscopy. *Br J Surg* 1993; **80**: 1593–1594.

32. Guillou P, Darzi A, Monson J. Experience with laparoscopic colorectal surgery for malignant disease. *Surg Oncol* 1993; **2** Suppl. 1: 43–49.

33. Ortega AE, Beart RW, Steele GD, Winchester DP, Greene FL. Laparoscopic bowel surgery registry – preliminary results. *Dis Colon Rectum* 1995; **38**: 681–686.

34. Monson J, Darzi A, Carey P, Guillou P.

Prospective evaluation of laparoscopic-assisted colectomy in an unselected group of patients. *Lancet* 1992; **340**: 831–833.

35. Hoffman G, Baker J, Fitchett C, Vansant J. Laparoscopic-assisted colectomy. Initial experience. *Ann Surg* 1994; **219**: 732–743.

36. Hartley JE, Qureshi A, Duthie GS, Lee PWR, Monson JRT. Laparoscopic surgery for colorectal cancer – a test of the surgeon not the equipment. *Br J Surg* 1995; **82**: 693 (Abstract).

37. Falk P, Beart R, Wexner S, *et al.* Laparoscopic colectomy: a critical appraisal. *Dis Colon Rectum* 1993; **36**: 28–34.

38. Milsom JW, Lavery IC, Church JM, Stolfi VM, Fazio VW. Use of laparoscopic techniques in colorectal surgery – Preliminary study. *Dis Colon Rectum* 1994; **37**: 215–217.

39. Van Ye TM, Cattey RP, Henry LG. Laparoscopically assisted colon resections compare favourably with open technique. *Surg Laparosc Endosc* 1994; **4**: 25–31.

40. Monson JRT, Guillou PJ. Complications of laparoscopic surgery for cancer and their avoidance. *Surg Oncol Clin N Am* 1994; **3**: 745–759.

41. Wexner S, Cohen S, Johansen O, Nogueras J, Jagelman D. Laparoscopic colorectal surgery: a prospective assessment and current perspective. *Br J Surg* 1993; **80**: 1602–1605.

42. Musser DJ, Boorse RC, Madera F, Reed III JF. Laparoscopic colectomy: At what cost? *Surg Laparosc Endosc* 1994; **4**: 1–5.

43. McArdle CS, Hole D, Hansell D, Blumgart LH, Wood CB. Prospective study of colorectal cancer in the West of Scotland: 10-year follow-up. *Br J Surg* 1990; **77**: 280–282.

44. Surtees P, Ritchie JK, Phillips RKS. High versus low ligation of the inferior mesenteric artery in rectal-cancer. *Br J Surg* 1990; **77**: 618–621.

45. Quirke P, Durdey P, Dixon M, Williams N. Local recurrence of rectal adenocarcinoma due to inadequate surgical resection. *Lancet* 1986; **8514**: 996–999.

46. Franlin ME, Rosenthal D, Norem RF. Prospective evaluation of laparoscopic colon resection versus open colon resection for adenocarcinoma. *Surg Endosc* 1995; **9**: 811–816.

47. Tucker JG, Ambroze WL, Orangio GR, Duncan TD, Mason EM, Lucas GW. Laparoscopically-assisted bowel surgery. Analysis of 114 cases. *Surg Endosc* 1995; **9**: 297–300.

48. Scott HJ, Spencer J. Colectomy: The role of laparoscopy. *Surg Laparosc Endosc* 1995; **5**: 382–386.

49. Tate JJT, Kwok S, Dawson JW, Lau WY, Li AKC. Prospective comparison of laparoscopic and conventional anterior-resection. *Br J Surg* 1993; **80**: 1396–1398.

50. Hartley JE, Qureshi A, Farouk R, Duthie GS, Lee PWR, Monson JRT. Total mesorectal excision – assessment of the laparoscopic approach. *Br J Surg* 1996; **83**: 694 (Abstract).

51. Blenkinsopp WK, Stewart-Brown S, Blesovsky L, Kearney G, Fielding LP. Histopathology reporting in large bowel cancer. *J Clin Path* 1981; **34**: 509–513.

52. O'Rourke N, Heald R. Laparoscopic surgery for colorectal-cancer. *Br J Surg* 1993; **80**: 1229–1230.

53. Darzi A, Lewis C, Menzies-Gow N, Guillou PJ, Monson JRT. Laparoscopic Abdominoperineal Excision of the Rectum. *Surg Endosc* 1995; **9**(4): 414–417.

54. Stone MD, Kane R, Bothe A, Jessup M, Cady B, Steele GD. Intraoperative ultrasound imaging of the liver at the time of colorectal cancer resection. *Arch Surg* 1994; **129**: 431–436.

55. Hartley JE, Gunn JM, Avery GS, Farouk R, Duthie GS, Monson JRT. Laparoscopic ultrasonography for the detection of hepatic metastases during laparoscopic surgery for colorectal cancer. *Br J Canc* 1995; **72** (Suppl xxv): 38 (abstract).

56. Hughes ES, McDermott FT, Polglase AI, Johnson WR. Tumour recurrence in the abdominal scar after large bowel cancer surgery. *Dis Colon Rectum* 1983; **26**: 571–572.

57. Ramos JM, Gupta S, Anthone GJ, Ortega AE, Simons AI, Beart RW. Laparoscopy and colon cancer: is the port-site at risk? *Arch Surg* 1994; **129**: 897–899.

58. Wexner SD, Cohen SM. Port site metastases after laparoscopic colorectal surgery for cure of malignancy. *Br J Surg* 1995; **82**: 295–298.

59. Nduka CC, Monson JRT, Menzies-Gow N, Darzi A. Abdominal wall metastases following laparoscopy. *Br J Surg* 1994; **81**: 648–652.

60. Lauroy J, Champault G, Risk N, Boutelier P. Metastatic recurrence at the cannula site: should digestive carcinomas still be managed by laparoscopy? *Br J Surg* 1994; **81** (suppl): 31 (Abstract).

61. Prasad A, Avery C, Foley RJE. Abdominal wall metastases following laparoscopy. *Br J Surg* 1994; **81**: 1697.

62. Gertsch P, Baer HU, Kraft R, Maddern GJ, Altermatt HJ. Malignant cells are collected on circular staplers. *Dis Colon Rectum* 1992; **35**: 238–241.

63. Leather AJM, Gallegos NC, Kocjan G, *et al*. Detection and enumeration of circulating tumour cells in colorectal-cancer. *Br J Surg* 1993; **80**: 777–780.

64. Ambrose NS, MacDonald F, Young J, Thompson H, Keighley MRB. Monoclonal antibody and cytological detection of free malignant cells in the peritoneal cavity during resection of colorectal-cancer – can monoclonal antibodies do better? *Eur J Surg Oncol* 1989; **15**: 99–102.

65. Taffinder NJ, Champault G. Port site metastases after laparoscopic colorectal surgery for cure of malignancy. *Br J Surg* 1996; **83**: 133.

66. Trokel MJ, Bessler M, Treat MR, Whelan RL, Nowygrad R. Preservation of immune response after laparoscopy. *Surg Endosc* 1994; **8**: 1385–1388.

67. Bessler M, Whelan RL, Halverson A, Treat MR, Nowygrad R. Is immune function better preserved after laparoscopic versus open colon resection? *Surg Endosc* 1994; **8**: 881–883.

68. Carey PD, Wakefield CH, Thayeb A, Monson JRT, Darzi A, Guillou PJ. Effects of minimally invasive surgery on hypocholorous acid production by neutrophils. *Br J Surg* 1994; **81**: 557–560.

69. Allendorf JDF, Bessler M, Kayton ML, *et al*. Increased tumor establishment and growth after laparotomy vs laparoscopy in a murine model. *Arch Surg* 1995; **130**: 649–653.

70. Allendorf JDF, Bessler M, Kayton ML, Whelan RL, Treat MR, Nowygrod R. Tumor growth after laparotomy or laparoscopy. *Surg Endosc* 1995; **9**: 49–52.

71. Da Costa ML, Flynn M, Redmond HP, Bouchier-Hayes D. Tumour growth is differentially accelerated by laparotomy and laparoscopy. *Br J Surg* 1995; **82**: 1554 (Abstract).

72. Nduka CC, Dye JF, Yong L, Mansfield AO, Darzi AW. CD11b expression in response to cancer cells spilled at laparotomy and laparoscopy. *Br J Surg* 1996; **83**: 1641 (Abstract).

73. Mathew G, Watson DI, Rofe AM, Baigrie CF, Ellis T, Jamieson GG. Wound metastases following laparoscopic and open surgery for abdominal cancer in a rat model. *Br J Surg* 1996; **83**: 1087–1090.

74. Dorrance HR, Oein K, O'Dwyer PJ. Laparoscopy promotes intraperitoneal tumour growth in an animal model. *Br J Surg* 1996; **83**: 1629 (Abstract).

75. Hoffman GC, Baker JW, Bradford Doxey J, Wilkens Hubbard G, Kirkland Ruffin W, Wishner JA. Minimally invasive surgery for colorectal cancer. Initial follow up. *Ann Surg* 1996; **6**: 790–798.

13b

The lower gastrointestinal tract: inflammatory bowel disease

S.D. Wexner, A.J.N. Iroatulam and G.H. Barsoum

Introduction

The success of laparoscopic cholecystectomy has kindled much interest in other types of laparoscopic abdominal surgery. Many enthusiasts have tried to reproduce the advantages reported in cholecystectomy. In some cases results have been similar while in others the advantages have not been achieved. There are several reasons for this problem. (Table 13b.1).

Firstly, the colon is a multiquadrant organ and therefore a colorectal procedure may involve dissection in several quadrants. This feature is in contrast with other

Table 13b.1 Differences between resectional laparoscopic colorectal surgery and other laparoscopic procedures

		Colon	**Gallbladder**	**Appendix**
Anatomy	Quadrants	Multiple	Single	Single
	Vascularization	Multiple	Single	Single
Procedures	Vascular ligation	Complex and cumbersome	Rapid	Rapid
	Resection	Variable	Consistent	Consistent
	Anastomosis	Required	Not required	Not required
	Specimen	Large (requires enlargement of port site for extirpation)	Small (can be retrieved from normal port)	Small (can be retrieved from normal port)

procedures in which the end organ (gallbladder or appendix) or defect (inguinal or diaphragmatic hernia) is confined to only one anatomic site. Access to various quadrants may require repositioning of monitors, instruments, personnel and the patient. Colonic vascular anatomy includes numerous large vessels in a fat encased mesentery. Vascular isolation and ligation may be cumbersome, especially in the presence of inflammation. The gallbladder and appendix each have only one artery which is easily and rapidly identified, isolated and quickly and inexpensively ligated. After a successful extirpation of the gallbladder or appendix, the procedure concludes. However, laparoscopic bowel surgery involves intestinal resection and restoration of continuity. Laparoscopic fashioning of a leak-free, well-vascularized and tension-free anastomosis requires a technical prowess which can only mature after a series of procedures. Colonic specimens are usually large and their retrieval normally requires either elongation of a port site or creation of a new incision on the abdominal wall. Conversely, the gallbladder and appendix are usually easily retrievable through 10–12 mm port sites and after repair of an inguinal or diaphragmatic hernia, no specimen needs removal. Lastly, whereas other laparoscopic surgery is generally undertaken for benign diseases, the primary indication for colorectal resection is malignancy. Therefore, while success of the former group of operations can be judged by short-term outcome, in the latter scenario long-term survival and recurrence rates are the crucial points. As yet such data are unavailable. The patient labelled in the short term as a 'success' may have a short-term morbidity-free hospital stay at a low cost with minimal disability. However, if that patient has an unexpected tumour recurrence or decreased survival the term 'failure' is more appropriate.

The application of laparoscopic technique in treating inflammatory bowel diseases was not heralded with enthusiasm because of the fragility of the inflamed intestinal tissues, thickened mesentery and presence of dense adhesions which are normally encountered in these patients during conventional open surgery.[1] However, since Peters[2] reported the results of laparoscopic proctocolectomy performed for mucosal ulcerative colitis in 1992, other series have been reported (Table 13b.2). Thibault et al.[3] reported a series of four laparoscopic-assisted total colectomies, three of which were performed for colonic Crohn's disease and one for mucosal ulcerative colitis. Liu et al.[1] reported a series of ten procedures, five of which were for Crohn's disease and the other five for mucosal ulcerative colitis. Milsom et al.[4] reported nine procedures, Bauer et al.[5] reported 18, Kreissler-Haag et al.[6] reported 20 and Ludwig et al.[7] reported 31 procedures all of which were performed for Crohn's disease. In their series, Reissman et al.[8] reported 49 procedures performed for Crohn's disease and 23 performed for mucosal ulcerative colitis. A thorough evaluation of these results demonstrates the feasibility of laparoscopic intestinal surgery for inflammatory bowel diseases.

For these reasons, we have chosen to focus upon the application of laparoscopic techniques for palliation of malignancy and for cure of benign disorders. Our practice includes a high volume of inflammatory bowel diseases allowing us to apply the techniques in these situations. Table 13b.3 shows the relative frequency of surgical indications and procedures laparoscopically performed in our department in the last five years.

Table 13b.2 Laparoscopic-assisted intestinal surgery for inflammatory bowel diseases reported in the literature

Authors	Crohn's disease (Number of patients)	Mucosal ulcerative colitis (Number of patients)
Peters[2]	–	2
Thibault *et al.*[3]	3	1
Liu *et al.*[1]	5	5
Milson *et al.*[4]	9	–
Bauer *et al.*[5]	18	–
Kreissler-Haag *et al.*[6]	20	–
Ludwig *et al.*[7]	31	–
Reissman *et al.*[8]	49	23

Table 13b.3 Laparoscopic procedures performed at Cleveland Clinic Florida for Benign Diseases through 1996

Procedures	
Segmental resection of colon or small bowel	84
Total abdominal colectomy	38
with ileonal reservoir	28
with ileorectal anastomosis	8
with end ileostomy	2
Total proctocolectomy	1
Diverting stoma procedures	41
Abdominoperineal resection of rectum	8
Adhesiolysis	8
Low anterior resection	5
Rectopexy	4
Hartmann's procedure or reversal	15

Pre-operative preparation

All patients should be given an accurate informed consent of the intended procedure, including conversion to laparotomy, if necessary. Consent is always obtained for stoma creation in all patients with inflammatory bowel disease regardless of expected operative findings. The stoma therapist selects the ileostomy site in the pre-operative period. If the patient has an iliac fossa phlegmon noted either during physical examination or by radiographic tests, then intra-operative ureteric catheters are scheduled to be placed by the urologist after the induction of anaesthesia. This decision should be explained to the patient and is the same if a laparotomy is planned instead of laparoscopy. All patients are advised to refrain from the use of aspirin or aspirin-containing compounds for at least 14 days before surgery.

Pre-operatively, the patient is completely evaluated. A colonoscopic study with biopsies and a small bowel series are mandatory to assess the nature and extent of the disease. Anal manometry is performed to document the condition of the sphincters in patients who are candidates for colectomy with ileoanal or ileorectal anastomosis. A variety of techniques of manometry are available and have been described elsewhere.[9-12]

General medical investigations _____

The majority of patients with inflammatory bowel diseases who are undergoing surgery have recently received doses of corticosteroids and immunosuppressive medications. It is therefore desirable to have a full pre-operative medical evaluation to exclude any complication consequent to these medications which could adversely affect the outcome of surgery. A careful history, physical examination and review of prior and present medical problems is crucial. Routine pre-operative investigation includes a complete blood count, serum electrolytes, albumin, calcium, magnesium, creatinine and blood serum urea and nitrogen, thrombin time and partial thromboplastin time, urine analysis, chest X-rays and electrocardiogram. A CT scan may be a useful adjunct if suspicion of a phlegmon or abscess exists. A small bowel series should be done to exclude Crohn's disease in patients labelled as having mucosal ulcerative colitis who are planning a restorative proctocolectomy. In patients with a history of Crohn's disease, a small bowel series should be undertaken to assess the extent of disease. However, even a well-planned enteroclysis may still fail to identify proximal strictures which can be found and treated by strictureplasty or resection during the laparoscopic procedure.

Bowel preparation consists of 45 cc of oral phosphosoda (C.B. Fleet Co., Lynchburg, VA) at 6 p.m. and a second dose at midnight, the night prior to surgery.[13-15] In addition, at 1 p.m., 2 p.m., and 10 p.m. the night prior to surgery, the patient is given 1 g each of metronidazole and neomycin;[16] patients are kept *nil per os* after midnight. Two grams of cefotaxine and 1 g of metronidazole are administered on call to the operating room. Five thousand units of heparin may be subcutaneously administered and steroids are given if necessary prior to the onset of surgery. The usual stress dose of steroids is 100 mg of hydrocortisone sodium succinate.

The patient is positioned on the operating table in a modified lithotomy position with the legs in Allen stirrups (Allen Medical, Bedford Heights, OH).[15] This position allows more flexibility for positioning of the surgical personnel and equipment (Fig. 13b.1). All patients require indwelling bladder catheters and gastric decompression prior to the establishment of pneumoperitoneum. Deep venous thrombosis prophylaxis should also be undertaken with pneumatic sequential compression stockings. If ureteric stents are required, they should be placed after induction of anaesthesia but before the incision is made. The nasogastric tube is removed before the patient is transferred to the recovery room. It is reinserted post-operatively only if the patient vomits more than 200 cc more than twice within any 24-hour period.

The abdomen is prepared and draped as for a laparotomy, exposing from the

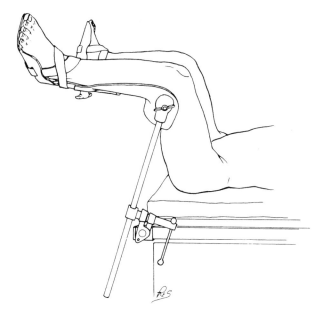

Fig. 13b.1   Lithotomy position with legs in Allen stirrups (Allen Medical, Bedford
Heights, OH).

pubis to the xiphoid and from one anterior superior iliac spine to the other. The
patient is then placed in steep Trendelenburg position and a 1 cm vertical incision
is made. The position of this incision will be dictated by the surgical indication
(Table 13b.4). For ileocolic resections, total proctocolectomies, small bowel resections, or strictureplasties, the midline infraumbilical position is selected. For
stoma creation a midline position midway between the xiphoid and the umbilicus
is utilized. For ileoproctostomy after total abdominal colectomy the stoma is
mobilized first and then the mid-epigastric position is employed under direct
intraperitoneal visualization. For small bowel obstruction secondary to suspected
adhesion, the Hasson technique is preferred. Furthermore, if a prior laparotomy
has been done, the Hasson technique or Verres needle through an alternate site
are safe alternatives. The Verres needle is then inserted through the incision into
the peritoneal cavity; an audible and palpable 'click' should be appreciated.
Furthermore, the free flow of sterile water or saline confirms the correct placement of the Verres needle. Failure to obtain free-flow indicates incorrect position
of the tip of the needle. Insufflation should not begin until proper needle placement is ascertained. A very rapid increase in pressure also denotes improper
needle placement and signifies that the needle should be repositioned. Insufflation
continues until the pressure reaches 15 mmHg after which the Verres needle is
removed and a 10–12 mm trocar is inserted. The camera is then introduced and a
thorough inspection of the peritoneal cavity is performed. Additional port sites
may vary according to the individual patient's body habitus, mobility of the
bowel, previous incisions and other factors.

Table 13b.4   Surgical indications and procedures performed for Crohn's disease

Indications	Procedures
Terminal ileal Crohn's disease	Ileocolic resection
Small bowel Crohn's disease	Small bowel resection/strictureplasty
Perineal Crohn's disease	Loop ileostomy Total proctocolectomy
Colonic Crohn's disease leading to total abdominal colectomy with ileostomy or Hartmann's procedure	Ileorectal anastomosis or Hartmann's reversal
Small bowel obstruction	Lysis of adhesions Small bowel resection

Post-operative management

All patients are placed in an intermediate care unit for frequent monitoring for the first 12 to 24 hours. Attention is obviously paid to pulse, blood pressure, temperature, and urinary output. All patients at this institution who undergo either a laparoscopic procedure or a laparotomy are given a clear fluid diet beginning from the day after surgery. In two prior prospectively randomized trials containing over 200 patients, even in the laparotomy setting 89 per cent of patients safely tolerated a diet on the day of surgery without adverse sequelae.[17–19] Appropriate peri-operative antibiotics and advancement to a solid diet should proceed in the standard fashion.[18] Ambulation is also commenced on the day of surgery.

Neither early oral feeding nor reduced post-operative hospital stay are peculiar to laparoscopic patients. In North America, the mean post-operative length of hospital stay is progressively decreasing. Some centres report a mean of five to seven days of hospitalization after laparotomy,[17,18] while others report a mean of seven to twelve days after laparoscopy.[19,20] A recent study from this institution showed that post-operative hospital stay after conventional open bowel resection decreased from a mean of ten days in 1988 to a mean of seven days in 1996 ($p < 0.0001$).[21] Much of the length of stay is very dependent upon both the expectations of the patient and the attitude of the surgeon.[22]

Metronidazole is administered for 24 hours in a regime of 500 mg IV with 1g Cefotaxime IV every eight hours. An intravenous patient controlled analgesia pump (PCA pump) is applied with meperidine hydrochloride up to 10–15 mg/h or morphine sulphate up to 6 mg/h for two to three days; a post-operative taper is employed.

Patients are discharged after they have tolerated a solid diet for at least 24 hours and had at least one normal bowel movement. If a stoma is present, the output should be 1.2 litres per day or less. Many times, the rate-limiting step for discharge is the need to adjust medications to reduce stoma output to an acceptable level. In addition, the patient must have received sufficient enterostomal therapy education prior to discharge even though home enterostomal education is routinely arranged for every patient. The abdomen should be soft, flat and non-tender with a clean wound; the patient should have no systemic signs of sepsis. The patient should return to normal activity as individually tolerated.

Crohn's disease

The prime objective of surgery for Crohn's disease is to treat the symptoms. Because of the young age of the majority of these patients, such interventions should ideally be accompanied by a short disability period, a low morbidity, and a long disease-free period. Complications of small bowel Crohn's disease include obstruction and sepsis (fistula or abscess). Colonic involvement may cause fistula or abscess, toxic megacolon, and very rarely, intestinal bleeding. In our practice small bowel stricture and obstruction accounts for 55 per cent of surgical intervention while fistulae and abscesses account for 32 per cent in patients with colonic disease.[23] In general, the most common indications for surgery are failure of medical management, fistula or abscess, toxic megacolon and perineal disease.[24] The most common indications reported in the literature are shown in Table 13b.5.

Laparoscopic ileocolic resection

In general port placement for laparoscopic right hemicolectomy should serve as a guideline for laparoscopic ileocolic resection for Crohn's disease (Fig. 13b.2).[25] In the routine setting, at least two and occasionally three additional 10–12 mm ports are required to mobilize the terminal ileum and right colon.

Ten mm diameter Babcock grasping instruments are then introduced; the colon should be gently grasped at the caecum and along the ascending colon with non-crushing intestinal clamps and retracted medially to expose the white line of Toldt along the lateral peritoneal reflection. Great care should be exercised to grasp only portions of bowel to be excised. Using a 10 mm electrocautery scissors or ultrasonic scissors (Ethicon Endosurgery Inc., Cincinnati, OH), dissection proceeds in an orderly fashion towards and beyond the hepatic flexure. Large vessels at the hepatic flexure are either divided between clips or with the ultrasonic scissors. The omentum can either be divided with electrocautery or ultrasonic scissors along the avascular plane or by dividing vessels in the lesser sac between clips.

It is crucial to examine the entire small bowel; this evaluation can be accomplished by a bimanual running of the bowel with two non-crushing bowel clamps. Careful handling of the bowel is imperative to avoid enterotomy. By this technique, the bowel is serially inspected over its entire length. This manoeuvre has led to the identification of proximal synchronous strictures missed by pre-operative small bowel radiographic studies. Synchronous strictureplasty or resection can be

Table 13b.5   Indications for laparoscopic surgery in Crohn's disease reported in the literature

Author	Terminal ileitis	Crohn's colitis	Perianal Crohn's	Stricture/ small bowel obstruction	Recto- urethral fistula	Recto- vaginal fistula	Enteric fistula
Thibault et al.[3]	–	3	2	–	–	2	–
Liu et al.[1]	3	1	–	1	–	–	–
Milsom et al.[4]	9	–	–	–	–	–	–
Bauer et al.[5]	17	–	–	1	–	–	–
Ludwig et al.[7]	15	3	7	–	6	–	–
Reissman et al.[8]	29	11	4	3	1	–	1

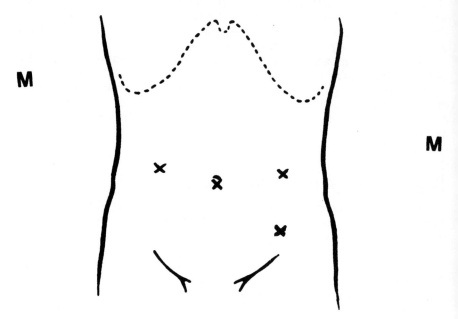

Fig. 13b.2   Port site placement for laparoscopic ileocolic resection.

performed in an extracorporeal fashion through the incision used for specimen delivery and anastomosis.[24–26]

After complete mobilization of the ileocolic region, the umbilical port is removed. That incision is then lengthened by 2–4 cm through or adjacent to the umbilicus through which the segment is delivered. Depending on the patient's body habitus, this incision may be extended superiorly or inferiorly.

We prefer to perform an extracorporeal ligation of the vessels, bowel resection and anastomosis in the same fashion as for a standard 'open' ileocolic resection. Resection margins should be limited to grossly normal appearing intestine. In most studies, microscopic disease at the margins does not correlate with the incidence of or interval to recurrence.[27–37] Conversely, performing frozen sections may lead to an unjustifiable, more extensive bowel resection leading to short bowel syndrome. Once the bowel is resected, the anastomosis is fashioned and the bowel returned to the abdomen. After the bowel is returned to the abdomen, pneumoperitoneum is re-established and further inspection is undertaken to verify haemostasis. Although it is technically possible to perform a completely intracorporeal laparoscopic mesenteric and bowel resection and anastomosis, the amount of time required and the expense for the additional ports and intracorporeal staplers is difficult to justify. Moreover, at the end of such a technical extravaganza an incision must be made to extract the specimen. Logic dictates performance of the additional steps through that same incision. The completely intracorporeal technique appears as a triumph of technology over common sense and an unconscionable financial expenditure.

After return of the anastomosed ileocolic segment into the peritoneal cavity, any concomitant strictured segment can be extracorporealized for strictureplasty or resection. If an ileostomy is necessary it can be formed through the previously identified right iliac fossa site as described elsewhere.[38,39]

Closure of all 10 mm or larger port sites is important. Initially, fascial closure was limited only to the umbilical port site because the abdominal wall muscles were believed to prevent incisional hernias at the lateral port sites. However, an increasing number of midline as well as lateral port sites have recently been reported.[40–42] For large ports such as 18 or 33 mm, the fascia may be exposed by retracting the skin and directly suturing the fascia in an ordinary fashion after completion of the procedure. For smaller (10 mm) ports, this option may not be feasible and therefore port site closure instruments have been designed.[42] The basic principle of these instruments is to place a fascial suture in each port under laparoscopic video guidance. After all the sutures are placed and the procedure is completed, they are tied in consecutive order after removal of the port under laparoscopic vision. Therefore, this device can be used after closure of the midline incision with reinsufflation of CO_2.

Results

Laparoscopic surgery for Crohn's disease at the Cleveland Clinic Florida has been undertaken in 31 patients with terminal ileitis. The mean operating time was 2.4 (0.6–4.5) hours, although the operating times have significantly decreased since the learning curve was surpassed. Specifically, during the first 15 cases, the mean length of time was 4.5 hours, whereas during the last 15 cases it was 2.5 hours ($p < 0.05$). The average duration of ileus was two days and patients were discharged on a mean post-operative day five (range: 3–18 days) (Table 13b.6). Several series of laparoscopic ileocolic resection for Crohn's disease have been reported in the literature and are shown in Table 13b.7; Table 13b.8 shows the overall results of laparoscopic surgery for inflammatory bowel disease reported to date.

Post-operative complications were noted in 14 per cent of patients including enterotomy and bleeding in two patients each. Some of the benefits of the laparoscopic approach to Crohn's disease included reduced post-operative pain, early resumption of normal activities, and enhanced cosmesis. Objective data supporting these subjective patient claims have been revealed in our recent study

Table 13b.6 Results of laparoscopic ileocolic resection for terminal ileitis at Cleveland Clinic Florida

Number of patients	31
Average age	36 (20–79) years
Mean operation time	2.5 (1.6–4.5) hours
First oral intake	1 (1–5) days
Mean duration of post-operative ileus	2 (1–5) days
Length of hospitalization	5 (1–15) days
Regular diet	3.5 (2–10)

Table 13b.7 Laparoscopic-assisted ileocolic resection for Crohn's disease, reports in the literature

Author	Number of cases
Reissman *et al.*[8]	30
Bauer *et al.*[5]	17
Ludwig *et al.*[7]	10
Milsom *et al.*[4]	9
Liu *et al.*[1]	3

which compared the results of laparoscopic-assisted and conventional open ileocolic resection for Crohn's disease.[43] A standard detailed questionnaire relative to patient's subjective recovery was also used. This questionnaire included inquiries regarding post-operative pain, medication use, cosmetic results, pre- and post-operative bowel function, sexual/social activity and post-operative return to full activity levels. The questionnaire was completed by 47 (66 per cent) patients. The percentage of returned questionnaires was identical in both the converted (64.6 per cent) and laparoscopic-assisted (69.5 per cent) groups. There were no statistically significant differences between the laparoscopic-assisted and converted groups relative to post-operative change in bowel habits, medication to assist bowel movements or dietary limitations ($p > 0.05$). However, patients in the laparoscopic-assisted group noted less use of pain medication, better cosmesis and faster return to both normal activity, and social/sexual interaction as compared to the converted group ($p < 0.05$). All patients who were employed prior to surgery returned to work after 3.7 ± 1.2 weeks in the laparoscopic-assisted group versus 8.02 ± 1.2 weeks in the converted group ($p < 0.001$). Although the duration of procedure was decreased in the open group, the difference in the duration of post-operative ileus (3.8 ± 0.2 versus 5.8 ± 0.2) and length of hospitalization (6.9 ± 0.8 versus 9.6 ± 0.6) between the two groups, respectively, were statistically significant.

In a separate study, we aimed to compare safety, outcome and disability of laparoscopic-assisted to conventional ileocolic resection with anastomosis for terminal ileal Crohn's disease (TICD). Specifically, the age, operative time, post-operative ileus, length of hospitalization and incidence of post-operative adhesions were compared. A questionnaire relative to patient's subjective recovery was also used. From August, 1991 to July, 1996, 74 patients underwent ileocolic

Table 13b.8   Results of laparoscopic-assisted bowel resection for inflammatory bowel diseases, reports in the literature

Author	Crohn's disease (*n*)	Mucosal ulcerative colitis (*n*)	Length of surgery (min)	Length of post-operative hospitalization (days)	Morbidity (%)
Reissman et al.[8]	49	29	180 (41–360)	6.5 (3–19)	18
Ludwig et al.[7]	31	–	195 (90–380)	6 (3–7)	3.3
Bauer et al.[5]	18	–	Not stated	6.6 (4–9)	11
Liu et al.[1]	5	5	175 (120–235)	7 (6–13)	20
Milsom et al.[4]	9	–	170 (150–210)	7 (5–12)	0

resection and anastomosis for TICD; 3 in the laparoscopic group were converted to a laparotomy and excluded from evaluation. Some 71 patients were divided into two groups: conventional group (CG) of 48 patients, and laparoscopic-assisted group (LAG) of 23 patients, and compared (**p = ns; *p < 0.05):

	LAG (n = 23)	CG (n = 48)
Mean age (years)	39.0 ± 3.2**	41.6 ± 2.4**
Mean operative time (minutes)	143 ± 10*	90.5 ± 3.7
Duration of post-operative ileus (d)	3.8 ± 0.2*	5.8 ± 0.2
Length of hospitalization (days)	6.9 ± 0.8*	9.6 ± 0.6
Laparotomy for adhesions (%)	8.8*	31

Duration of follow-up was 1–59 (mean 30 ± 1.9) months. The number of returned questionnaires was similar in both groups. No significant differences between the LAG and CG were noted relative to change in bowel habits, assisted bowel movements or dietary limitations. LAG showed greater improvement in pain medication use, cosmesis, and return to normal social activity (LAG: 4.4 ± 0.7 weeks vs CG: 9.3 ± 1.7 weeks) and social/sexual interaction (LAG: 50% vs CG: 15%) compared to the CG (p < 0.05). We concluded that laparoscopic-assisted ileocolic resection for TICD is safe, associated with better cosmesis, decreased post-operative ileus and laparotomy for adhesions, 50% reduction in length of disability and improvement in social–sexual interaction than is conventional surgery.[43]

Colonic Crohn's disease

Involvement of the colon by Crohn's disease may be segmental, however, the entire colon is involved in approximately 60 per cent of cases of colonic Crohn's disease, half of which have rectal sparing. These latter patients may be candidates for total abdominal colectomy with either ileostomy or ileoproctostomy. Similarly, patients with indeterminate colitis are often best served by preliminary colectomy prior to restorative proctocolectomy.[44] Regardless of the condition of the small bowel, patients with a confirmed diagnosis of colonic Crohn's disease should not undergo either restorative proctocolectomy or continent ileostomy. Thus, preliminary total colectomy may be helpful in these patients.

Laparoscopic-assisted total abdominal colectomy with Brooke ileostomy or total proctocolectomy

Indications

These procedures may be indicated for Crohn's colitis, mucosal ulcerative colitis and indeterminate colitis. Contra-indications to the laparoscopic technique include acute toxic colitis and perforation, bleeding disorders, pregnancy, and curable colonic malignancy.

Surgical procedure

A mushroom-tipped catheter is inserted in the rectum and a complete washout with normal saline and betadine is performed. Normally two 10–12 mm ports are placed in the left and right upper quadrants as well as one each in the left and right lower quadrants. All ports are placed lateral to the rectus muscles (Fig. 13b.3). After the patient is placed in the steep Trendelenburg position, the bowel

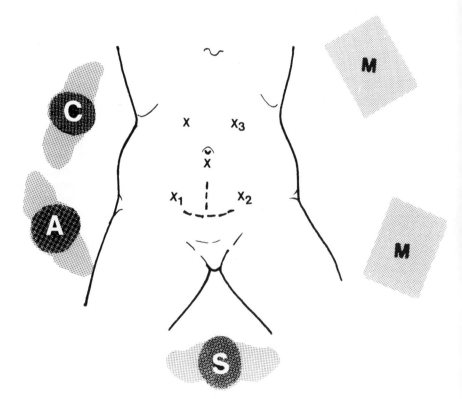

Fig. 13b.3 Port placement for laparoscopic-assisted total abdominal colectomy with Brooke ileostomy. (x and x_1 ports are used for left-sided mobilization and x_2 and x_3 ports for right-sided mobilization.)

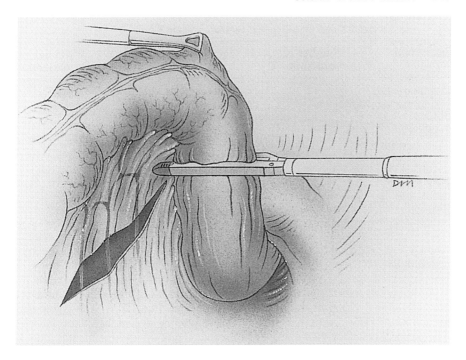

Fig. 13b.4   Laparoscopic division of the restosigmoid junction.

is gently grasped and medially retracted with 10 mm diameter Babcock retractors. Electrocautery or ultrasonic scissors mobilization of the colon commences at the right iliac fossa and proceeds beyond the hepatic flexure. It is important to identify both the right ureter and the duodenum. The left colon is mobilized by grasping and retracting it medially, exposing the white line of Toldt for dissection from the iliac fossa to the splenic flexure; care must be taken to identify the left ureter. The gastrocolic omentum is then divided, either along its avascular plane or by dividing vessels with clips, electrocautery, or ultrasonic scissors. After complete mobilization of the entire colon, a Pfannensteil incision is made through which the entire colon is delivered. Mesenteric vessels are divided and ligated in the usual manner. The colon is resected at the rectosigmoid junction and the rectal stump is returned into the abdomen. An ileoproctostomy can then be performed with a circular stapler. Alternatively, pneumoperitoneum can be re-established to allow an intracorporeal anastomosis.[45] Lastly, if time and resources are available, intracorporeal vascular division can be followed by delivery of the specimen through a 33 mm port and an intracorporeal ileoproctostomy can be fashioned.

To perform a Brooke ileostomy, the right iliac fossa ileostomy site is prepared and the entire specimen is delivered through that site. Specifically, after division of the rectosigmoid junction with a laparoscopic 60 mm stapler (Fig. 13b.4), the terminal ileum is delivered in continuity at the end of the specimen. The bowel is then divided extracorporeally with a 75 mm linear cutter. Pneumoperitoneum is re-established to verify the orientation of the terminal ileum and its mesentery as well as to verify

Table 13b.9 Laparoscopic-assisted total proctocolectomy for inflammatory bowel disease: indications and procedures at Cleveland Clinic Florida

Indication	Number of patients	Procedure	Number of patients
Crohn's colitis	12	Total proctocolectomy with ileoanal reservoir	22
Mucosal ulcerative colitis	23	Total abdominal colectomy with ileorectal anastomosis	7
		Total abdominal colectomy with end ileostomy	2
		Reversal of end ileostomy with ileorectal anastomosis	3
		Total proctocolectomy	1
Total	35		35

haemostasis. After port sites are closed, the stoma is matured. Laparoscopic-assisted ileoproctostomy can be performed either at the time of colectomy or at a later date contingent upon the condition of the patient and disease activity.

If total proctocolectomy is performed, all vascular control is achieved intracorporeally after division of the rectosigmoid junction (Fig. 13b.4). The pelvic dissection is undertaken with the ultrasonic scissors to the level of the levator muscle. The perineal operator then makes a skin incision and divides the levator muscle to deliver the rectal specimen. The remainder of the colon is delivered in continuity with the ileum through the ileostomy site as detailed above. Stoma maturation and perineal wound closure are effected in the usual manner.[46] The only difference between laparoscopy and laparotomy is that the pelvic suction/irrigation drain is delivered to the level of the levators through the iliac fossa port under direct vision.[47]

Results

At Cleveland Clinic Florida, 12 patients who presented with Crohn's colitis and 23 patients with mucosal ulcerative colitis underwent laparoscopic-assisted total colectomy. Twenty-two patients underwent total proctocolectomy with ileoanal reservoir. Seven patients with rectal sparing disease underwent total abdominal colectomy with ileorectal anastomosis. Two patients had colectomy with end ileostomy. Three patients who had previously undergone a total abdominal colectomy with end ileostomy underwent a reversal procedure with take down of ileostomy and performance of laparoscopic ileorectal anastomosis, and one patient underwent laparoscopic total proctocolectomy (Table 13b.9).

Hartmann's reversal

Prior to restoring intestinal continuity, a thorough investigation of both the rectal stump and the proximal colon are mandatory. This assessment is to exclude previously undiagnosed premalignant transformation, new pathology such as stricture formation, and residual pathology such as advancement of Crohn's disease. Colonoscopy, rectosigmoidoscopy, and contrast enemas are valuable in this appraisal process; intra-operative ureteric catheter insertion is extremely helpful.[48] The initial step is to dissect the stoma free from the abdominal wall using ordinary surgical technique. Subsequently, any adhesions in the proximity of the fascia are lysed under direct vision to ensure a free space before the introduction of the laparoscope. After sufficient mobilization of the stoma is achieved, the edges are trimmed and the anvil of a 29–33 mm circular stapler device is secured into the proximal bowel (Fig. 13b.5a). Subsequently, the proximal bowel containing the anvil is placed into the abdominal cavity (Fig. 13b.5b). Several 0 polydioxane fascial sutures are placed, but not tied. A 10–12 mm port is placed in the standard peri-umbilical camera position. A 33 mm port is introduced through the incision and one or two of the fascial sutures are tied to prevent CO_2 leak; an additional 10/12 mm port is placed under direct vision in the supraumbilical position through which the peritoneal cavity is insufflated. Through the periumbilical port, as in any other laparoscopic procedure, the abdominal pelvic cavities are inspected. Adhesions from the previous procedures are very frequently present and should be carefully divided.

Two to three additional 10–12 mm ports are placed under direct laparoscopic visualization. After adequate exposure is achieved by lysis of adhesions and the small bowel is retracted out of the pelvis, attention is paid to both the proximal bowel and the rectal stump. The proximal bowel is inspected for sufficient mobilization to ensure a tension-free anastomosis. Additional mobilization is frequently required by incising the lateral peritoneal attachments, including mobilization of the splenic flexure or transverse colon. For ileoproctostomy, the ileal mesentery needs to be liberated to the superior mesenteric axis. The rectal stump is identified and freed from adhesions to other organs. Rigid proctoscopy may be performed to facilitate the rectal stump dissection.

After both the rectal stump and the proximal bowel are cleared and confirmed safe and well-vascularized, the anvil is grasped with a modified Allis clamp (Ethicon Endosurgery, Cincinnati, OH). The circular stapler is introduced transanally and guided laparoscopically to reach the end of the rectal stump and the previous staple line. After the shaft is completely exposed, the anvil is guided towards the pelvis and attached (Fig. 13b.6). After securely attaching the anvil to the circular stapler, the laparoscope is placed in the right iliac fossa port for better visualization while the circular stapler device is approximated. In women, care must be taken to prevent injury to the vagina.

After the anastomosis is performed, the stapler is gently removed and the proximal and distal doughnuts are carefully inspected for integrity (Fig. 13b.7). The pelvis is irrigated with saline to immerse the anastomosis and a straight atraumatic Dennis clamp is used to occlude the proximal colon while the anastomosis is tested for air leak by transanal air insufflation. If no leak is found, the fluid is aspirated. The ports are removed, the fascia at all port sites is closed, and the skin at the stoma site is left open to heal by secondary intention. If a completion proctectomy is to be performed, then it proceeds as already described in the previous section.

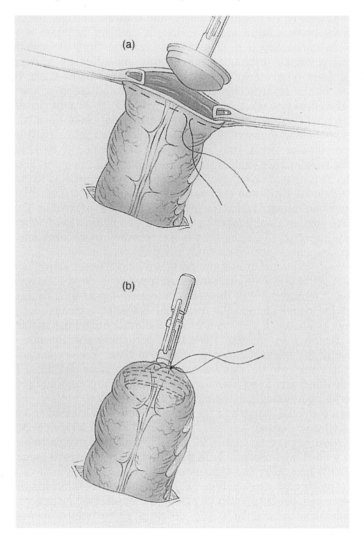

Fig. 13b.5 (a) The anvil of a 29 or 33 mm circular stapler is secured into the proximal bowel. (b) The bowel containing the anvil is placed in the abdominal cavity.

Results

A review of our experience in laparoscopic restoration of intestinal continuity showed that this technique was attempted in 15 and completed in 9 (60 per cent) patients (Wexner 1996, personal communication). The other 6 patients had their procedure converted because of severe adhesions. The median time between the initial procedure and closure was six months in all the groups. The median operative time was statistically different between the laparoscopic and converted

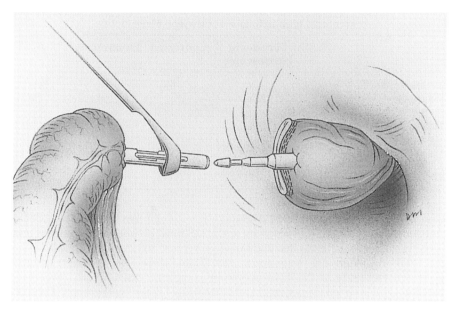

Fig. 13b.6 The anvil is guided towards the pelvis and attached to the receptor of the circular stapler.

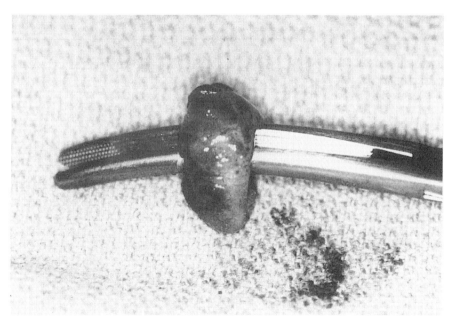

Fig. 13b.7 Proximal and distal doughnuts are carefully inspected for integrity.

Table 13b.10   Results of laparoscopic-assisted (n = 15) Hartmann's reversal compared to conventional open technique at Cleveland Clinic Florida

	Successful laparoscopic	Converted	Laparotomy	p
Number of cases	9	6	15	NS
Median operative time (minutes)	135	185	160	NS
Median post-operative ileus (days)	3	5	4	> 0.05
Median post-operative hospitalization (days)	4	10	7	> 0.05
Morbidity (%)	22	33	39	

groups (135 versus 185 minutes, respectively; $p < 0.05$). We have not recorded a statistically significant difference in operative time between laparoscopic and open Hartmann's reversal techniques (135 versus 160 minutes, respectively; $p > 0.05$). Although not statistically significant, there was a trend towards decreased morbidity in the laparoscopically completed cases (22 per cent) compared to the converted (33 per cent) and laparotomy (39 per cent) groups. The first bowel movement occurred at a median of day three, four and five days for the laparoscopic, laparotomy and converted groups, respectively. The median post-operative length of stay was four, seven and ten days for the laparoscopic, laparotomy and converted groups, respectively ($p < 0.05$) (Table 13b.10).

Perineal Crohn's disease _____

Faecal diversion may be required in patients with severe perineal Crohn's disease as these patients can have complications such as incontinence or complex recurrent or chronic sepsis. We prefer the use of a loop ileostomy for temporary faecal diversion.[49] The use of the laparoscopic technique for ileostomy creation has had the advantages of minimal post-operative pain, rapid return of bowel function, early oral intake, low morbidity and excellent cosmesis.

Technique

The camera port is situated midway between the umbilicus and the xiphoid. If the standard peri-umbilical position is used, the camera is then too close to the stoma site port to allow adequate manoeuvrability. The second 10–12 mm port is placed at the site previously marked for ileostomy. An optional third port is used only if necessary to inspect or mobilize the bowel or to divide adhesions, if required. The third port is placed in a mirror image position to the stoma site, opposite the second port. After exploration of the abdominal cavity, a laparoscopic 10 mm diameter Babcock clamp is used to grasp the selected intestinal loop. For the creation of a loop ileostomy, the most distal segment of ileum that can be delivered without tension is utilized. For an end sigmoid colostomy, a stapler is

Table 13b.11   Results of laparoscopic faecal diversion at Cleveland Clinic Florida

Number of stomas	41
Loop ileostomy	31
Loop colostomy	4
End colostomy	6
Mean length of surgery	93 (35–210) minutes
Time to stoma/bowel function	2.3 (1–6) days
Time to oral intake	2.0 (0–2) days
Length of hospital stay	5.3 (2–22) days
Conversion to open technique	5 (12%)

used to divide the sigmoid colon and the proximal end is then exteriorized by gently grasping the appropriate segment of bowel through the stoma site port. The port is then withdrawn over the Babcock clamp shaft. The shaft is maintained with the insufflated sleeve well within the abdomen. Two crescents of skin are then excised to allow for a 2 cm diameter skin aperture. With the aid of right-angled retractors for exposure, the anterior fascia is divided, the rectus fibres are spread in a cephalad to caudad direction and the posterior rectus fascia and peritoneum are divided. The camera is used to visualize the underside of the stoma site during this process to ensure safe use of electrocautery. Finally, the bowel loop is withdrawn through the site; camera verification of appropriate intestinal orientation is essential.[38] For a loop ileostomy, a rod is placed under the mesenteric margin and after closure of the camera (and if used optional third) port the stoma is matured.

Results

Among the 41 patients who underwent laparoscopic faecal diversion, 31 had a loop ileostomy, 4 a loop colostomy and 6 an end colostomy (Table 13b.11). Indications for faecal diversion included 24 patients with perineal Crohn's disease and 17 without Crohn's disease. Conversion was required due to thick adhesions in two cases, due to an enterotomy in one, a colotomy in one, equipment failure in one and unclear anatomy in another. Post-operative complications consisted of outlet and small bowel obstruction in three cases. One patient required reoperation and at laparotomy a rotation of the terminal ileum was observed. The other patient had a narrow fascial opening which was successfully managed by two weeks of self-intubation of the stoma. The mean operative time was 93 (range 35–210) minutes and the mean length of hospitalization was 5.3 (range 2–13) days. Stoma function started after a mean period of 2.3 (range 1–6) days. The reason for the long hospital stay was the requirement for stoma therapy education. After sufficient time has passed and if the perineal problem improves, the stoma can be taken down and intestinal continuity restored. The reasons for conversion reported in the literature are reviewed in Table 13b.12. These same 41 patients are then compared to 11 patients who underwent faecal diversion by laparotomy during the same time period. All patients who underwent faecal diversion without any resectional abdominal procedures were studied. Prior to laparotomy, inflammatory bowel disease, recurrent or metastatic cancers were not absolute contra-indications. Parameters evaluated included age, indications, previous

Table 13b.12   Laparoscopic-assisted bowel resection for inflammatory bowel disease: rates of conversion

Author	Rate of conversion (%)	Reason for conversion
Reissman *et al.*[8]	18	Large inflammatory mass; fistula; bleeding; enterotomy
Ludwig *et al.*[7]	19	Dense adhesions; mesenteric thickening; perforation; small bowel dilation
Bauer *et al.*[5]	22	Fixed intra-abdominal mass; severe recurrent disease
Liu *et al.*[1]	10	Technical reason
Milsom *et al.*[4]	0	None

abdominal surgery, operative time, time until stoma function, length of post-operative hospitalization and cosmetic results. Patients were divided into a laparoscopy group (LG) and open group (OG). Choice of the procedure was at the surgeon's discretion; one surgeon routinely performed laparoscopy while two others did not. Between March 1993 and October 1996, 41 laparoscopic and 11 conventional open intestinal stomas for faecal diversion were performed. There were no significant differences between the two groups relative to mean age of patients (LG = 46, range 19–80 versus OG = 58, range 36–81 years) or number of patients with previous abdominal surgery (LG = 9 (22 per cent) versus OG = 3 (27 per cent). There was a statistically significant difference in the mean duration of surgery (LG 93 , range 35–210 minutes versus OG = 74, range 50–113 minutes; $p = 0.001$), while no significant differences were noted when patients with prior abdominal surgery were compared separately (LG = 98, range 85–200 minutes versus OG = 95, range 65–115 minutes; $p > 0.05$). Morbidity rates were not statistically different between the 2 groups (8 (19.5 per cent) versus 2 (18.2 per cent)), respectively. There were statistically significant differences relative to time to stoma function (2.3, range 1–4 days versus 4.5, range 3–8 days; $p < 0.05$), and length of post-operative hospitalization (5.3, range 2–12 days versus 7.6, range 5–19 days; $p < 0.05$) in the LG and OG groups, respectively. We concluded that although laparoscopic stomas take longer to create than do stomas by laparotomy, the stomas begin to function more rapidly allowing a more expeditious hospital discharge.[50]

Ulcerative colitis

In an elective setting the most frequent indication for surgery is intractability of disease. Patients in this group have their lifestyle altered due to the persistent symptoms and frequently have the disease controlled only with prohibitive doses of medical agents with unacceptable side effects. Moreover, the true morbidity, cost and disability of medical therapy for ulcerative colitis are seldom known and are even less frequently compared to analogous parameters associated with surgical therapy.[51] We have assessed and compared medical and surgical therapy for patients hospitalized due to severe ulcerative colitis.[52] These patients were matched for age, duration and severity of disease based upon Truelove and Witts' activity index, colonoscopic and histologic appearance and Acute Psychological and Chronic Health Evaluation (APACHE) II scores. Morbidity, cost and disability of 20 medically treated patients who required at least one hospital admission were compared to 20 patients treated by restorative proctocolectomy. Demographic data, number of hospital admissions, length of stay, total hospital charges including consultant's, surgeon's, and anaesthetist's fees, morbidity of each approach and disability were addressed. Statistical analysis was performed using Mann–Whitney and Fisher's exact tests. The mean patient ages were similar – 53.6 years in the medical group versus 48.1 years in the surgical group (p = NS) and the average duration of disease 10.5 years and 9.5 years, respectively (p = NS). The same variety of pancolitis was noted in both groups; APACHE scores of 13 and 14 were noted in the medical and surgical groups, respectively. No significant differences were noted between the two groups relative to total number of hospital admissions and combined length of stay per patient. The total mean hospital cost for the medical group was \$28,477.00 per patient versus \$33,041.00 for the surgical group (p = NS). Post-operative disability was six months in the medical group versus five months in the surgical group (p = NS). However, patients in the medical group required more transfusions (25 per cent) than did those in the surgical group (0 per cent) (p < 0.05) and significant weight loss was more common in the medical group (45 per cent) compared to the surgical group (5 per cent) (p < 0.01). All patients in the surgical group were permanently weaned from steroids. Furthermore, while 65 per cent of patients in the medical group had significant related complications, the major surgical complication rate was 15 per cent (p < 0.01). These results demonstrate clearly that medical treatment for ulcerative colitis is associated with higher overall morbidity than surgical therapy. Surgery may also be necessary for dysplasia and surgical options include laparoscopic-assisted total colectomy with end ileostomy or ileoproctostomy or laparoscopic-assisted restorative proctocolectomy with ileal 'J' pouch. The former two procedures have already been described earlier in this chapter.

Laparoscopic-assisted restorative proctocolectomy with ileal 'J' pouch

This operative technique is the same as that described for the laparoscopic-assisted total abdominal colectomy with ileostomy for Crohn's colitis. Since the bowel is very inflamed, great care must be taken to avoid injury during mobilization. Both ureters must be identified before any vascular ligation is undertaken. Failure to identify the ureters in any colorectal procedure warrants conversion to laparotomy. After mobilization of the entire colon, a Pfannensteil incision is made through which the entire colon is delivered. The mesentery is scored and vessels are divided and ligated in the usual manner. After rectal mobilization, the anus is transected 1 cm cephalad to the dentate line with a 30 mm stapling device. The terminal ileum is delivered in continuity and an extracorporeal bowel division is done with a 75 mm linear cutter. The 'J' pouch is formed by stapling the terminal 30–40 cm of ileum together through an apical enterotomy using either a 75 mm or

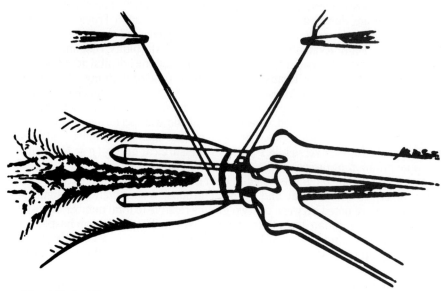

Fig. 13b.8   The terminal 30 to 40 cm of ileum is stapled together to form a 'J' pouch.

100 mm linear cutting stapler (Fig. 13b.8).[53,54] After the stapler is fired, a purse-string suture is applied to the apical enterotomy. The anvil of a 29 mm circular stapler is introduced in the bowel lumen through the purse string suture (Fig. 13b.5b). After the anastomosis is fashioned, the doughnuts are inspected for integrity (Fig. 13b.7) and an air insufflation test is undertaken. The loop ileostomy is then delivered through the previously selected site in the right iliac fossa. Alternatively, that site may have been used for one of the ports.

Results

Of the 28 laparoscopic ileoanal restorative proctocolectomies with ileal 'J' pouch performed at this institution, 23 (82 per cent) were undertaken for mucosal ulcerative colitis.[45] Other diagnoses included Familial Adenomatous Polyposis in four cases and juvenile polyposis in one. We compared these patients with 20 age, gender and diagnosis-matched controls who underwent restorative procto-colectomy using a standard midline incision (Table 13b.13).[53] The length of ileus was similar in both groups. The mean time to resolution of ileus was 3.6 (2–11) days in the laparoscopic-assisted colectomy and 3.3 (2–5) days in the standard colectomy group. The mean time until oral intake was 2.5 (0–7) days in the laparoscopic-assisted colectomy group and 4.3 (3–8) days in the standard colect-omy group. In analysing the length of hospitalization, the groups were similar. The mean length of hospitalization was 7.1 (2–30) days in the laparoscopic-assisted colectomy group and 8.9 (6–18) days in the standard colectomy group. However, a difference was noted in the two groups with respect to the length of operation. The mean length of operation in the laparoscopic-assisted colectomy group was 240 (120–330) minutes while the mean length of surgery was 140

Table 13b.13 Results of laparoscopic-assisted proctocolectomy with ileal 'J' pouch for mucosal ulcerative colitis compared to open restorative proctocolectomy

	Laparoscopic-assisted	Open
Number of patients	23	20
Length of surgery (min)	240 (120–330)	140 (120–300)
Mean time to resolution of ileus (days)	3.6 (2–11)	3.3 (2–5)
Mean time to oral intake (days)	2.5 (0–7)	4.3 (3–8)
Mean post-operative length of stay (days)	7.1 (2–30)	8.9 (6–8)
Number of transfused patients	16	7
Number of transfusions per patient (units)	2 (1–15)	2 (2–5)
Morbidity	12 (43%)	6 (30%)
Mortality	0	0

(120–300) minutes in the standard colectomy group. Interestingly, the ranges are basically identical, highlighting that the surgeon may encounter both simple and difficult cases, regardless of the surgical techniques applied. Transfusion was required in 16 patients in the laparoscopic-assisted colectomy group and in only 7 in the standard colectomy group ($p < 0.05$). However, the mean number of transfusions in each group was 2 (laparoscopic-assisted: range 1–15; standard: range 2–5). These patients were not stratified for either pre-operative haemoglobin or steroid dose. This result is consistent with that published by Peters and Bartels.[55] Their group measured both pre-operative and 24-hour post-operative haemoglobin levels as an indirect indicator of operative blood loss. They did not demonstrate any statistically significant difference, although they did observe a trend towards a greater fall in the laparoscopic group (more intra-operative blood loss using the laparoscope). Thus, the only two studies that have quantified blood loss have documented a higher loss with laparoscopic than with open surgery. These data refute the subjective claims made by others.[56]

Although no post-operative mortality occurred, 12 of the 28 patients (43 per cent) and 6 of the 20 (30 per cent) experienced post-operative morbidity (Table 13b.14) ($p < 0.05$). The two most common complications were ileus and wound infection. One patient in the laparoscopic-assisted colectomy group required reoperation in the immediate post-operative period because of intra-abdominal haemorrhage. The incidence of complications was much higher than that seen in patients who have undergone segmental colectomy.

Conclusions ———————————————————

As more experience is gained with the use of the laparoscope, surgeons will continue to attempt larger and more complicated procedures. However, enthusiasm must be tempered with reality. Basic proven surgical tenets should not be abandoned in favour of inadequate and cumbersome technology or unacceptable cost. We must continue to evaluate the parameters in a meaningful prospective fashion to perform the necessary statistical evaluations needed to decide what role laparoscopic colon surgery will have in our future armamentarium. Laparoscopic resection for cure of colorectal malignancy is unproven relative to its merits. Conversely, the same technology is clearly advantageous when applied by appropriately trained individuals in selected patients with benign pathology including inflammatory bowel disease. Within that latter group, neither total abdominal colectomy nor restorative proctocolectomy appear routinely justifiable. Conversely, ileocolic resection and stoma creation are excellent laparoscopic indications. Patients who undergo these procedures via the laparoscope have significantly improved outcome as compared to their counterparts who undergo laparotomy.[23,38,51,57,58]

References

1. Liu CD, Rolandelli R, Ashley SW, Evans B *et al.* Laparoscopic surgery for inflammatory bowel diseases. *Am Surg* 1995; **61**: 1054–1056.
2. Peters WR. Laparoscopic total proctocolectomy with creation of ileostomy for Ulcerative colitis: report of 2 cases. *J Laparoendosc Surg* 1992; **2**: 175–178.
3. Thibault C, Poulin EC. Total laparoscopic proctocolectomy and laparoscopic assisted proctocolectomy for inflammatory bowel disease: operative techniques and preliminary report. *Surg Laparosc Endosc* 1995; **5**: 475–476.
4. Milson JW, Lavery IC, Bohm B, Fazio VW. Laparoscopically assisted ileocolectomy in Crohn's disease. *Surg Laparosc Endosc* 1992; **3**: 77–80.
5. Bauer JJ, Harris MT, Grumback NM, Gorfine SR. Laparoscopic assisted intestinal resection for Crohn's disease. *Dis Colon Rectum* 1995; **38**: 712–715.
6. Kreissler-Haag D, Hildebrandt U, Pistorius G, *et al.* Laparoscopic surgery in Crohn's disease. *Surg Endosc* 1994; **8**: 1002 (Abstract).
7. Ludwig KA, Milsom JW, Church JM, Fazio VW. Preliminary experience with laparoscopic intestinal surgery for Crohn's disease. *Am J Surg* 1996; **171**: 52–56.
8. Reissman P, Salky BA, Pfeifer J, *et al.* Laparoscopic surgery in the management of inflammatory bowel disease. *Am J Surg* 1996; **171**: 47–50.
9. Jorge JM, Wexner SD. Anorectal manometry: techniques and clinical applications. *S Med J* 1993; **86**: 924–931.
10. Jorge JM, Wexner SD. A practical guide to anorectal physiology. *Contemp Surg* 1993; **43**: 214–224.
11. Wexner SD (guest ed.). Practical colorectal physiology: investigation and intervention. *Seminars in Colon and Rectal Surgery* 1992; **3**(2): 63–151.
12. Wexner SD, Bartolo DCC (eds). *Constipation: aetiology, evaluation and management.* Butterworth–Heinemann, Oxford, 1995.
13. Oliveira L, Daniel N, Bernstein M, *et al.* Mechanical bowel preparation for elective colorectal surgery. A prospective randomized surgeon blinded trial comparing sodium phosphate (SP) and polyethyline glycol (PEG) based oral lavage solutions. *Dis Colon Rectum* 1997; **40**: 585–591.
14. Cohen SM, Wexner SD, Binderow SR, Nogueras JJ, Daniel N, Ehrenpreis ED, Jensen J, Bonner GF, Ruderman WB. Prospective, randomized, endoscopic-blinded trial comparing precolonoscopy bowel cleansing methods. *Dis Colon Rectum* 1994; **37**: 689–696.
15. Beck DE, Wexner SD (eds). *Fundamentals of Anorectal Surgery.* McGraw-Hill, New York, 1992.
16. Wexner SD, Beck DE. Sepsis prevention in colorectal surgery. In: Fielding LP, Goldberg SM (eds). *Operative Surgery: Colon, Rectum, and Anus*, 5th edn, But-

terworth–Heinemann, London, 1993; 41–46.

17. Binderow SR, Cohen SM, Wexner SD, Nogueras JJ. Must early postoperative oral intake be limited to laparoscopy? *Dis Colon Rectum* 1994; **37**: 584–589.

18. Reissman P, Wexner SD. Is oral feeding safe after elective colorectal surgery? *Ann Surg* 1995; **222**: 73–77.

19. Monson JRT, Darzi A, Carey PD, Guillou PJ. Prospective evaluation of laparoscopic assisted colectomy in an unselected group of patients. *Lancet* 1992; **340**: 831–833.

20. Guillou PJ. Laparoscopic surgery for diseases of the colon and rectum: quo vadis? *Surg Endosc* 1994; **8**: 669–671.

21. Iroatulam A, Alabaz O, Chen H, Potenti F, Weiss E, Nogveras J, Wexner SD. A decrease in the length of hospitalization after segmented non-laparoscopic colectomy during a 9 year period. *Dis Colon Rectum* 1997; **40**(6): A43.

22. Rajagopal HS, Thorson AG, Sentovitch JM *et al.* Decade trends in length of postoperative stay following abdominal colectomy. *Dis Colon Rectum* 1994; **37**: 26 (abstract).

23. Reissman P, Salky B, Edye M, Wexner SD. Laparoscopic surgery in Crohn's disease: indications and results. *Surg Endosc* 1996; **10**: 1201–1204.

24. Wexner SD, Reissman P, Bernstein M. Surgery of Crohn's disease including stricturoplasty. In: Nyhus LM, Baker RJ, Fischer JE (eds). *Mastery of Surgery*, 3rd edn, Little, Brown and Company, Boston, 1996, pages 1384–1399.

25. Cohen SM, Wexner SD. Laparoscopic right hemicolectomy. *Surg Rounds* 1994; 627–635.

26. Wexner SD. General principles of surgery in ulcerative colitis and Crohn's disease. *Seminars Gastroenterol* 1991; **2**: 90–98.

27. Adloff M, Arnaud JP, Ollier JC. Does the histologic appearance at the margin of resection affect the postoperative recurrence rate in Crohn's disease? *Am Surg* 1987; **53**: 543–546.

28. Heuman R, Boeryd B, Bolin T, Sjodahl R. The influence of disease at the margin of resection on the outcome of Crohn's disease. *Br J Surg* 1983; **70**: 519–521.

29. Cooper JC, Williams NS. The influence of microscopic disease at the margin of resection on recurrence rates in Crohn's disease. *Ann Roy Coll Surg Engl* 1986; **68**: 23–26.

30. Pennington L, Speranza V, Simi M, Leardi S, Del Papa M. Recurrence of Crohn's: are there any risk factors? *J Clin Gastroenterol* 1986; **8**: 640–646.

31. Chardavoyne R, Flint GW, Pollack S, Wise L. Factors affecting recurrence following resection for Crohn's disease. *Dis Colon Rectum* 1986; **29**: 495–502.

32. Pennington L, Hamilton SR, Bayless TM, Cameron JL. Surgical management of Crohn's disease: influence of disease at the margin of resection. *Ann Surg* 1980; **192**: 311–317.

33. Williams JG, Wong WD, Rothenberger DA, Goldberg SM. Recurrence of Crohn's disease after resection. *Br J Surg* 1991; **78**: 10–19.

34. Hamilton SR, Reese J, Pennington L *et al.* The role of resection margin frozen section in the surgical management of Crohn's disease. *Surg Gynecol Obstet* 1985; **160**: 57–62.

35. Papaioannou N, Piris J, Lee ECG, Kettlewell MGW. The relationship between histological inflammation in the cut ends after resection of Crohn's disease and recurrence. *Gut* 1979; **20**: A916.

36. Hamilton SR, Rees J, Pennington L *et al.* No role for resection margin frozen section in the surgical management of Crohn's disease. *Gastroenterology* 1982; **82**: 1078.

37. Fazio VW, Marchetti F, Church JM, Goldblum JR, Lavery IC, Hull TL, Milson JW, Strong SA, Oakley JR, Secic M. Effect of resection margins on the recurrence of Crohn's disease in the small bowel. A randomized controlled trial. *Ann Surg* 1996; **224**: 563–573.

38. Oliveira L, Reissman P, Wexner SD. Laparoscopic creation of stomas. *Surg Endosc* 1997; **11**: 264–267.

39. Teoh TA, Reissman P, Cohen SM, Weiss EG, Wexner SD. Laparoscopic loop

240   *The lower gastrointestinal tract: inflammatory bowel disease*

ileostomy. *Dis Colon Rectum* 1994; **37**: 514 (letter).

40. Reissman P, Shiloni E, Gofrit O *et al.* Incarcerated hernia in a lateral port site: an unusual early postoperative complication of laparoscopic surgery. *Eur J Surg* 1994; **160**: 191.

41. Storms P, Stuyven G, Vanhemelen G, Sebrechts R. Incarcerated trocar-wound hernia after laparoscopic hysterectomy. *Surg Endosc* 1994; **8**: 901.

42. Reissman P, Bernstein M, Verzaro R, Wexner SD. Port site fascia closure in laparoscopic assisted colectomy. *J Laparoendosc Surg* 1995; **5**(5): 335–337.

43. Alabaz O, Iroatulam A, Nessim A, Weiss EG, Nogveras JJ, Wexner SD. Comparison of laparoscopic-assisted and conventional ileocolic resection in Crohn's disease (Abstract). *Int J Colorect Dis* 1997; **12**(3): 182.

44. Wexner SD, Johansen OB, Nogueras JJ, Jagelman DG. Laparoscopic total abdominal colectomy: a prospective trial. *Dis Colon Rectum* 1992; **35**: 651–655.

45. Cohen SM, Wexner SD. Laparoscopic restorative proctocolectomy. In: Jager R, Wexner SD (eds). *Laparoscopic Colorectal Surgery.* Churchill-Livingstone, New York, 1996; 201–205.

46. Nogveras JJ, Wexner SD. Stoma Prolapse. In: Mackeigan JM and Cataldo PA (eds). *Intestinal Stomas*, Quality Medical Publishing, St Louis, 1993; 268–277.

47. Reissman P, Cohen SM, Weiss EG, Wexner SD. Simple technique for pelvic drain placement in laparoscopic abdominoperineal resection. *Dis Colon Rectum* 1994; **37**: 381–382.

48. Paramesweran S, Gilliland R, Iroatulam A, Daniel N, Kirby K, Nogveras JJ, Wexner SD. Role of elective ureteric catheterization in colorectal surgery. *Dis Colon Rectum* 1997; **40**(6): A48–A49.

49. Wexner SD, Taranow DA, Johansen OB

et al. Loop ileostomy is a safe option for fecal diversion. *Dis Colon Rectum* 1993; **36**: 349–354.

50. Iroatulam A, Wexner SD. Laparoscopic versus conventional open stoma creation for fecal diversion. (Abstract) *Int J Colorect Dis* 1997; **12**(3): 181.

51. Sher ME, Agachan F, Weiss EG, Nogueras JJ, Wexner SD. Laparoscopic surgery for diverticulitis. *Surg Endosc* 1997; **11**: 19–23.

52. Sher ME, Sands LR, Agachan F, Nogveras JJ, Weiss EG, Wexner SD. Morbidity, cost and disability of medical therapy for ulcerative colitis: what are we really saving? *Int J Colorect Dis* 1996; **11**(3): 143.

53. Schmitt SL, Cohen SM, Wexner SD, *et al.* Does laparoscopic assisted ileal pouch anal anastomosis reduce the length of hospitalization. *Int J Colorectal Dis* 1994; **9**: 134.

54. Reissman P, Piccirillo M, Ulrich A, Daniel N, Nogueras JJ, Wexner SD. Functional results of the double stapled ileoanal reservoir. *J Am Coll Surg* 1995; **181**: 444–450.

55. Peters WR, Bartels TL. Minimally invasive colectomy: are the potential benefits realized? *Dis Colon Rectum* 1993; **36**: 751–756.

56. Senagore AJ, Luchtefeld MA, Macheigan JM *et al.* Open colectomy versus laparoscopic colectomy: are there differences? *Am Surg* 1993; **59**: 549–553

57. Joo JS, Agachan F, Wexner SD. Laparoscopic surgery for lower gastrointestinal fistulas. *Surg Endosc* 1996; **136**: 576 (abstract).

58. Chen H, Alabaz O, Iroatulam A, Nessim A, Joo J, Weiss EG, Nogveras JJ, Wexner SD. Laparoscopic colectomy for benign colorectal disease is associated with a significant reduction in disability compared with laparotomy. *Dis Colon Rectum* 1997; **40**(6): A20.

13c

The lower gastrointestinal tract: laparoscopic rectopexy

R.J. Stacey and A. Darzi

Introduction

Rectal prolapse is uncommon and its true incidence is unknown. Prolapse may occur at any age but is most common at the extremes of life. In children most prolapse occurs within the first three years of life and with an equal sex distribution. In adults, the majority of patients are female. The descent of the rectum through the anal canal is of two types. Prolapse involving the mucous membrane only is termed partial. Where the full thickness of rectal wall descends, the prolapse is termed complete. Internal or 'hidden' prolapse occurs when the rectum intussuscepts but does not protrude beyond the anal canal.

Partial prolapse is the more common type seen in children and is a self-limiting disease. In the adult patient mucosal prolapse may occur as a result of sphincter damage following childbirth or operation for perianal fistula. In addition the development of prolapsing haemorrhoids ultimately predisposes to a more extensive mucosal prolapse.

The aetiology of complete prolapse remains unclear although it seems likely that it is related to pelvic floor weakness, borne out by the common occurrence in patients with spinal cord injuries and in the elderly with poor sphincter tone. It has also been shown that resting activity of the sphincteric and levator ani muscles is reduced during defecation in patients with prolapse.

The management of rectal prolapse is surgical. Although many procedures have been described only a small number remain in active use. Operations for rectal prolapse are conventionally divided into two groups on the basis of anatomical approach. Transabdominal repairs involve rectal fixation, or large bowel resection, or a combination of the two. Perineal procedures include resection, rectal reefing (Delorme), anal encirclement or even perineal rectosigmoidectomy.

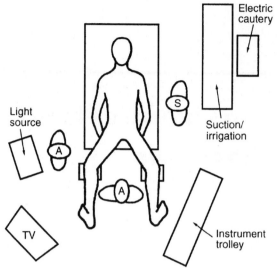

Fig. 13c.1   Theatre set-up

This chapter is concerned with the treatment options in complete rectal prolapse with special reference to the new technique of stapled laparoscopic rectopexy.

Video-assisted colorectal surgery is one of the latest additions to the range of operations being performed laparoscopically. For colonic resection, colonic mobilization, division of mesenteric vessels and bowel are usually carried out intracorporeally. A small incision is then made to deliver the specimen and fashion the anastomosis. However, without the need for bowel resection, laparoscopic procedures for treating rectal prolapse may constitute some of the best applications of laparoscopic colorectal techniques.

Operative technique

A nasogastric tube and urinary catheter are passed when the patient is anaesthetized. All procedures are performed with the patient in the Lloyd–Davies position. The theatre set-up is shown in Fig. 13c.1. Pneumoperitoneum is created using a standard technique. A 10 mm zero degree telescope is inserted through a subumbilical port and initial laparoscopy is performed.

The operator stands on the left side of the patient, and two video screens are positioned on either side of the knees. Three 12 mm trocars are introduced into the abdomen to facilitate use of the laparoscopic stapling instruments (Endo–Hernia, Autosuture, Ascot, UK) (Fig. 13c.2).

The camera is inserted into the right iliac fossa port and a Babcock is passed through the left iliac fossa port holding the recto-sigmoid junction anteriorly and to the left. A second Babcock grasping instrument is passed through the suprapubic port to elevate the middle third of the rectum. This provides tension on the

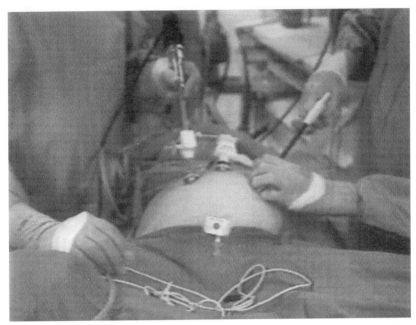

Fig. 13c.2   Insertion of ports: 12 mm at umbilicus; 10 mm port to the right of the umbilical port; 10 mm port at left iliac fossa; 10 mm suprapubic port. This figure is also reproduced in colour between pages 276 and 277.

peritoneal reflection on the right side of the recto-sigmoid junction. Identification of both ureters is established early in the dissection, with the aid of illumination from fibre optic ureteric stents;[1] the use of diathermy is restricted until the ureters are identified in order to reduce the risk of thermal injury (Fig. 13c.3 a,b). The peritoneal reflection is divided using scissors and, by careful dissection, the avascular plane between the fascial capsule of the rectum anteriorly and the fascia of Waldeyer posteriorly is dissected under direct vision (Fig. 13c.4).

Division of the lateral ligaments is easily performed under direct vision. Posteriorly the pelvic nerves are identified and preserved. Close and magnified views of the mesorectum ensure the dissection continues within the correct planes with minimal bleeding (Fig. 13c.5). In a female, retraction of the pouch of Douglas is facilitated by holding the cervix upwards with a blunt Hulka cervical forceps (Rocket Ltd, Watford, UK) held through the vagina by an assistant. This elevates the cervix and body of the uterus, allowing anterior dissection to be completed.

Having mobilized the rectum down to the pelvic floor, a strip of polypropylene mesh (Surgipro Mesh, Autosuture, Ascot, UK), approximately 10 × 6 cm is introduced into the abdomen through the sub-umbilical port for placement in the presacral space. The endoscopic stapler is then introduced into the right iliac fossa port, and the mesh is initially stapled to the sacrococcygeal area. On average three to four staples are then inserted cephalad to the initial staple to fix the mesh to the sacrum (Fig. 13c.6). After fixation of the mesh, the rectum is held on light

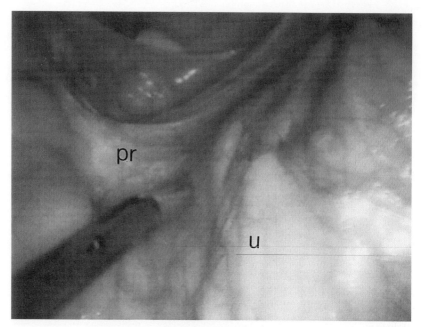

Fig. 13c.3(a) Laparoscopic identification of the right ureter (u). Peritoneal reflection divided (pr). This figure is also reproduced in colour between pages 276 and 277.

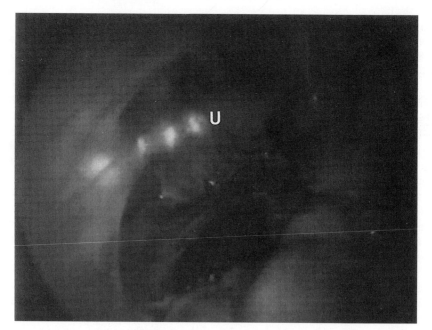

Fig. 13c.3(b) Visualization of ureters (u) with the aid of fibro-optic light source. This figure is also reproduced in colour between pages 276 and 277.

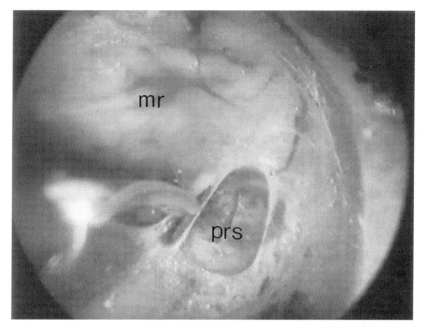

Fig. 13c.4 Development of the plane between the sacrum (s) and mesorectum (mr), using sharp dissection (prs, pre-rectal space). This figure is also reproduced in colour between pages 276 and 277.

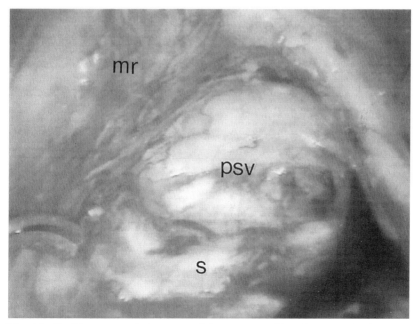

Fig. 13c.5 Mesorectum (mr) separated from sacrum (s) and presacral veins (psv). This figure is also reproduced in colour between pages 276 and 277.

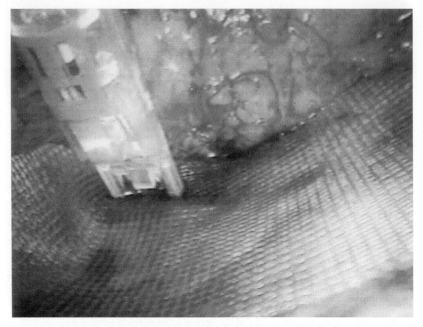

Fig. 13c.6   Prolene mesh being stapled to sacral fascia using the hernia stapler. This figure is also reproduced in colour between pages 276 and 277.

tension using the laparoscopic Babcock forceps and the right limb of the mesh is sutured to the serosa of the rectum using 2:0 silk on a curved needle.

Sutures are placed only along the superior and inferior mesh edges. The rectum is then retracted to the right, and the left limb of the mesh brought around the rectum and secured to the rectal wall in a similar fashion at the upper and lower mesh edges. On average two or three sutures are required on either side (Fig. 13c.7). The Szabo–Berci needle holder and Flamingo forceps (Storz Ltd, Germany) are used to facilitate suturing and knot tying.

The stapler is used to re-approximate the peritoneal edges before the operation is completed. The laparoscopic ports are removed, followed by closure of the fascial defects with interrupted sutures. Peri-operative antibiotics are employed in all cases.

Patients and results

We have carried out this procedure on 29 patients. All were carried out by a single surgeon (AD). In one case the laparoscopic procedure had to be converted to open due to difficulty in ventilation. The post-operative course has been uneventful, with rapid resumption of normal bowel function. The mean hospital stay was 5 days (4–15) and early mobility was a marked feature in these patients. The complications included single cases of urinary tract infection, incisional hernia

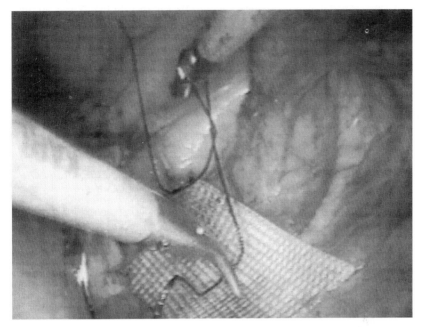

Fig. 13c.7   Mesh being sutured to the side of the rectum using the Szabo–Berci needle holder and Flamingo. This figure is also reproduced in colour between pages 276 and 277.

through a port hole and a large extra-peritoneal haematoma at the port site. The mean follow up to date is 8 months. One patient developed mucosal prolapse at 3 months which required injection with phenol in almond oil.

Discussion

As patients presenting with rectal prolapse are frequently old and infirm, many surgeons have tended to favour the low morbidity, local perineal approaches.[2] Such local procedures include the Thiersch wire, Delorme's plication or a silastic sling around the anal canal.[3] In contrast, some surgeons advocate radical operations such as anterior resection[4] or combined abdomino-perineal pelvic floor repair[5,6] for those patients who are fit to undergo major procedures. Where resection is not indicated others have advocated rectal fixation or rectopexy. Graham[7] was the first to mobilize the rectum down to the levator muscles, a manoeuvre which is still considered the most important element required for a successful outcome. Most currently preferred operative techniques represent a modification of Graham's approach in which fixation procedures are performed on the mobilized rectum. Originally these procedures relied on the use of a polyvinyl alcohol sponge[8] inserted in the presacral space to fix the rectum to the sacrum, or on suturing an inert sling to fix the mobilized rectum to the sacral promontory.

The irritant properties of the sponge help to fix the rectum firmly but predispose to infection. Fixation of an inert polypropylene mesh in front of the rectum was described by Ripstein but this has been associated with acute kinking of the bowel or even intestinal obstruction if too tight.[9] Early experience with these complications has led us to adopt a modification of the procedure whereby the polypropylene mesh is inserted behind the rectum and attached to the sacrum to achieve posterior fixation.

Our own preliminary experience with laparoscopic rectopexy has been encouraging. Early mobilization and discharge from hospital has been a marked feature. Although follow up is short the functional results have been excellent.

Laparoscopic colonic surgery has the same potential benefits as laparoscopic cholecystectomy with potentially a shorter post-operative stay and less post-operative pain. The recent introduction of a commercially available endoscopic stapler for use in laparoscopic hernia repair, and a specifically designed needle holder has provided us with the tools necessary for laparoscopic rectopexy.

Patients with normal bowel habit (or diarrhoea) and no history of constipation or obstructed defaecation are probably ideal candidates for laparoscopic rectopexy without resection, especially if there is no significant redundancy of the sigmoid colon. In patients with massive procidentia, the presence of a large mesorectum and redundant sigmoid will more likely mandate a resective procedure and simple rectopexy should be avoided. As laparoscopic experience increases it may be that those patients requiring resection for rectal prolapse may undergo this procedure laparoscopically. In benign disease such as this, concerns over adequacy of colonic resection margins are not an issue and simple trans-anal delivery of the specimen with subsequent intracorporeal anastomosis may be a suitable option.

Our preliminary experience leads us to suggest that as laparoscopic technology advances and surgical expertise is gained this minimally invasive approach will soon have a major impact on the practice of colorectal surgery. The benefit of such a minimally invasive approach to rectal prolapse becomes especially obvious in the elderly or physiologically disabled patient with prolapse.

References

1. Sackier JM Visualisation of the ureter during laparoscopic colonic resection. *Br J Surg* 1993; **80**: 1332.

2. Goligher JC *Surgery of the Colon, Anus and Rectum*, 4th edn, Baillière Tindall, London, 1980.

3. Jackman FR, Francis JN, Hopkinson BR. Silicon rubber band treatment of rectal prolapse. *Ann R Coll Surg Engl* 1980; **62**: 386–387.

4. Porter NH Collective results of operations for rectal prolapse. *Ann R Coll Surg Engl* 1962; **55**: 1087.

5. Goligher JC. The treatment of complete prolapse of the rectum by the Roscoe Graham operation. *Br J Surg* 1957; **45**: 323–333.

6. Hughes ESR, Gleadell LW. Abdomino-perineal repair of complete prolapse of the rectum. *Proc R Soc Med,* 1962; **55**: 1077–1080.

7. Henry MM. Rectal prolapse. *J Hosp Med* 1980; **24**: 302–307.

8. Wells CA. Polyvinyl-alcohol sponge. An inert plastic for use as a prosthesis in the repair of large hernias. *Br J Surg* 1955; **42**: 618.

9. Miller RL. Ripstein procedure for rectal prolapse. *Am Surg* 1979; **45**: 531–534.

10. Monson JRT, Darzi A, Carey PD, Guillou PJ. Prospective evaluation of laparoscopic assisted colectomy in an unselected group of patients. *Lancet* 1992; **340**: 831–833.

14a

Hernia repair: inguinal hernia

R.C.G. Russell

Introduction

The introduction of laparoscopic surgery has been of the greatest benefit to surgery as a whole. For the first time for many years the surgeon has been allowed to think about technique and discussions on technique have become respectable. What is more, common operations which were of low interest have come to occupy centre stage. The benefit to the patient of this interest will be great. Nowhere is this more important than in the area of laparoscopic hernia repair. The debate about endoscopic surgery becoming the pre-eminent surgical approach will be won or lost around the question of whether or not the endoscopic repair of hernia is better than the traditional open repair. The importance is far greater than is at first apparent. Hernia repair has been the traditional training ground for the surgeon, and is essential for maintaining technical skills as it is the most common general surgical procedure. If the open hernia repair proves preferable, then that skill in endoscopic manipulation will be lost, and without that skill the will to learn and achieve technical endoscopic excellence to apply to other intra-abdominal conditions will be decreased. On the other hand, if hernia repair is advantageous to the patient when performed endoscopically, the skills of dissection, ligating, clipping and suturing will become second nature, and will be rapidly applied in other areas.

The challenge, however, is great. The criteria for efficacy of inguinal hernia repair are recurrence rates, post-operative complications, patient acceptability, pain, time off work, length of hospital stay, and costs. Recent results with the Lichtenstein repair performed as a day case under local anaesthesia show that a 2-year recurrence rate of 0.1 per cent can be achieved, as well as a sepsis rate of 0.4 per cent, 25 per cent having no medication for pain post-operatively, and a mean return to work on day 10 for office workers and day 17 for manual workers.[1] The cost advantage for the operation remains with the open method, and will always do so.

In approaching this debate it is useful to consider the anatomic basis of the hernia repair, the exact procedure performed during traditional open procedures, the laparoscopic techniques and more carefully the comparison between the two methods for hernia repair.

Adult anatomy[2]

The problem in understanding the anatomy of the inguinal canal is that many descriptions have varied from the standard texts, many terms are used, often inaccurately, and the concept of the inguinal canal as a dynamic three-dimensional structure with relationships altering in different body positions is ill understood. It is only since the advent of endoscopic hernia repair that the surgeon has paid attention to the intra-abdominal aspect of the groin.

The inguinal canal is an oblique space measuring 4 cm in length, and extending 2–4 cm above the inguinal ligament between the internal and external openings. The subcutaneous external inguinal ring is a triangular opening in the aponeurosis of the external oblique lateral to and above the pelvic crest. The opening is formed by the two crura, the medial and the lateral, and the lateral is inserted into the pubic tubercle. The deep inguinal ring is an opening in the transversalis fascia, level with the mid-point of the inguinal ligament.

The anterior wall is formed by the aponeurosis of the external oblique muscle and laterally by participation of the internal oblique muscle, which at this point is muscular and not aponeurotic. The superior wall is formed by the internal oblique and transversus abdominis muscles and their aponeuroses, and the inferior wall by the inguinal ligament and lacunar ligament.

The posterior wall is formed by fusion of the aponeuroses of the transversus abdominis muscle and transversalis fascia in 75 per cent, and by only the transversalis fascia in 25 per cent (Fig. 14a.1).

External oblique muscle

The external oblique fascia (innominate fascia of Gallaudet) is a thin tissue like membrane covering the external oblique muscle and aponeurosis. At the superficial ring this fascia forms the intercrural fibres between the crura on its way down to the scrotum as the external spermatic fascia. The external oblique aponeurosis which is formed by a deep superficial layer merges medially with the anterior rectus sheath medial to the lateral border of the rectus muscle. Below, the inguinal ligament (of Poupart) marks the inferior edge of the external oblique aponeurosis. This ligament extends from the anterior superior iliac spine to the pubic tubercle where the lacunar ligament (of Gimbernat) and the reflected inguinal ligament are formed. The inguinal ligament is related to the iliopsoas muscle and its fascia, to the femoral vessels indirectly, to the femoral ring, to the iliopubic tract, and to other thickenings of the transversalis fascia.

The lacunar ligament

The lacunar ligament (Gimbernat's) is formed before the inguinal ligament reaches the pubic tubercle and is a triangular extension of the inguinal ligament;

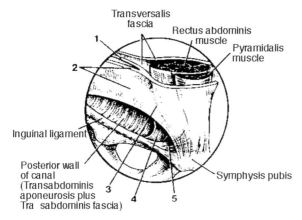

Fig. 14a.1   An idealized view of the inguinal canal: 1 – transversus abdominis
aponeurosis; 2 – inferior fibres of internal oblique, muscular or
aponeurotic; 3 – lateral border of rectus sheath; 4 – reflected inguinal
ligament; 5 – ligament of Henle.

it is inserted at the pecten pubis and its lateral end meets the proximal end of
Cooper's ligament.

Cooper's ligament
Cooper's ligament is the thickened periosteum along the pectineal border of the
superior pubic ramus, and may well be formed with fibres from the tendinous
origin of the pectineus muscle.

Internal oblique and transversus abdominis muscle

McVay[3] regarded this muscle as arising from the iliopsoas muscle fascia; it does
not arise from the inguinal ligament. The muscle is inserted into the anterior
rectus sheath. The fibres do not strengthen the posterior inguinal wall.

Transversus abdominis muscle arises from the iliopsoas fascia, and is inserted
below onto Cooper's ligament and above into the anterior lamina of the rectus
sheath. The integrity of the transversus abdominis muscle prevents the formation
of a hernia.

The conjoint tendon
The conjoint tendon is the fusion of the lower fibres of the internal oblique
aponeurosis with similar fibres from the aponeurosis of the transversus abdominis as they insert into the pubic tubercle and superior ramus of the pubis. This
arrangement is said to exist in only 3 per cent of subjects.[4] Thus, an inguinal
hernia is not repaired with the conjoined tendon, but with the internal oblique
muscle and aponeurosis, the ligament of Henle, the interfoveolar ligament and the
reflected inguinal ligament.

The ligament of Henle
The ligament of Henle is the lateral expansion of the tendon of the rectus abdominis or an expansion of the rectus sheath, which inserts into the pubic bone. This ligament is present in 30–50 per cent of patients and is fused with the transversalis fascia.

The interfoveolar ligament
The interfoveolar ligament (of Hesselbach) is an apparent thickening of the transversalis fascia at the medial end of the internal inguinal ring.

The reflected inguinal ligament
The reflected inguinal ligament is composed of aponeurotic fibres from the inferior crus of the external inguinal ring reaching medially and upward to the linea alba.

Thus, it is preferable to drop the term conjoint tendon in place of *conjoined area* which contains the ligament of Henle, the transversus abdominis aponeurosis, the inferior medial fibres of the internal oblique, the reflected inguinal ligament and the lateral border of the rectus tendon and sheath.

Transversalis fascia
Transversalis fascia is now used to describe the entire connective tissue sheet lining the musculature of the abdominal cavity. It is thin and closely adherent in the portion covering the transversus abdominis aponeurosis, and as such forms an adequate layer for use in hernia repair (Fig. 14a.2).

The intra-abdominal anatomy
Space of Bogros
Fat and other connective tissue lies within a space between the peritoneum and the transversalis fascia, and held in place by the posterior lamina of the transversalis fascia. It is a lateral extension of the retropubic space. Within this space is a venous network composed of the deep inferior epigastric vein, the iliopubic vein, the retropubic vein, and the communicating vein. The importance of these veins is that they bleed during dissection of this space in preparation for the various mesh repairs, such as those performed by Stoppa.[5]

Hesselbach's triangle
Hesselbach's triangle is defined as having the inferior (deep) epigastric vessels as its superior and lateral border, the rectus sheath as its medial border and the inguinal ligament as its lateral and inferior border. Most direct and external hernias occur in this area (Fig. 14a.3).

Fossae of the anterior abdominal wall
Because the endoscopist looks from the inside out, these fossae have become of importance. Located on either side of the midline these fossae are marked by the obliterated embryonic urachus extending from the dome of the bladder to the

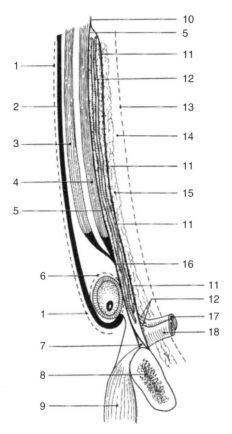

Fig. 14a.2   A vertical section of the abdominal wall at the level of the femoral artery; the space of Bogros: 1 – innominate fascia; 2 – external oblique aponeurosis; 3 – internal oblique muscle; 4 – transversus abdominis muscle; 5 – transversalis fascia anterior; 6 – external spermatic fascia; 7 – Cooper's ligament; 8 – pubic bone; 9 – pectineus muscle; 10 – transversalis fascia; 11 – transversalis fascia posterior lamina; 12 – vessels; 13 – peritoneum; 14 – space of Bogros; 15 – pre-peritoneal fat; 16 – transversus abdominis aponeurosis and anterior; lamina of transversalis fascia; 17 – femoral artery; 18 – femoral vein.

umbilicus (median umbilical ligament). Laterally, the fossae are separated by the medial umbilical ligaments (obliterated umbilical arteries) and the lateral umbilical ligaments (inferior or deep epigastric arteries). The fossae are:

1. The lateral fossae are lateral to the inferior epigastric arteries and contain the internal ring – the site of an indirect inguinal hernia.
2. The medial fossae lie between the inferior epigastric arteries and the medial umbilical ligaments, the site of a direct inguinal hernia.

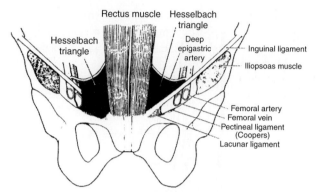

Fig. 14a.3   Stylized view of the anterior abdominal wall from within.

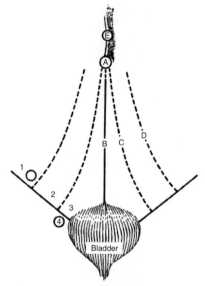

Fig. 14a.4   Diagram of the fossae of the abdominal wall and their relation to the sites of groin hernias: A – umbilicus; B – median umbilical ligament (obliterated urachus); C – medial umbilical ligament (obliterated umbilical arteries); D – lateral umbilical ligament containing inferior (deep) epigastric arteries; E – falciform ligament; 1 – lateral fossa (site of indirect inguinal hernia); 2 – medial fossa (site of direct inguinal hernia); 3 – supravesical fossa (site of supravesical hernia); 4 – femoral ring (site of femoral hernia).

3. The supravesical fossae lie between the medial and median umbilical ligaments, the site of an external supravesical hernia.

Thus a hernia through either the medial or the supravesical fossa is a direct hernia and in Hesselbach's triangle (Fig. 14a.4).

Myopectineal orifice

Myopectineal orifice is a weak area bounded by the internal oblique muscle, the transversus abdominis muscle, iliopsoas muscle, rectus muscle and sheath and the pubis. Through this area pass all direct hernias. Thus, a direct hernia will pass through Hesselbach's triangle, the medial fossa, the space of Bogros, a defect in the transversalis fascia and aponeurosis and the myopectineal orifice before breaking out through the posterior inguinal wall into clinical awareness. It is the plethora of names and concepts that has led to such anatomical confusion amongst clinicians whose knowledge of anatomy continues to decrease.

Pathophysiology

The integrity of the abdominal wall is dependent on the oblique orientation of the inguinal canal, the sphincter-like structure of the internal ring and the transversalis fascia. Development of a groin hernia depends on numerous factors. Obesity, obstructive pulmonary airways disease, hyperplasia of the prostate, ascites, pregnancy, constipation and colonic stenosis each predispose to chronically raised intra-abdominal pressure. The increase in incidence with age points to alteration of collagen metabolism as a possible cause for weakening of the fascial structures. Other factors include loss of fat with age, an insufficiency of the sphincter mechanism of the internal ring and the presence of a processus vaginalis.[6] The pampiniform plexus serves as an additional plug during straining. Rarely if ever is the cause trauma or strenuous physical activity. Although the aetiology remains unknown, it is presumed that an inguinal hernia is due to one or more of the above factors together with an individual predisposition.[7]

Clinical approach

Classification

The results of hernia repair are clearly related to the location and size of the fascial defect. For example, the risk of recurrence in a large direct hernia is at least five times as high as in a small indirect hernia. In order to compare results of hernia repair, it is necessary to have a precise and uniform terminology to make clinical studies reproducible and comparable. Nyhus[8] introduced a classification of four different types (Table 14a.1). An alternative classification is that of Gilbert[9] in which types I–III are differentiated by the size of the internal ring, and type IV and V are direct hernias differentiated by the size of the posterior wall defect.

Diagnosis

Most inguinal hernias can be diagnosed by palpation; however, even an experienced surgeon cannot easily distinguish a direct from an indirect hernia. In patients who report symptoms but do not have appropriate signs, sonography

Table 14a.1   Classification of inguinal hernias[8] (Nyhus)

Type I	Indirect hernias in which the internal abdominal ring is of normal size, configuration and structure.
Type II	Indirect hernias in which the internal ring is enlarged and distorted without impinging on the floor of the inguinal canal.
Type IIIa	Direct hernia in which the protrusion does not herniate through the internal ring. *All direct hernias are of this type.*
Type IIIb	Indirect hernias which have expanded medially and encroach on the posterior inguinal wall.
Type IV	Recurrent hernias – may be direct (A), indirect (B), or femoral (C), or a combination of these types (D).

is indicated. With ultrasound examination in the supine and upright positions supported by a Valsalva manoeuvre, an inguinal hernia can be diagnosed in 90 per cent of instances.[10] In rare cases of inguinal pain without clinical or sonographic findings, computed tomography is indicated to rule out an obturator hernia. Finally, herniography, or even resorting to laparoscopy, may be of value excluding a hernial sac.

Indications for surgery

Generally, the diagnosis of a groin hernia implies surgical repair. The only exceptions are terminally ill patients with hernias not complicated by incarceration or strangulation. It is widely accepted that direct hernias, especially those presenting as broad direct bulges, are ten times less prone to strangulation than indirect hernias. Indeed the Royal College of Surgeons of England guidelines suggested that these direct 'bulges', if asymptomatic did not require operation.[10] (These 'bulges' are not to be confused with Malgaigne's bulges, which are not hernias at all.) Nevertheless, if there is doubt that the hernia is or is not direct, operation should be advised, especially in patients over 65 years as incarceration and strangulation are more common in this group of patients.

Assessment of surgical results

Criteria for assessing hernia repair are safety (absence of morbidity and mortality), convenience for the patient (day case, absence of pain, mobility, return to work) and recurrence rate. The average recurrence rate is about 10 per cent after a primary hernia repair and more than 20 per cent after repair of recurrent hernias. Most published studies are unreliable because of one of the following deficits:

1. Inadequate length of follow-up: about 40 per cent of recurrences appear within the first year, but 35 per cent are discovered as late as five or more years after operation.
2. Patients lost to follow-up: dissatisfied patients move to another surgeon.
3. Unreliable methods of follow-up: up to 50 per cent of patients are unaware of recurrence, hence a telephone follow-up is inadequate.

Complications

Any procedure performed for inguinal hernia must have a low complication rate. The fact that 80,000 hernias are repaired annually in the United Kingdom and around 500,000 in the United States of America implies that any debilitating problem would have long-term implications. Elective hernia repair carries a mortality rate of less than 0.01 per cent, but the risk of a fatal outcome can be as high as 5 per cent in emergency procedures, and if bowel resection is required in those over 80 years, the mortality rate climbs to 20 per cent.

With local anaesthesia, and immediate post-operative mobilization, the commonest complication is haematoma. The frequency of infection is about 1.2 per cent, irrespective of whether prosthetic meshes or antibiotics are used.[11] Specific complications are associated with injuries to nerves and vessels of spermatic cord. Entrapment of the ilioinguinal or genitofemoral nerve is followed by a distinct neuralgia syndrome. Genitofemoral neuropathy results in pain and paraesthesia from the inguinal region to the scrotum and upper thigh. The ilioinguinal syndrome is characterized by pain and paraesthesia with extension to the back. Resection of the nerve is the only treatment.

A painful swelling of the testis within two days of the operation indicates the onset of an ischaemic orchitis. Remission is spontaneous in 60 per cent of cases while the remainder progress to testicular atrophy.

The incidence and consequences of these complications must be taken into account when the balance is weighed between merits and disadvantages of a particular procedure.

Surgical procedure

When considering a surgical procedure, it is wise to define the exact operation which is performed, so that it can be compared to the new laparoscopic approaches.

The open technique

Bassini repair
The Bassini repair was described in 1884,[12] and involved the division and suture of the transversalis fascia and aponeurosis; but all three layers, namely, the transversalis fascia, transversus muscle and the internal oblique muscle were sutured with a single layer of interrupted non-absorbable material. As the technique entered common use, the importance of the division of the transversalis fascia was neglected and only the internal oblique muscle was sutured to the inguinal ligament. Even when the traditional technique is employed, the results are not as good as the Shouldice technique; namely a recurrence rate of 10.4 per cent at 30 months compared with 3 per cent for the Shouldice procedure.[13]

Shouldice repair

The Shouldice repair was introduced in 1945 and has been the only procedure practised at the Shouldice Clinic in Toronto, so that by 1992, 200,000 operations for hernia had been performed.[14] In a study of 6000 hernia repairs with a minimum follow-up of 10 years the recurrence rate was 0.6 per cent.[15] Despite this low rate of recurrence in the hands of the Clinic, it has been less well done by the generality of surgeons, with a recurrence rate of up to 6 per cent.[16]

The technique consists of herniotomy with clearing of the cremasteric fibres from the cord, division of the transversalis fascia to the pubic tubercle, and suture of the posterior wall in four layers using polypropylene. The lower leaf of the cut transversalis fascia is sutured to the undersurface of the transversus aponeurosis as a continuous suture to the internal ring; the suture continues medially to the pubic tubercle taking the upper leaf to the front of the lower leaf adjacent to the inguinal ligament. With the same suture the internal oblique is sutured to the inguinal ligament in two layers without tension. The external oblique is finally plicated in front of the cord to complete the inguinal canal (Fig. 14a.5).

The nylon darn

The nylon darn is probably still the most common repair performed in the United Kingdom. It was introduced by Maloney[17] and has the advantage of being rapidly and easily taught, but with the disadvantage of a recurrence rate in the region of 10–15 per cent.

The sac is dissected from the surrounding structures, opened, ligated and divided. The posterior wall is not divided but plicated with nylon. The repair is undertaken with a tension free interlocking darn between the internal oblique and the inguinal ligament. The external oblique is closed in a single layer.

The mesh repair

Perhaps the most important development in hernia repair has been the acceptance of non-absorbable mesh as a safe, risk free, and effective method of repairing the posterior abdominal wall. The technique of using mesh in the preperitoneal position was conceived by Stoppa in France.[5] He has shown the mesh to be safe and trouble free in the long term.

Lichtenstein in the United States has pioneered the use of mesh from the anterior approach.[18,19] The technique has the merit of great simplicity. Under a local anaesthetic block, the inguinal canal is opened and the hernia identified. If there is an indirect sac, it is opened and the inguinal canal assessed with a finger. The sac is simply inverted into the abdomen without excision, suture or ligature. A sheet of prosthetic mesh is fashioned measuring 5 × 10 cm. The lower edge is tacked in place by a continuous prolene suture which secures the mesh medially to the lacunar ligament and then proceeds laterally along the inguinal ligament beyond the internal ring. A slit in the mesh at the internal ring allows emergence of the spermatic cord. The superior edge of the mesh is loosely secured by a similar continuous suture to the rectus sheath and internal oblique above. A single suture approximates the tails of the mesh to the inguinal ligament lateral to the internal ring. The external oblique is sutured in front of the cord (Fig. 14a.6).

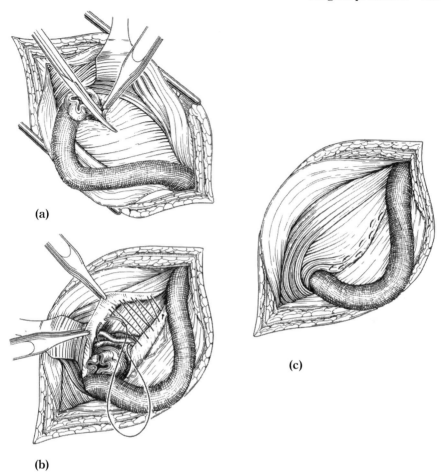

(a)

(b)

(c)

Fig. 14a.5   The Shouldice repair: (a) – division of the transversalis fascia; (b) – plicating the transversalis fascia; (c) – completion of the transversalis fascia suture.

In an experience of 4000 operations, there has only been one major complication, a case of orchitis. There has been no neuralgia or seroma. Only four recurrences have been encountered.[20] Results with this operation are impressive and bring out into the open the debate of whether a laparoscopic approach is justified.

The laparoscopic method

Ligation of the sac
In 1982 Ger described the repair of inguinal hernias during major abdominal surgery.[21] The sac was left undisturbed and the peritoneal opening closed by

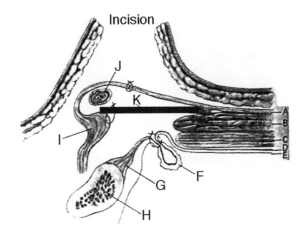

Fig. 14a.6 The Lichtenstein repair – sagittal view of the completed repair: A – External oblique aponeurosis; B – Internal oblique muscle; C – Transversus aponeurosis; D – Transversalis fascia; E – Peritoneum; F – Inverted direct sac; G – Cooper's ligament; H – Pubis; I – Inguinal ligament; J – Spermatic cord; K – Mesh patch bridging defect.

2–10 interrupted stainless steel clips. The procedure was successful in 11 of the 12 patients followed-up for 26–44 months. The success of the method led to the development of a laparoscopic technique using a specially designed clip applier for closing the neck of the sac. This approach was used in one patient with a right inguinal hernia; it is the first reported case of laparoscopic treatment for a hernia. Using a slightly different technique, Mann *et al.* reported 20 laparoscopic repairs for indirect hernias in 19 young patients (mean age 22 years) ligating the neck with an endoloop. There were no recurrences after 1–22 months.[22]

These techniques have been largely abandoned in favour of the preperitoneal approach. Nyhus type I and II hernias should be managed by a herniotomy using an anterior open approach with or without closing of the transversalis fascia; the laparoscopic approach is not appropriate.

Plug technique

Using a transperitoneal approach the musculofascial defect is identified, and a prosthetic mesh is placed into the defect to obliterate the space, and the edges of the peritoneum re-approximated. In a series of 100 hernia repairs, there were 8 recurrent hernias in the first 50 repairs followed for 1–28 months. Six were direct and two indirect. The authors have now abandoned this technique and use a preperitoneal mesh.[23] It is no longer acceptable to use plugs in hernia repair laparoscopically as the results have been poor, but the Lichtenstein group continue to use a plug as part of their repair for recurrent hernias.[19]

Patch technique

Three types have been described; *intraperitoneal* where the patch is applied directly onto the peritoneum within the peritoneal cavity; *pre-peritoneal* where the peritoneum is opened over the inguinal region and the patch placed over the musculofascial defect followed by closure of the peritoneum; and *extraperitoneal* where the pre-peritoneal space is entered in the lower midline and dissected down to the inguinal region, the patch being introduced into and applied within the pre-peritoneal space.

Intraperitoneal The first laparoscopic inguinal hernia repair was performed by Popp, during a myomectomy.[24] He used three interrupted sutures to narrow the internal ring and then placed a patch of dehydrated dura mater over the repair, fixing it to the peritoneum with seven catgut sutures. Fitzgibbons (Filipi *et al.*) has been the main proponent of the intraperitoneal method,[25] suggesting that a prosthesis would be rapidly peritonealized and that such positioning would avoid the need for extensive pre-peritoneal dissection. Further, the mesh would be easier to position so that larger mesh coverage could be achieved to ensure support for the weak area of the abdominal wall. Despite considerable experience and some good results, the main disadvantage of this technique is that small bowel becomes adherent to the mesh, and intestinal obstruction occurs. For this reason, the technique has been abandoned and indeed should not be performed.

Pre-peritoneal or TAPP procedure The pre-peritoneal or TAPP procedure was developed by Arregui *et al.*[26] The hernial sac was excised at its neck and the pre-peritoneal space entered through the defect. Blunt dissection was used to separate the pre-peritoneal fat and peritoneum from the fascia transversalis, epigastric vessels and spermatic cord, Cooper's ligament, iliopubic tract, rectus muscle, transversus abdominis aponeurotic arch and the fascia transversalis lateral to the internal ring. This is a wide area and an extensive dissection, but it is critical to the successful treatment of hernia by this pre-peritoneal and retroperitoneal route. In indirect hernias, the internal ring was tightened using an absorbable suture and in direct or recurrent hernias the fascia transversalis was loosely sutured in order to prevent fluid gathering in the empty sac, thereby creating a bulge like the original hernia. This bulge takes several weeks to resolve and is disturbing to the patient. Non-absorbable polypropylene mesh (5×10 cm) was fashioned to fit over the inguinal and femoral areas overlapping the ring laterally, Cooper's ligament inferiorly, the pubic tubercle medially, and the transversus abdominis aponeurotic arch superiorly. The mesh is laid as a complete sheet over the femoral vessels as well as the testicular vessels and spermatic cord. The mesh was anchored with three absorbable sutures to the fascia transversalis and transversus abdominis aponeurotic arch superomedially, the iliopubic tract or Cooper's ligament inferomedially, and the fascia transversalis and transversus abdominis lateral to the internal ring. The peritoneum was closed over the mesh with absorbable suture (Fig. 14a.7).

Alternative techniques have used staples, often in large number to position the mesh, and initial experience was based on the use of a small mesh. The lessons learnt with this technique are the need to place a large mesh, to suture with as few sutures as possible, and to maintain the position of the mesh as the pneumoperitoneum is evacuated. It is essential to close the peritoneum to minimize adhesion formation and the possibility of intestinal obstruction. Finally, care must be taken to close the abdominal wall defect at the site of the ports.

Typical of the results achieved with the transabdominal pre-peritoneal approach (TAPP) are those of Royston from England[27] and Geis *et al.* from

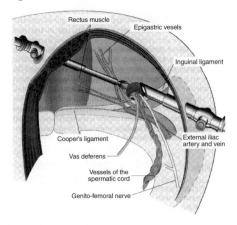

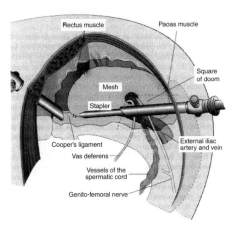

Fig. 14a.7   (a) The laparoscopic view of an indirect inguinal hernia; (b) The mesh in place and the positioning of staples. No staple should be placed in the 'square of doom' for fear of damaging vital structures.

Chicago.[28] The former presented a series of 409 repairs: 94 per cent were discharged from hospital within 24 hours, 54 patients (15 per cent) had minor complications such as fluid collections (23), spontaneously resolving testicular pain (9), and nerve pain (11), while seven patients had major complications such as urinary retention (5), small bowel obstruction (2), port site hernia (1) and mesh infection (1). Convalescent time was short (return to work at 12 (2–95) days). Three recurrences have been noted at a median time of 7 months. In the Chicago experience of 450 procedures there were similar results but no intestinal or mesh-related complications occurred.

Extraperitoneal   The extraperitoneal technique was pioneered by Kerman in order to overcome the disadvantages of the transperitoneal approach with its possible complications affecting the intraperitoneal structures. It is discussed at length in the next chapter. Experience with the technique has emphasized the points learned with the transabdominal approach, namely careful dissection, a large mesh and avoidance of staples. In expert hands the results are good.

Conclusion

The advantages of the laparoscopic approach are that it is more comfortable for the patient, the post-operative pain is less and the return to full activities and work is quicker,[29] but the comparison with the Lichtenstein approach has yet to be submitted to a controlled trial. It is probable, but not yet documented, that the recurrence rates will be similar. The argument will centre around cost and complications. The procedure will inevitably be more expensive as the technology employed is more expensive than that used by the open techniques. Nevertheless this may be an acceptable price to pay for the improved comfort.[30] The major debate will revolve around the incidence of major and even life threatening complications which can occur with the laparoscopic technique, namely, damage to the intra-abdominal structures with perforation, obstruction and even strangulation of the bowel. There is no doubt that the expert will reduce these complications to an acceptable level, but most hernias are not repaired by experts, and the occasional hernia surgeon will undoubtedly have problems with the laparoscopic technique. Perhaps the answer is that all hernias should be done by hernia experts in laparoscopic institutes. Until that Utopian day arrives, the position for today is clear, namely that hernias in patients under the age of 50 should be repaired by the open approach using the Shouldice technique, on the basis that it is better to avoid foreign material in the younger patient, but in the patient over 50 using a Lichtenstein mesh repair. Such a policy will ensure effective treatment with low cost, and minimal chance of any major intra-abdominal event which is life-threatening. Any such incident is an unacceptable risk in the management of a minor surgical condition.

References

1. Kark AE, Kurzer M, Waters KJ. Laparoscopic hernia repair [letter]. *Lancet* 1994; **344**: 54.
2. Skandalakis JE, Colborn GL, Androulakis JA, Skandalakis LJ, Pemberton LB. Embryologic and anatomic basis of inguinal herniorrhaphy. *Surg Clin N Am* 1993; **73**: 799–836.
3. McVay CD. *Surgical anatomy*, 6th edn, WB Saunders, Philadelphia 1984, pages 484–584.
4. Condon RE. The anatomy of the inguinal region and its relationship to groin hernia. In: Nyhus LM, Condon RE, (eds) *Hernia*, 2nd edn, JB Lippincott, Philadelphia, 1978, pages 14–78.
5. Stoppa RE, Rives JL, Warlamont CR, *et al.* The use of dacron in the repair of hernias of the groin. *Surg Clin N Am* 1984; **64**: 269–285.
6. Hahn-Pedersen J, Lund L, Hansen Hojhus J, Bojsen-Moller F. Evaluation of direct and indirect inguinal hernia by computed tomography. *Br J Surg* 1994; **81**: 569–572.
7. Schumpelick V, Treutner KH, Arlt G. Inguinal hernia repair in adults. *Lancet* 1994; **344**: 375–379.

8. Nyhus LM. Individualisation of hernia repair: a new era. *Surg* 1993; **114**: 1–2.
9. Gilbert A. An anatomic and functional classification for the diagnosis and treatment of inguinal hernia. *Am J Surg* 1989; **157**: 331–333.
10. Clinical guidelines on the management of groin hernia in adults. London, Royal College of Surgeons of England, July 1993.
11. Gilbert AI, Felton II. Infection of inguinal hernia repair considering biomaterials and antibiotics. *Surg* 1993; **177**: 126–130.
12. Bassini E. Ueber die behandlung des Liestenbruches. *Arch Klin Chir* 1890; **40**: 429–476.
13. Kux M, Fuchsjäger N, Schemper M. Shouldice is superior to Bassini inguinal herniorrhaphy. *Am J Surg* 1994; **168**: 15–18.
14. Bendavid R. The rational use of mesh in hernia repairs. A perspective. *Int Surg* 1992; **77**: 229–231.
15. Glassow F. Inguinal hernia repair using local anaesthesia. *Ann R Coll Surg Engl* 1984; **66**: 382–387.
16. Kingsnorth AN, Gray MR, Nott DM. Prospective randomised trial comparing the Shouldice technique and plication darn for inguinal hernia. *Br J Surg* 1992; **79**: 1068–1070.
17. Maloney GD. Darning inguinal hernias. *Arch Surg* 1972; **184**: 129.
18. Lichtenstein IL, Shulman AG, Amid AP, Montllor MM. The tension-free hernioplasty. *Am J Surg* 1989; **157**: 188–193.
19. Shulman AG, Amid PK, Lichtenstein IL. Patch or plug for groin hernia – which? *Am J Surg* 1994; **167**: 331–336.
20. Amid PK, Shulman AG, Lichtenstein IL. A critical comparison of laparoscopic hernia repair with Lichtenstein tension-free hernioplasty. *Med J Austr* 1994; **161**: 239–240.
21. Ger R. The management of certain abdominal herniae by intra-abdominal closure of the neck of the sac. Preliminary communication. *Ann R Coll Surg Engl* 1982; **64**: 342–344.
22. Mann DV, Hershman MJ, Rosin RD. Laparoscopic inguinal hernia repair [abstract]. Third International meeting of the Society of Minimally Invasive Surgery, Boston, Mass, 1991.
23. Schultz L, Graber J, Pietrafitta J, Hickok D. Laser laparoscopic herniorrhaphy: a clinical trial. Preliminary results. *J Laparoendosc Surg* 1990; **1**: 41–45.
24. Popp LW. Endoscopic patch repair of inguinal hernia in a female patient. *Surg Endosc* 1990; **4**: 10–12.
25. Filipi CJ, Fitzgibbons RJ, Salerno CM, Hat RO. Laparoscopic herniorrhaphy. *Surg Clin N Am* 1992; **72**: 1109–1114.
26. Arregui ME, Davis CJ, Yucel O, Nagan RF. Laparoscopic mesh repair of inguinal hernia using a preperitoneal approach. A preliminary report. *Surg Laparosc Endosc* 1992; **2**: 51–53.
27. Milkins RC, Lansdown MJR, Wedgwood KR, Brough WA, Royston CMS. Laparoscopic hernia repair: a prospective study of 409 cases. *Min Inv Ther* 1993; **2**: 237–242.
28. Geis WP, Crafton WB, Novak MJ. Laparoscopic herniorrhaphy: Results and technical aspects in 450 consecutive procedures. *Surg* 1993; **114**: 765–774.
29. Stoker DL, Spiegelhalter DJ, Sing R, Wellwood JM. Laparoscopic versus open inguinal hernia repair: randomised prospective trial. *Lancet* 1994; **343**: 1243–1245.
30. Notaras MJ. Laparoscopic hernia repair [letter]. *Lancet* 1994; **344**: 54–55.

14b

Hernia repair: extraperitoneal laparoscopic inguinal hernia repair

S.S. Mudan, H. Gajraj and R.S. Taylor

Background

Laparoscopic hernia repair is now increasingly widely practised throughout Europe and in the United States. Acceptance of the concept has been much slower in the United Kingdom and many surgeons remain unconvinced of the superiority of the method when compared with well-established conventional open techniques. The reasons against a more general acceptance are said to be:

1. Availability of excellent conventional open techniques.
2. Increased complication rate.
3. Unknown recurrence rate.
4. Requirement for a general anaesthetic.
5. Technical difficulty (longer learning curve for extraperitoneal approach).

Some of these considerations are based more on prejudice than fact and will be addressed briefly below.

Recurrence rates

If open herniorrhaphy is as successful as many claim, it might be asked why such a wide variety of repairs have already been described and continue to be described. Although excellent long-term recurrence rates of 3 per cent and less for primary hernia repair have been reported these are largely from specialized centres and cannot be considered as representative of overall results. They are also open to the criticism that often not all the patients are examined, they are not always followed up for a sufficient period and it is recognized that around 50 per cent of patients with recurrent hernias are unaware of them.[1] In Britain, where tradition employs hernia repair as a vehicle for basic surgical training, there is increasing evidence that the realistic recurrence rate for primary hernias is at least 15 per cent at five years. The experience is probably not much different in Europe[2] or Canada.[3] A study of papers randomly selected from presentations at three recent International meetings showed that between 7 and 35 per cent of patients having laparoscopic hernia repair were for recurrences after open repair. The recurrence rates for open repair of recurrent hernias are even more alarming.[4]

One explanation of these findings may be that a large number of surgeons are still employing 'modifications' of established techniques which bear no resemblance to the original descriptions. As Bendavid[4] has aptly stated 'corruption of well established operative procedures represents probably the single most important sin committed by (hernia) surgeons'.

The results of the 'tension free' open mesh repairs are better even in inexpert hands and perhaps represent a fairer standard to which laparoscopic repair should be compared.[5,6] While 40 to 50 per cent of recurrences after conventional open operations do not appear until 15 or more years post-operatively, this is not the case for the mesh repairs where most recurrences present within the first six months.[1] It seems probable that the same situation will apply to laparoscopic mesh repair so that the definitive recurrence rate will soon declare itself. Early data for the equivalent transperitoneal laparoscopic procedures indicate recurrence rates of 1.7 per cent[7] despite the inclusion of many repairs of open recurrences. These are very encouraging results and bettered only by the figure of less than 0.5 per cent recurrence rate for the entirely extraperitoneal laparoscopic technique.[8]

In this context it is important to remember that a new and developing procedure still only a little way along the 'learning curve' is being compared with well-established techniques. It is interesting to note that the Shouldice clinic reported a recurrence rate of 17 per cent in 1945 falling to only 1 per cent by 1950 and it may well be that this target can be more readily achieved with laparoscopic repair even for recurrent hernias.

Complications _____

The incidence of complications which have been reported for laparoscopic repair[9] has been perceived by many as being much higher than for open repair. To a large extent this is a misconception and there is no doubt that the complications of open hernia repair in everyday surgical practice are much higher than generally thought.[10] Problems relate largely to haematoma formation, infection, testicular atrophy and neuralgias. Nerve injury is the commonest problem and occurs in 10–15 per cent of patients after primary hernia repair with an even higher incidence for recurrent hernias.[10,11] This complication is much less common in laparoscopic procedures, most often involves the lateral cutaneous nerve of the thigh and almost certainly relates to inappropriate staple placement (see below).

Testicular atrophy has not been reported, but scrotal haematomata may be as frequent as 5 per cent particularly if extensive dissection of the indirect sac is always carried out. Infection is exceedingly rare even in the transperitoneal procedure.[8] Further details are beyond the scope of this chapter, but are readily obtained from the already quite extensive literature on the subject.

Recovery and patient satisfaction

To date there have been very few randomized controlled prospective studies comparing open against laparoscopic hernia repair in terms of patient satisfaction and rapidity of recovery. Those available are small series, but have been favourable to laparoscopic repair in terms of reduced post-operative pain[12,13] and early resumption of normal working activity within 7–10 days.[14,15,16] In contrast some 20 per cent of manual workers and 16 per cent of office workers have an ongoing work disability following the Lichtenstein open mesh repair.[6] The average period off work for non-mesh procedures is 7 weeks[17] and written recommendations from one of the foremost British day case units advises waiting 10 weeks before returning to heavy work.

General or local anaesthetic, in-patient or day case

In the United Kingdom hernia repair under local anaesthesia has still failed to achieve widespread popularity (less than 10 per cent) despite some enthusiastic reports and encouragement by the hospital authorities.

For day cases local anaesthesia is not without complications and there seems little reason to avoid a general anaesthetic except for those patients who represent a high risk. It is tempting to suggest that perhaps surgeon satisfaction exceeds patient satisfaction and that this accounts for the unpopularity of the technique in the public perception. Certainly some recent reports have indicated that recovery is by no means as uneventful as is sometimes claimed and in a series of 35 patients 74 per cent would have preferred in-patient treatment while half experienced considerably more pain than they had expected.[18] There is also a significant incidence of wound complications identified (28 per cent) when community surveillance is included in the follow-up.[19]

The American figure of around 60–80 per cent for day cases may well be more insurance company- rather than patient-dictated and evidence from the Royal College of Surgeons of England[20] suggests that only up to one-third of hernia patients are suitable for day case treatment. However, in our own unit, with a dedicated day case facility we have been able to increase the percentage of day case hernia repairs from 10 to over 70 in a period of five years using a laparoscopic approach.

Reviewing all the available evidence on conventional hernia repair it is quite clear that there is no room for complacency about the present situation and, in view of the now well proven benefits of laparoscopic cholecystectomy, it seems entirely reasonable to continue to investigate the extension of laparoscopic techniques for hernia repair.

Technical considerations

Following initial unsatisfactory experience with various techniques including ring closure,[21] sac ligation, plugging[22] and application of small patches,[23] the techniques of laparoscopic hernia repair have evolved considerably in parallel with experience and the surgical equipment. The majority of surgeons now use a transabdominal approach for the placement of a pre-peritoneal patch (TAPP) with a lesser number using a totally extraperitoneal approach (TEPP) and only a few the intraperitoneal onlay mesh repair (IPOM).

Common to all techniques is the establishment of a tension-free repair by the placement of a patch to cover the entire groin area including the indirect, direct and femoral hernia sites, thus completely reinforcing Fruchaud's myopectineal orifice.[24,25] The effectiveness of this type of repair, first described in 1920 by Cheatle[26] has been well-established by the open operations of Nyhus[27] and Stoppa.[28] The laparoscopic-assisted insertion of a prosthetic patch mimics this and can, therefore, be considered as a new way of performing an old operation rather than a wholly new procedure. Critics would argue that the average size of the patch employed laparoscopically does not start to compare with that, for example, of Stoppa. However, this argument does not stand close examination since a large portion of his patch is clearly designed to protect the open incision from herniation and is situated well away from actual or potential inguinal defects. Furthermore, the results of the laparoscopic patch procedures are at least as good as any open patch procedure. Indeed, it is possible to insert a much bigger patch with the extraperitoneal approach than either the open or transperitoneal methods due to the greater availability of space.

Technique of the totally extraperitoneal laparoscopic hernia repair

Patient selection and information

At present we have no strict exclusion criteria with the exception of unsuitability for a general anaesthetic. In keeping with the French opinion, age and previous lower abdominal surgery are not necessarily regarded as contraindications.[29] Most of our patients are entered into an ongoing trial of open tension-free mesh repair (Lichtenstein) against extraperitoneal laparoscopic repair. This is carefully explained to the patients in the outpatient clinic and upon admission for surgery they are randomized to one of the two groups. Unless there are specific medical or social contraindications all patients are informed that they can expect to be discharged the same day.

Prophylaxis

Deep venous thrombosis prophylaxis is achieved through the use of pneumatic calf compression and for high risk patients subcutaneous heparin is administered. A single dose of a broad spectrum antibiotic is given peroperatively, although there is no controlled trial evidence to show that omitting this increases the infection rate.

Patient preparation

Prior to arrival in the operating theatre care must be taken to ensure that the patient has an empty bladder. We do not routinely pass a catheter since this resulted in some problems of urinary retention early in our experience and is unnecessary except for recurrent and femoral hernias. The procedure is performed under general anaesthesia with the patient supine on the operating table and the head end tilted slightly downward. The operating surgeon usually stands on the side opposite to the hernia with his assistant and the scrub nurse directly opposite. Some surgeons (including the senior author) prefer to reverse this arrangement and operate from the same side, thereby avoiding the requirement to reach across the patient when manipulating two instruments. The television monitor is placed at the foot of the table. The abdomen is examined to ensure that the bladder is not palpable and the skin prepared from the xiphoid cartilage to the groin and including the penis and scrotum.

Creation of the retroperitoneal space

The extraperitoneal approach is made possible by the fact that the peritoneum in the suprapubic region can be easily separated from the anterior abdominal wall, thereby creating sufficient space to enable dissection of the hernial sac and the insertion of a mesh. Several methods can be used to develop this space and the following is a largely personal account of our experience with a variety of techniques.

The authors' preferred method is based on that described by Dulucq.[30,31] In this approach the Verres needle is first inserted in the midline just above the pubis. Slight resistance is felt as it penetrates the anterior rectus sheath (linea alba) and the needle need only be inserted a little further to enter the suprapubic space of Retzius (Fig. 14b.1). With the CO_2 turned on at a pressure of 10–12 mmHg and maximal flow, the needle is then manipulated gently in all directions until flow is achieved and approximately 1.5 litres are insufflated. On occasions it can be quite difficult to start the CO_2 flowing, usually due to the needle being situated too deeply, but this becomes easier with practice.

Next a small transverse or vertical (according to individual surgical preference) sub-umbilical incision as described by McKernan[8] is made down to the level of the

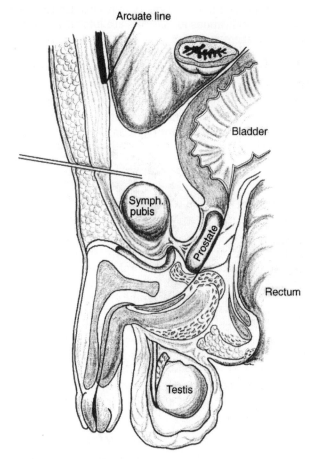

Fig. 14b.1   The Verres needle can be seen penetrating the linea alba and extending into the space of Retzius. Development of the pre-peritoneal space is already well advanced.

anterior rectus sheath which is incised just lateral to the linea alba on the ipsilateral side to the hernia. The medial edge of the rectus muscle is then retracted laterally just enough to permit the passage of a 10 mm trocar which is directed towards the pubis in a situation deep to the rectus muscle, but superficial to the posterior rectus sheath. Dulucq differs in that he passes the trocar subcutaneously to a point roughly on a level with the anterior superior iliac spine where it is angled to point 60° downwards towards the sacrum and, with a well-controlled push, penetrates through the fused midline layers of the transversalis fascia into the newly created operating space. The gas supply is connected to this cannula at a pressure of about 10 mmHg and the laparoscope inserted.

Both techniques run the risk of tearing the periotoneum particularly if the gas dissection has been inadequate. This problem can be avoided by opening the posterior rectus sheath just below the umbilicus and inserting a blunt trocar into the space between the peritoneum and the posterior rectus sheath. This does not present any great difficulties, but the plane is best developed initially by finger dissection rather than blindly and must be slightly to the side of the midline. This approach has the advantage that a wider field of view is obtained and subsequent lateral dissection is easier without the restrictions of the posterior rectus sheath. Whichever method is employed the procedure is facilitated by the use of a laparoscope with an operating channel.

The space can also be expeditiously developed using a balloon dissector. Two currently available models are the GSI Spacemaker Balloon Dissector (General Surgical Innovations Inc., Portola Valley, CA) and the Origin Balloon (Origin Medsystems Inc., Menlo Park, CA). The latter is transparent and has the advantage of enabling direct vision with the telescope within the balloon whilst inflation and dissection are proceeding. Both instruments may save a little time, but have the drawback of incurring significant additional fixed expenditure. There are two further potential problems common to the balloons. Firstly the inferior epigastric vessels may be dissected off the anterior abdominal wall or secondly the fibres of the rectus muscle can be split. The authors are presently experimenting with a much simpler balloon of our own prototype.

A fundamental and important difference we have noted between the McKernan approach with or without balloon assistance, and the Dulucq technique is the exact plane into which the telescope enters. With the former technique the telescope lies superficial to the posterior lamina of the transversalis fascia[31] (Fig. 14b.2). The trocar in the Dulucq approach pierces the posterior lamina of the transversalis fascia to enter the true pre-peritoneal space and thus is one layer closer to the peritoneum and hernia sac (Fig. 14b.3). This posterior lamina is very variable in density and, if thick, subsequent identification of the anatomy and dissection of the sac is much simpler with the Dulucq approach. We find his method perfectly satisfactory and upon entry the telescopic view consists of fine arachnoid connections between the outer surface of the peritoneum and the deep surface of the transversalis fascia. The telescope is advanced slowly sweeping from side-to-side against the posterior surface of the anterior abdominal wall until

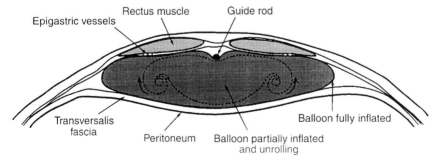

Fig. 14b.2   The diagram of a Spacemaker Balloon inflated *in situ* showing its location between the epigastric vessels and the posterior lamina of the fascia transversalis. (By permission of Radcliffe Medical Press[31])

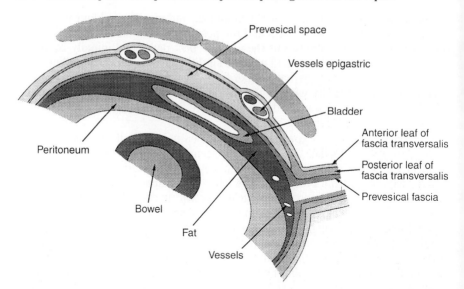

Fig. 14b.3   Schematic diagram of lower abdominal wall showing the relationship of the various layers at the internal ring. By the Dulucq approach a working space is created as shown in this figure – the prevesical space. Through the McKernan approach the working space is created between the two layers of the transversalis fascia, i.e. immediately deep to the inferior epigastric vessels.

the pubis is reached (and easily felt) and the reflective white of Cooper's ligament seen. Alternatively, this dissection can be carried out using a Lahey swab inserted through the second midline trocar.

Demonstration of the anatomy, trocar placement and dissection technique

Excellent descriptions of the detailed anatomy as seen through a laparoscope are available[32,33] and merit very careful study by the aspiring hernia laparoscopist. Fig. 14b.4 is reproduced from Rosser's article and depicts all the important structures that can be encountered and which must not be damaged. At this stage the operation is similar to the transperitoneal approach and once learnt the anatomy is clearer.[34] The back of the pubis, Cooper's ligament, iliopubic tract and the inferior epigastric vessels need to be identified clearly. A 10 mm trocar is then inserted under direct vision approximately midway between the umbilicus and the pubis. We prefer to use an Apple trocar since this is easier to suture through than most alternative ports and can be re-autoclaved (GU Manufacturing Co. Ltd, 841 Coronation Road, Park Royal, London NW10 7QL). If a stapler is to be employed, which the authors do not recommend because of the risk of more damage and the cost, this trocar must be 12 mm in diameter.

McKernan places this trocar in the immediate suprapubic position, but in our

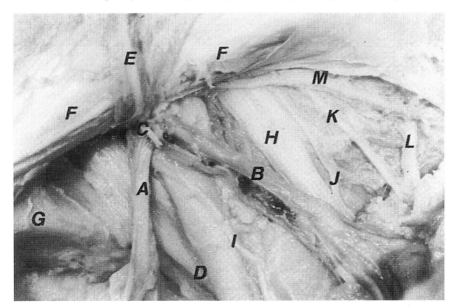

Fig. 14b.4 Left inguinal area viewed from the abdominal aspect. (By permission of *Surgical Laparoscopy and Endoscopy*.)
Key: A, vas deferens; B, gonadal vessels; C, internal ring; D, Triangle of Doom (external iliac artery and vein); E, inferior epigastric vessels; F, transversus abdominis arch and aponeurosis; G, Cooper's ligament; H, femoral nerve; I, genital branch of genito-femoral nerve; J, nerve to iliacus muscle; K, anterior branch of the lateral femoral cutaneous nerve; L, posterior branch of the lateral femoral cutaneous nerve; M, deep circumflex iliac artery.

opinion this interferes with subsequent patch placement. Once the landmarks are seen, dissection can proceed in a lateral direction on a fairly superficial plane ignoring the hernial orifices for the time being. Using a combination of sharp and blunt dissection the peritoneum is gently stripped off the anterior abdominal wall to a level 3–4 cm above the anterior superior iliac spine. It may be very adherent at this level, especially on the left side from previous diverticulitis or on the right after appendicectomy, and it is important to keep very close to the abdominal wall during dissection and to ensure it is adequately separated. Accidental opening of the peritoneum will cause troublesome pneumo-peritoneum and hamper further dissection. This can be rectified by reducing inflation pressure and inserting an open intraperitoneal Verres needle. Only rarely is it necessary to suture the peritoneum. A 5 cm trocar is then inserted 2 cm above the iliac spine on a level with the lateral margin of the ipsilateral rectus sheath.

Attention is now re-directed to the hernia sites. Most direct sacs are already at least partially reduced or can be easily reduced by external pressure. It is generally a simple matter to demonstrate the junction with the transversalis fascia and reduce the hernia entirely. The margins of the defect should be cleared completely with particular attention to the medial aspect where bladder may be

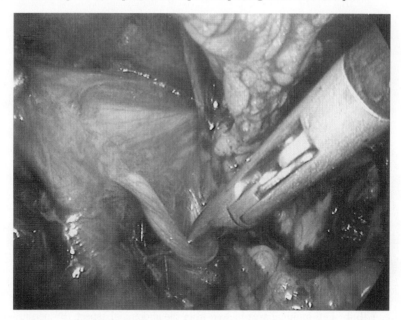

Fig. 14b.5 The vas deferens is being separated from the postero-medial aspect of the indirect sac of a left-sided hernia. The inferior epigastric vessels are seen just to the left of the forceps. This figure is also reproduced in colour opposite page 277.

present. To avoid bladder damage, the tissues should be swept out of the sac in a medial direction without cutting. If the hernia is large, the transversalis fascia lining the defect can be grasped with forceps, drawn inwards and sutured to the abdominal wall, so eliminating 'pseudo-sac' formation which can worry patients. However, this manoeuvre is not strictly necessary as the condition will always settle spontaneously after a few weeks. No attempt should be made to close the defect as this inevitably creates unacceptable tissue tension and pain. At this stage the presence of a femoral hernia should be checked by visualizing the medial border of the femoral vein, although full dissection of this vessel is not necessary. Passing more laterally the site of an indirect hernia can be identified by locating the inferior epigastric vessels. In the obese patient this can be a problem. At this stage confusion can arise if the vessels have been dissected by a balloon. They will be seen hanging down as a curtain obstructing the view and are best ligated and divided. Beginning at a point close to the inferior epigastric vessels superomedial to the internal ring and using a mixture of sharp and blunt dissection to tease the tissues apart, it is usually possible to identify the indirect sac. This is then separated from the cord structures, the vas deferens on the medial side (Fig. 14b. 5) and the spermatic vessels on the lateral side, but lying behind the sac as seen through the laparoscope. Once mobilized the sac can be drawn cephalad with the rest of the peritoneum (Fig. 14b.6). For a scrotal hernia no attempt is made to reduce the sac completely. Wantz has very clearly demon-

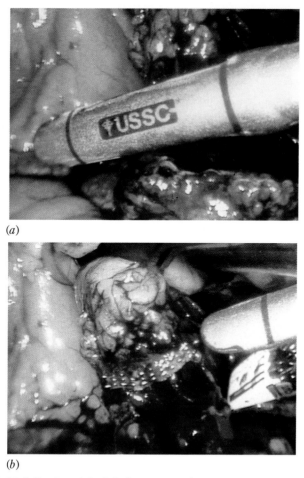

(a)

(b)

Plate 13a.6 High ligation of the inferior mesenteric artery during laparoscopic anterior resection using an endoscopic linear stapler; (a) about to fire and (b) division completed between rows of staples.

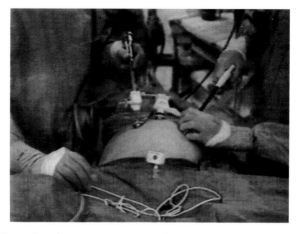

Plate 13c.2 Insertion of ports: 12 mm at umbilicus; 10 mm port to the right of the umbilical port; 10 mm port at left iliac fossa. 10 mm suprapubic port.

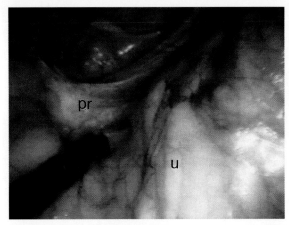

Plate 13c.3 (a) Laparoscopic identification of the right ureter (u). Peritoneal reflection divided (pr).

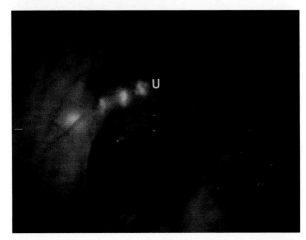

Plate 13c.3 (b) Visualization of ureters (u) with the aid of fibro-optic light source.

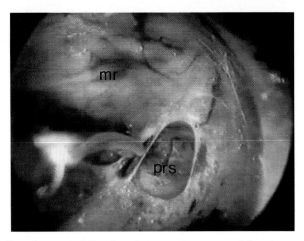

Plate 13c.4 Development of the plane between the sacrum (s) and mesorectum (mr), using sharp dissection. (prs, pre-rectal space.)

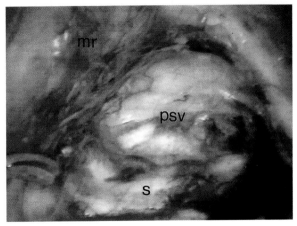

Plate 13c.5 Mesorectum (mr) separated from sacrum (s) and presacral veins (psv).

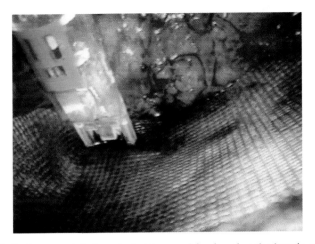

Plate 13c.6 Prolene mesh being stapled to sacral fascia using the hernia stapler.

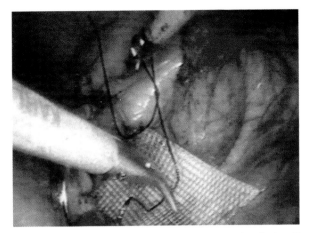

Plate 13c.7 Mesh being sutured to the side of the rectum using Szabo–Berci needle holder and Flamingo.

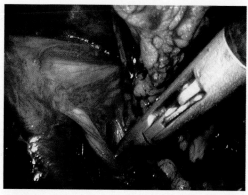

Plate 14b.5 The vas deferens is being separated from the postero-medial aspect of the indirect sac of a left-sided hernia. The inferior epigastric vessels are seen just to the left of the forceps.

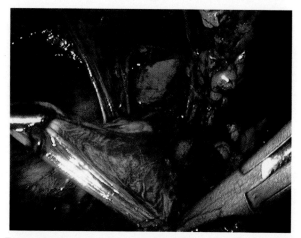

Plate 14b.6 The sac of the left indirect inguinal hernia has been fully mobilized and is being separated from the vas deferens and spermatic vessels.

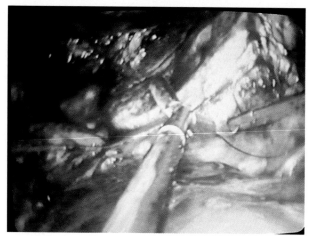

Plate 14b.7 A 2/0 prolene suture is about to be passed through the peritoneum over Cooper's ligament.

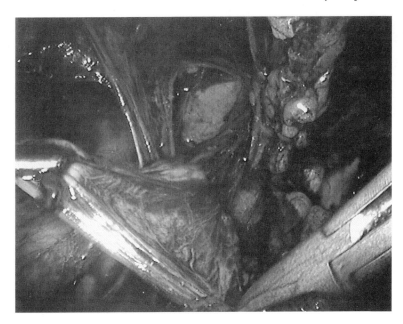

Fig. 14b.6   The sac of the left indirect inguinal hernia has been fully mobilized and is being separated from the vas deferens and spermatic vessels. This figure is also reproduced in colour opposite this page.

strated that further dissection beyond the level of the external ring or pubic tubercle will greatly increase the risk of nerve or testicular damage and is likely to lead to a high incidence of haematomata. The sac should be ligated, after confirmation of no contents, with a 2/0 vicryl suture and an extra-corporeal knot. Distally the sac should be left open to avoid hydrocoele formation, but held carefully after division to ensure there is no bleeding from the cut edge. If this is not done the distal sac will disappear down the inguinal canal and be impossible to retrieve with the risk of haematoma formation. No concern need be attached to the development of a pneumo-scrotum often seen at this stage. If bilateral herniation is present the procedure is duplicated on the other side. Recurrent hernias require special care, but rarely is the peritoneum very adherent except at the point where high sac ligation has been carried out.

Choice and size of the patch ————

Ideally the prosthesis should be non-immunogenic, tolerant of body fluids, sterilizable, non-carcinogenic, resistant to infection, and should retain an adequate tensile strength. We prefer polypropylene mesh which is a monofilament patch with an open weave and find that it has good handling characteristics and memory.

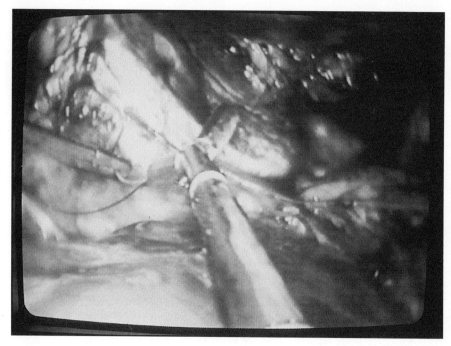

Fig. 14b.7   A 2/0 prolene suture is about to be passed through the peritoneum over Cooper's ligament. This figure is also reproduced in colour opposite page 277.

The most important lesson that has been learnt from a study of recurrences in early laparoscopic hernia experience is the necessity to employ a large patch giving adequate overlap and to adequately expose the solid landmarks of the region. For this purpose we believe a size of 12 × 15 cms or a little wider, correctly placed, is probably adequate for most patients. We use a single suture fixation technique since this enables rapid correct spatial orientation of the patch and is more reliable, safer and much less expensive than staples.[34] A 2/0 prolene suture is passed via the midline trocar, through Cooper's ligament (Fig. 14b.7), but not the periosteum, and brought out through the same trocar. The needle holder should operate through the lateral trocar. The two ends are then threaded through the appropriate point on the patch which can be 'parachuted' into position along the stitch prior to external knotting. Orientation is further facilitated by marking the patch with a horizontal line and a stitch to indicate the supero-lateral corner.

For bilateral herniae a similar technique is employed utilizing a large single patch measuring 28 × 10 cm or sometimes two *separate* patches. The size of the single patch can make placement troublesome and this can be helped by the use of the following method. Firstly the mesh is clearly marked with a vertical line in the midline and a transverse line 2 cm above the lower margin. Next a vicryl suture is attached to the mid-point of the upper margin and the end left long. The patch is now rolled from above downwards in its long axis leaving a 2 cm strip at the lower edge. A stitch in the middle and at each end will hold it rolled up and is easy to insert down a 10 mm trocar running along a previously placed Cooper's ligament suture as described above. A second suture is then placed in the opposite Cooper's ligament and the stitches holding the patch in the rolled position are cut. By grasping the loose end of the mid-point suture through the suprapubic trocar the patch is then very easily unrolled.

Fixation of the patch

It is mandatory that sufficient dissection is carried out to enable the mesh to lie flat without any tendency for the margins to curl over. If the patch is large enough and dissection adequate, fixation at other points is probably not required, but if used supero-laterally it is very important to keep above the level of the anterior superior iliac spine to avoid damage to the lateral cutaneous nerve of thigh or the ilio-inguinal nerve (Fig. 14b.4). No fixation should take place below the level of the ilio-pubic tract. Inappropriate application of an excessive number of staples will inevitably result in nerve or vascular damage and should be avoided. Fixation at one point only allows the mesh to adapt to the contours of the abdominal wall in a more satisfactory manner. For large direct hernia it is our practice to slit the patch and pass it under the cord structures, and this quite widely used technique does ensure that the lower margin stays in place. Theoretical objections relate to possible fibrosis around the cord structures with the risk of sterility[35] and the potential weakness in the patch created by slitting.[36] However, we are careful to parietalize the cord structures and place the patch sufficiently low to prevent recurrence from the inferior border.[37] Where there is a very large direct defect an additional suture may be inserted between the mesh and the medial border of the defect for additional security.

Many, even experienced laparoscopic surgeons, perceive suturing techniques as difficult or impossible, often without even trying. This attitude is conceptual rather than real and laparoscopic suturing is little different from the 'no touch' techniques commonly used in open orthopaedic surgery some years ago. With a little practice it is very easy to develop suturing skills and indeed in a small personal trial comparing laparoscopic peritoneal closure with staples and suturing, the latter was slightly faster and achieved a much sounder looking closure. Arguably, the sutures are more reliable than staples which can become detached.

Although we routinely use a single suture to orientate the patch it is probable that a simple onlay patch, unfixed, is just as effective and has the advantages of avoiding the second 10 mm trocar and reducing operating time.

Closure

Following patch placement haemostasis is checked and 50 cc of dilute bupivicaine solution instilled. The space is then gradually desufflated under direct vision, making sure that the edges of the mesh do not curl and the peritoneum rolls down and holds it firmly in place. Indirect sacs should be held up behind the mesh. The

Table 14b.1   Incidence of complications in 152 cases of extraperitoneal laparoscopic hernia repair

	Number
Recurrence	2
Cord/scrotal haematoma	6
Pseudo-sac (transient)	9
Nerve trauma	5
Genito-femoral	3
Ilio-inguinal	1
Lateral cutaneous nerve of the thigh	1
Pubic discomfort	1
Testicular pain	2
Intestinal obstruction	0
Testicular atrophy	0
Retention of urine	1
Trocar site herniation	0

port sites should be closed deeply although the risk of herniation is probably much less than with transperitoneal trocar penetration.

Results

In a series of over 600 laparoscopic hernia repairs over 500 have been carried out using an entirely extraperitoneal approach. This relates to the fact that for teaching purposes it is felt that the transperitoneal approach is more appropriate to be learnt first (see below). Patients are kept on long-term follow-up and seen at 6 weeks, 6 months and then yearly. There have been two recurrences to date with a maximum follow-up of 72 months. The first occurred within 2 weeks of surgery and at re-operation was found to be related to the use of too small a patch. The second arose 4 months after operation and repeat laparoscopy showed the lower margin of the mesh to have folded upwards, almost certainly due to inadequate dissection. The incidence of complications is shown in Table 14b.1.

All instances of cord haematoma related to complete dissection of large indirect scrotal sacs, a practice now discontinued. Two of the three patients with genito-femoral neuralgia also occurred in this group and no explanation was apparent for the third. One patient suffered discomfort in the region of the lateral cutaneous nerve of the thigh and one in the distribution of the ilio-inguinal nerve. All these patients settled spontaneously after a maximum of 8 weeks. A single patient with persistent pain in the region of the pubic tubercle has been helped, but not completely relieved, by a local injection of dopamedrone.

Discussion

Table 14b.1 illustrates the main pros and cons of the open pre-peritoneal patch (OPP), the transabdominal pre-peritoneal patch (TAPP) and the totally extra-peritoneal (TEP) approaches and several points merit consideration. The intra-peritoneal onlay mesh technique (IPOM) has not been listed since we consider this to be both dangerous and inappropriate since there is a proven incidence of adhesion formation and fistulation of bowel has also been recorded. The excep-tion to this is the Toy–Smoot PTFE repair and a literature search has failed to find any such problems with this technique for which excellent results have been reported.[41] However, the use of any other type of patch for IPOM repair is absolutely contra-indicated and it is very difficult to see the advantage of using a more expensive intraperitoneal patch which requires quite extensive fixation with the attendant potential risk of nerve damage.

The situation regarding TAPP is somewhat different. It is probably true to say that most of the problems seen with the transperitoneal repair relate to the peritoneal suture line. The integrity of this is often suspect when the closure is carried out with staples. Several cases have been described where loops of bowel have penetrated through defects in the closure with the development of intestinal obstruction and in some instances gangrenous bowel. In contrast, the extraper-itoneal approach allows the placement of a pre-peritoneal patch without the requirement of a peritoneal incision. If the TAPP approach is employed the present authors consider stapling to be an unacceptable way of closing the peritoneum and believe that the use of a continuous suture which requires only a few minutes for insertion is much better. It seems very unlikely that this will become undone as can happen with staples since bigger and more controlled bites of peritoneum can be taken with a needle than with a staple.

Strongly in favour of the TAPP approach is the fact that an indirect sac can be circumcised with no need for dissection. This helps to avoid the potential com-plications of damage to the testicular vessels or genito-femoral nerve and scrotal or cord haematomata which are very definite problems even with limited extra-peritoneal sac dissection.

The extraperitoneal approach is considerably more difficult to learn than the transperitoneal and it is strongly recommended that the technique of trans-peritoneal repair should be fully mastered first. Indeed, this may partly account for the very low recurrence rates reported which are mostly from units with experienced surgeons who have already completed their 'learning curves' with the transperitoneal approach. Another reason for the low recurrence rate may relate to the splinting effect of the peritoneum in fixing the mesh. Although a similar effect is achieved with the transperitoneal method, the altered tensions created by the peritoneal closure line may render it less effective.

Conclusions

Just as the jury is still out for primary laparoscopic repair, so it is for the extraperitoneal technique. However, available evidence would suggest that, at

282 Hernia repair: extraperitoneal laparoscopic inguinal hernia repair

least for some cases, the extraperitoneal approach offers certain advantages over the transperitoneal operation. The authors believe that it is wrong to consider that all hernias should necessarily be treated by the same method. There is little doubt that for direct and probably small indirect hernias, the extraperitoneal technique is superior. For large indirect hernias we have reservations and it may well be that the transperitoneal approach with circumcision of the sac and suturing of the peritoneal incision is better and certainly quicker. It also reduces the risk of complications associated with extensive sac dissection. For bilateral direct and recurrent hernias the extraperitoneal approach is excellent and has far fewer complications than conventional repair.

A final comment on costs is merited. The opponents of laparoscopic hernia repair constantly cite increased costs compared with open surgery. However, most of the arguments do not stand close examination. It is entirely realistic to carry out laparoscopic hernia repair without the use of disposables and in the knowledge that patients will usually return to normal activities, including work, in about half the time of the best alternative techniques.

References

1. Van Steensel, Professor of Surgery, Delft, Holland. Personal communication.
2. Bendavid R. Proceedings of 'Expert Meeting on Hernia Surgery', St Moritz, Switzerland, February 1994.
3. Ijzermans JNM, de Wilt H, Hop WCJ, Jeekel H. Recurrent inguinal hernia treated by classical hernioplasty. *Arch Surg* 1991; **126**: 1097–1110.
4. Bendavid R. Expectations of hernia surgery. In: *Surgical Laparoscopy* Patreson-Brown, Garden (eds) WB Saunders Co. Ltd, London 1994, page 387.
5. Amid PK, Schulman AG, Lichtenstein IL. The Lichtenstein open tension free hernioplasty. In: *Inguinal Hernia: Advances or Controversies?* Arregui ME, Nagan RF (eds), Radcliffe Medical Press, Oxford.
6. Lichtenstein IL, Shulman AG, Amid PK. The cause, prevention and treatment of recurrent groin hernia. *Surg Clin N A* 1993; **73**: 529.
7. Phillips EH, Carroll BJ, Fallas MJ, Arregui ME, Corbitt J, Fitzgibbons RJ, Pietrafitta J, Sewell RW, Seid AS, Schultz LS, Toy FK, Waddell RL. Reasons for recurrence following laparoscopic hernioplasty. In: *Hernia*, 3rd edn, JB Lippincott, Philadelphia, PA, 1989, pages 253–264.
8. Tetik C, Arregui ME, Castro D, Davis CJ, Dulucq JL, Fitzgibbons Jr RJ, Franklin ME, Hammond JC, McKernan JB, Rosin RD, Schultz LS, Toy FK. Complications and recurrences associated with laparoscopic repair of groin hernias: a multi-institutional retrospective analysis. In: *Inguinal Hernia: Advances or Controversies?* Arregui ME, Nagan RF (eds), Radcliffe Medical Press, Oxford, 1994.
9. Wantz GE. Complications of inguinal hernia repair. *Surg Clin N Am* 1993; **64**: 287–298.
10. Wantz GE. Testicular atrophy and chronic residual neuralgia as risks of inguinal hernioplasty. *Surg Clin N Am* 1993; **73**: 571–581.
11. Kathouda N. Complications of laparoscopic hernia repair. In: *Inguinal Hernia: Advances or Controversies?* Arregui ME, Nagan RF (eds), Radcliffe Medical Press, Oxford, 1994, pages 277–282.
12. Sewell RW, Waddell RL. Complications of laparoscopic inguinal hernia repair. In: *Inguinal Hernia: Advances or Con-*

troversies? Arregui ME, Nagan RF (eds), Radcliffe Medical Press, Oxford, 1994, pages 489–493.

13. Riner JK, Jager R. Outpatient laparoscopic herniorrhaphy. In: *Inguinal Hernia: Advances or Controversies?* Arregui ME, Nagan RF (eds), Radcliffe Medical Press, Oxford, 1994.

14. Payne JH, Grininger LM, Izawa MT, Podoll EF, Lindahl PJ. A randomised prospective comparison between laparoscopic, pre-peritoneal and the anterior 'tension-free' repair of inguinal herniation with mesh. In: *Inguinal Hernia: Advances or Controversies?* Arregui ME, Nagan RF (eds), Radcliffe Medical Press, Oxford, 1994.

15. Seid AS, Deutsch H, Jacobsen A. Laparoscopic herniorrhaphy. *Surg Laparosc Endosc* 1992; **2**: 59–60.

16. Hawasli A. Laparoscopic inguinal herniorrhaphy: the mushroom plug repair. *Surg Laparosc Endosc* 1992; **2**: 111–116.

17. Taylor RS, Fiennes AGTW. A tension-free modification of the Dulucq pre-peritoneal laparoscopic hernioplasty. *Min Invas Ther* 1992; **1** (supp 1): 100.

18. Robertson GSM, Burton PR, Haynes IG. How long do patients convalesce after inguinal herniorrhaphy? Current principles and practice. *Ann Roy Coll Surg End* 1992; **75**: 30–33.

19. Michaels JA, Reece-Smith H, Faber RG. Case-control study of patient satisfaction with day-case and inpatient inguinal hernia repair. *J R Coll Surg Edin* 1992; **37**: 99–100.

20. Bailey IS, Karran SE, Toyn K, Brough P, Ranaboldo C, Karran SJ. Community surveillance of complications after hernia surgery. *Br Med J* 1992; **304**: 469–471.

21. Royal College of Surgeons of England. Commission on the Provision of Surgical Services. Guidelines for Day Case Surgery. Royal College of Surgeons of England, London, 1985.

22. Ger R, Monroe K, Duvivier R, Mishrick A. Management of indirect inguinal hernias by laparoscopic closure of the neck of the sac. *Am J Surg* 1990; **159**: 370–373.

23. Schultz L, Graber J, Pietrafitta J, Hickok D. Laser laparoscopic herniorrhaphy: a clinical trial preliminary results. *J Laparosc Endosc Surg* 1991; **1**: 41–45.

24. Corbitt JD. Laparoscopic herniorrhaphy. *Surg Laparosc Endosc* 1991; **1**: 23.

25. Fruchaud H. Anatomie chirurgicale des hernie de l'aine. C Dion, Paris, 1956, page 169.

26. Cheatle GL. An operation for the radical cure of inguinal and femoral hernia. *Br Med J* 1920; **2**: 68.

27. Nyhus LM, Condon RE, Hawkin HN. Clinical experiences with pre-peritoneal hernia repair for all types of hernia of the groin. *Am J Surg* 1960; **100**: 234.

28. Stoppa R, Rives JL, Warlaumont C, Palot JP, Verhaege PF, De Lattre JF. The use of dacron in the repair of hernias of the groin. *Surg Clin N Am* 1984; **64**: 269.

29. Begin G-F. Laparoscopic extra-peritoneal treatment of inguinal hernias in adults. A series of 200 cases. *End Surg* 1993; **1**: 204–206.

30. Dulucq JL. The treatment of inguinal hernias by insertion of mesh through retroperitonoscopy. *Postgrad Gen Surg* 1992; **4**(2): 173–174.

31. Dulucq JL. Traitment des hernie de l'aine par mise en place d'un patch prosthetique sous-peritoneal en retroperitoneoscopie. *Cahiers de Chirurgie* 1993; **79**: 15–16.

32. McKernan JB, Laws HL. Laparoscopic pre-peritoneal prosthetic repair of inguinal hernias. *Surg Rounds* 1992; 597–610.

33. Read RC. Cooper's posterior lamina of transversalis fascia. *Surg Gynaecol Obst* 1992; **174**: 426–434.

34. Spaw AT, Ennis BW, Spaw LP. Laparoscopic hernia repair: the anatomic basis. *J Laparoendosc Surg* 1991; **1**: 269.

35. Rosser J. The anatomical basis for laparoscopic hernia repair revisited. *Surg Laparosc Endosc* 1994; **4**(1): 36–44.

36. Litwin D. Risks to fertility with laparoscopic mesh repair. In: *Inguinal Hernia: Advances or Controversies?* Arregui ME, Nagan RF (eds), Radcliffe Medical Press, Oxford, pages 223–225.

37. Cameron AEP. Accuracy of clinical diagnosis of direct and indirect inguinal hernia. *Br J Surg* 1994; **81**: 250.
38. Ralphs DNL, Brain AJL, Grundy DJ, Hobsley M. How accurately can direct and indirect hernias be distinguished? *Br Med J* 1980; **280**: 1039–1040.
39. Mudan SS, Thomas PRS, Read RC, Fiennes AGTW. Extra-peritoneal hernia repair: Role of the Fascia Transversalis. BACA Annual Meeting, June 1994, Sheffield, UK.
40. Castro D, Arregui ME, Tetik C, Nagan RF. Laparoscopic inguinal hernia repair. Total extra-peritoneal laparoscopic hernia repair with prosthetic replacement. In: *Inguinal Hernia: Advances or Controversies?* Arregui ME, Nagan RF (eds), Radcliffe Medical Press, Oxford, pages 423–427.
41. Toy FK, Smoot Jr RT. Toy–Smoot laparoscopic hernioplasty. *Surg Laparosc Endosc* 1991; **1**: 151–155.

15

Totally extraperitoneal endoscopic surgery

A.G.T.W. Fiennes

Introduction

The totally extraperitoneal approach for laparoscopic groin hernia repair[1-3] has been discussed elsewhere in this volume (p. 264) and has among other advantages the virtue of logic: operation is carried straight to the anatomical plane of the lesion and remains either contained within that plane or very close to it.

A similar concept has, for a quarter of a century, attracted attention to the surgery of the retroperitoneal organs:[4-9] to operate on intra-abdominal or intrathoracic viscera with minimal invasion of the body wall is an accepted rationale of minimal access surgery. To invade and expose to risk of injury the peritoneum and its contents, when the surgical target is retro- or extraperitoneal, may by the same token seem illogical.

Just as with transparietal access to the body cavities, however, logic has to be tempered with an understanding of the useful and of the technically feasible. Not all that is possible is useful and not all that is desirable is yet possible: limits are imposed by our anatomical understanding (which needs revision), by our faculties of orientation (which need technical support) and by current instrumentation (which requires development).

Accordingly this overview will identify by organ system those procedures which have been demonstrated or seem feasible, consider issues of surgical access and instrumentation and finally point to limits of our anatomical understanding.

Organ systems

If the abdominal organ systems are considered in sequence from the sagittal plane to the parietes, it can be seen that none is entirely intraperitoneal. Parts of the upper and lower digestive tract and a great part of its appended glands occupy the retroperitoneum. The genito-urinary system is entirely retroperitoneal, alongside important endocrine and lymphatic elements. The option to approach the major blood vessels either trans- or extraperitoneally is well known from standard vascular surgery, where an extraperitoneal approach to the abdominopelvic autonomic nervous system is also standard practice. Finally, particular attention is due to the musculoskeletal elements of the parietes themselves, where significant new prospects arise.

Digestive surgery

As is well known from standard surgical procedures, most of the duodenum and parts of the right and left colon are either retroperitoneal or have at least a bare posterior aspect. From the same experience these organs are notoriously easy to mobilize toward the sagittal plane, because their blood supply arises near the ventral midline of the aorta.

Duodenum

It is thus not surprising that the second and third parts of the duodenum are easily visualized from their posterolateral aspect[10] when an extraperitoneal approach is made to the right adrenal gland (see below): with the patient in the extended lateral position the duodenum pushes anteriorly off the inferior vena cava, initiating an endoscopic Kocher's manoeuvre, which may be performed as an adjunct to a minimally invasive mobilization of the stomach or for access to the duodenum per se. The debate over laparoscopic versus retrograde endoscopic common bile duct clearance continues,[11–13] but not every papilla can be cannulated and not every bile duct entered. The retroperitoneal approach to the duodenum offers either transduodenal sphincter surgery or an opportunity to support endoscopic cannulation, for example in the presence of a duodenal diverticulum, which, depending on location, may also be most conveniently operated by this route.

Liver

The same approach provides excellent access to the right lobe of the liver, specifically to its posterolateral aspect, which may be difficult to reach transperitoneally and classically requires wide exposure. Laparoscopic decortication of simple cysts,[14] drainage of abscesses,[15,16] hydatid cyst drainage[17] and enucleation of tumours[18,19] have been demonstrated. Depending on location of the lesion, retroperitoneoscopy may be the approach of choice.

Lesser sac

The fourth part of the duodenum and the posterior aspect of the body of the pancreas can be developed into the anterior confine of the dissection space when a retroperitoneoscopic approach is made to the left adrenal (see below). This may therefore be the convenient approach to a gut endocrine tumour at this location. In the same approach the roof of the dissection space is constituted by the inferior, lateral floor of the lesser sac, through which the hilar aspect of the spleen is visible. Although as yet undemonstrated, to approach thus the posterior wall of the stomach may be of utility in endoscopic[20–23] morbid obesity surgery.[24–25]

Ligation of the splenic vessels on the superior border of the pancreas is desired during open surgery precisely when the spleen is largest and the vessels hardest to reach and has not been demonstrated by transperitoneal laparoscopy at all. A left retroperitoneal approach offers this manoeuvre[10] as an adjunct to open or laparoscopic[26,27] splenectomy and may also offer a means of isolating the short gastric vessels.

Pancreas

McMahon[28] has demonstrated laparoscopic enucleation of endocrine tumours of the pancreas. Depending on their location, a right or left retroperitoneoscopic approach may be the approach of choice for these and other benign lesions,[29] offering significant advantages over both a fairly extensive epigastric incision or a transperitoneal laparoscopic access which may approach the pancreas from the wrong aspect. A right retroperitoneal approach enables mobilization of the entire head of the pancreas[10] and offers at least a theoretical avenue of dissection for pancreaticoduodenectomy, with the advantage that the critical determinants of resectability could be assessed early. Note that the location of the inferior mesenteric vein would make this harder to achieve from the left.

Colon

During the approach from the flank the retroperitoneal aspect of the descending colon is traced proximally and the splenic flexure swept forward. It follows that exteriorization of the descending or sigmoid colon could be assisted from a retroperitoneal approach, but the utility has yet to be demonstrated.[30,31]

Genito-urinary tract

The genito-urinary tract has, by reason of embryology, the retroperitoneum as its natural habitat. It is therefore no surprise that retroperitoneal endoscopic surgery has been demonstrated in respect of virtually its every organ. In this regard the landmark achievement of Gaur,[32] who demonstrated balloon dissection of the perinephric space over two years ago,[33] ranks alongside that of Dulucq[1] in relation to groin hernias two years previously.

Kidney and renal pelvis

With the patient in the lateral position Gaur[34] made a finger-sized incision below the twelfth rib and entered the fascia of Gerota. A home-made, low-cost, air-inflated elastomere balloon[33] was then inserted into the fascial space and inflated to 30 mmHg. After waiting a few minutes the balloon was deflated and a standard laparoscopy cannula inserted into the wound. The fascial contents of the perinephric space had been compressed, leaving the kidney free within it. The ureter could be ligated and divided and its proximal stump used as a retractor to reveal the vessels entering the renal hilum. The pragmatism of this approach is undiminished by the issue of organ retrieval and morselation[35] which is shared by the transperitoneal laparoscopic surgery of solid organs and lies beyond the scope of this chapter.

The technique is anatomical and can therefore be as bloodless as the transperitoneal approach is difficult and bloody. Both techniques may have similar advantages over the open approach,[36] but meet their limits when there is marked inflammatory change around the kidney and in neither case is the oncological efficacy proven. Although the method of Gaur may offer much superior access to the renal vein and cava, instrumental control for tumour dissection within the venous lumen remains an unanswered challenge.

Pyelolithotomy by the Gaur approach offers a demonstrable alternative[37] to nephroscopy or lithotripsy.

Ureter

The ureter is easily cannulated from the bladder and the technology for intraluminal ureteric lithotripsy is well developed. Thus, although extraperitoneal approaches to the ureter from below (by extension of the Dulucq approach to the groin), from the flank (as when initiating an approach to the adrenal) or posteriorly and superiorly (as for Gaur's approach to the kidney) are all equally feasible, in practice they remain reserve procedures for ureteric stones[9,38,39] where lithotripsy is either unavailable or unsuccessful. Ureterolysis[40] is an obvious application, with a lateral approach – offering access to the entire length of the ureter – perhaps the most rational. The palliative procedure of ureterostomy in situ[41] has not been described using this technique, but offers very clear advantages over open surgery in the palliative care setting, where the pain and morbidity of a muscle cutting incision in the flank is a real issue. As a general proposition, intra-operative ultrasound may be of value in locating the ureter in the retroperitoneum of an obese subject.[42]

Bladder

Anterior bladder injury is a recognized pitfall of laparoscopic hernia surgery.[43] From this fact, and from the ease with which, in the Dulucq hernia approach, the Cave of Retzius is opened, it follows that dissection may be carried down the pelvic side-wall, medial to the iliac vessels. Bladder diverticula in either location can be easily isolated – if necessary in a combined transurethral and retroperitoneal procedure – and excised, for example by stapling. The approach should be born in mind as an immediate remedy to inadvertent endoscopic bladder perforation. Inflammatory change in the Cave of Retzius will render any such approach a certain impossibility within a very few days.

The anterior bladder neck is equally easily accessible by pre-peritoneoscopy. With increasing focus on the morbidity of very prolonged transurethral prostatectomy,[44] a real alternative thus exists for the surgery of large hyperplastic prostates. In the female pre-peritoneoscopic bladder neck surgery is more advanced,[45] with totally extraperitoneal laparoscopic Burch colposuspension[46,47] gaining ground rapidly in the treatment of female incontinence. Surprisingly, this procedure has become dominated by advocates of balloon dissectors[46] (see below, page 296).

Spermatic cord

The totally extraperitoneal approach for laparoscopic groin hernias provides an opportunity for concomitant vasectomy and varicocoele ligation: [32,48,49] the vas deferens and the testicular pedicle are critical landmarks easily reached prior to hernia dissection and the magnified view of testicular artery and vein[32] aids their distinction. The wide exposure afforded by the approach enables accessory venous channels[50] to be pursued.

Endocrine organs

Open adrenalectomy is a hallowed preserve of dissection technique[51] based on surgical anatomy: it is not surprising that, as already indicated, its endoscopic counterpart has also come to serve as a road map of surgical anatomy, retaining the same, numerically restricted but definite set of indications in the treatment of hypertension (Conn's tumour, nodular hyperplasia)[52,53] and of Cushing's Disease.[53,54] The role of laparoscopic surgery for phaeochromocytoma is less certain, but is probably restricted by the size issue alone to tumours less than 6 cm in diameter.[54–57]

The feasibility of a retroperitoneoscopic approach to the adrenal was presented in an animal model by Brunt in 1992.[58] Human retroperitoneal endoscopic adrenalectomy was undertaken shortly afterwards by Taylor[59] and published approximately simultaneously by Mandressi.[42] The author's own approach is similar, placing the patient in the lateral position, with loin extension to widen access between costal margin and iliac crest. Initial puncture is below the tip of the eleventh rib in the mid-axillary line and the telescope seeks a trajectory anterior to the upper half of the kidney. This approach provides a useful angle of access to the vascular axis of the gland, unlike the posterior, prone approach[42] for nephrectomy. The prone approach does permit bilateral[60] operation without turning the patient.

Transperitoneal laparoscopic adrenalectomy[61] has also been demonstrated, through the hepatorenal recess on the right, where in the author's view anterior retraction of the liver may be difficult, and via infra-, supra- and retrocolic approaches[57,62,63] on the left, where the multiple anterior relations of the gland may be a source of difficulty. It is worth noting that modern pharmacology and anaesthesia render the time-honoured manoeuvre of initial adrenal vein ligation a superfluous source of engorgement of the gland.

With patients leaving hospital 2–4 days after surgery,[64,65] there seems little doubt that the laparoscopic approach offers advantages of patient comfort over the open – although this is occasionally disputed by those who have not suffered a muscle cutting incision in the loin. The vasculature is excellently seen and the extraperitoneal approach offers a closed space able to tamponade venous oozing. A successful retroperitoneoscopic approach on either side requires precise understanding of the retroperitoneal fascia (see the section on anatomy below, page 299): the gland occupies the renal compartment[10] and must be approached accordingly (see also Surgical Access, page 293). Doubt has been expressed about the oncological efficacy of laparoscopic as compared to open adrenalectomy, but so long as the tumour is so small as to permit the organ boundaries to be reached at all, this criticism begs foundation in audit of the open procedure. The retro-peritoneoscopic approach may be paradoxically harder in the very thin, whose tissue planes are more condensed. In this regard the trans- and retroperitoneal approach may be complementary.

Lymphoreticular system

Laparoscopic pelvic lymphadenectomy[49,66,67] is well established in the management of genito-urinary malignancy.[68] The advantage to this undertaking of a pre-peritoneoscopic approach to the spaces of Retzius and Bogros lies in laying bare the entire plane along internal and external iliac axes without peritoneal incision or intrusion by loops of intestine. Its disadvantage lies in the relative difficulty of obtaining access to the correct pre-peritoneal plane and in the greater demands of anatomical orientation from an unaccustomed perspective. However, these problems have effectively been resolved for the incomparably commoner indication of groin hernia.[69]

The para-aortic nodes are relatively easy to access laparoscopically by pneumoperitoneum, but this approach may be rendered difficult by adhesions, concomitant splenomegaly, obesity or distended loops of intestine. Once again, a lateral extraperitoneal approach offers direct access to the para-aortic plane[66] and may pose less physiological threat[36,70,71] in compromised patients. The combination of such a manoeuvre with laparoscopic-assisted splenectomy[72–74] may be attractive as an alternative to staging laparotomy, although changes in treatment regimes for many lymphomas have considerably restricted the indications for the latter.[75–77]

Major blood vessels

With the excellence of access afforded by the pre-peritoneal approach to the groin on the one hand and with the demonstration of access to the para-aortic region on the other, it comes as no surprise that reconstructive surgery to the aorto-iliac tree has also been successfully undertaken.[78]

Dulucq[79] has demonstrated both aorto-iliac and iliofemoral bypass surgery with hand-sutured anastomoses by the totally extraperitoneal approach. The patients were ambulant on the day of surgery and discharged within two days. Clearly such procedures make the three-fold demand of high expertise in vascular surgery, anatomical understanding of the extraperitoneal approach and technical mastery of laparoscopic suture techniques. The apprenticeship may thus be long and it is not clear whether this work will be eclipsed by endoluminal techniques or whether it will come to complement them.[80]

Lumbar sympathectomy

Upward extension of a pre-peritoneal groin approach or a direct lateral retro-peritoneoscopic approach both offer good access to the lumbar sympathetic chain and are more logical than the transperitoneal laparoscopic approach which has also been demonstrated. Extraperitoneal approaches, in common with the traditional approach, offer a closed space around minor bleeding from lumbar veins, but, in addition, minimize incapacity. This represents a bonus in patients who are nearly always frail.[81,82] The procedure also has an advantage of anatomical efficacy over phenol ablation, which is notoriously partial.

The real problem attached to the procedure is that of dwindling or entirely absent indication, since its failure to conserve tissue in peripheral vascular disease is now amply known.[5,83] Nevertheless, where an indication does exist and especially where skilled radiological resources are lacking, lumbar sympathectomy by retroperitoneoscopy may survive as a rarity.[84]

Parietes

The above review of procedures may seem exhaustive. Nevertheless, both muscle and skeleton are worth consideration.

Hernias

This chapter is not concerned with groin hernia, but these are not the only herniae of the abdominal wall: Spigelian hernia has been successfully operated by laparoscopy.[85] The tension-free insertion of mesh and the lack of muscle-cutting exploration both offer significant advantages over open exploration and suture closure. An extraperitoneal technique would lend itself equally to incisional[86] and ventral hernias, but a sufficiency of peritoneum is required to cover the mesh: the application may be ideally suited to a suitably designed balloon dissector.

Spine

Spinal fusion by the anterior and anterolateral route needs an extensive surgical access conferring morbidity that often favours the biomechanically less satisfactory posterior procedure.[87] It has been reasoned that, if retroperitoneal endoscopy can reach the paramedian organs applied to the posterior abdominal wall, then it can also expose the anterolateral surface of the lumbar spine sufficiently to permit anterolateral plate fixation. This procedure has been demonstrated in the sheep but its feasibility and usefulness in humans remains to be established.[88–90]

Surgical access ⎯⎯⎯⎯⎯⎯⎯⎯⎯⎯⎯⎯⎯⎯⎯⎯

Totally extraperitoneal endoscopic access may be anatomically less invasive than transperitoneal, but invasiveness is not limited to anatomy: with less effect on venous return and more localized body wall distension, extraperitoneal access may also be less injurious haemodynamically.

This issue has not yet been formally studied. Nevertheless it should now be clear that, with its repertoire of procedures, retroperitoneoscopy offers a panel of potential advantages to weigh against its perceived difficulties: while the latter are partly indeed just perceived (because the technique is unaccustomed) there are also real issues of surgical anatomy and of technical support.

A distinction may be made between problems of surgical access (the siting of access cannulae and the dissection manoeuvres required to create and reach an operating space related to the target organ) and those of instrumental access, the means by which instruments can so be introduced into this space to enable correct tissue manipulation. Inevitably these issues overlap.

A further distinction may be made between initial access to the extraperitoneal plane and the way in which an appropriate operating space is to be created in that plane.

Initial access to the extraperitoneal plane

Three distinct routes of access to the extraperitoneum have been demonstrated: from the hypogastrium into the spaces of Retzius[91] and Bogros,[92] into the flank in the mid-axillary line and posteriorly below the twelfth rib. Each presents its own balance of virtues and specific difficulties. Naturally this balance alone cannot direct a choice of access: it must rather be weighed against the site, relations and orientation of the target organ.

Hypogastric approach

Endoscopic access to the retropubic and retro-inguinal spaces was developed to permit totally extraperitoneal hernia repair and two variants exist, as follows.

1. Via the rectus abdominis sheath: a sub-umbilical incision exposes the anterior rectus sheath, which is incised transversely near the midline and the muscle retracted laterally. The posterior and medial recess of the sheath appears to offer an easy conduit for blunt dissection to reach the pre-peritoneal plane caudal to the Arcuate Line of Douglas and thence into the spaces of Retzius and Bogros. This dissection may be pursued by the finger, with a blunt sound,[2] with an operating laparoscope,[3] by balloon dissection[93] or with an 'optical scalpel'.[10]
2. By insufflation and direct puncture: a Verres needle can be used to puncture the abdominal wall in the suprapubic notch, entering the roof of the Cave of Retzius in the base of the median umbilical ligament. Carbon dioxide insufflation at 12 mmHg distends the ligament, which can now be cannulated either with a sharp trocar passed subcutaneously from the umbilicus to the level of the arcuate line and then thrust through the linea alba or by direct cut-down at this level.[94]

These two basic methods lead the surgeon to different anatomical planes, separated by a posterior leaf of fascia transversalis.[95] The consequences become apparent when the access space is enlarged into an operating space. The posterior leaf of fascia transversalis is much tougher lateral to the epigastric vessels: it will be of little significance as an obstacle to surgery near the midline or down the pelvic sidewall (e.g. bladder, bladder neck, iliac lymph nodes, vas deferens), for which the techniques may be considered nearly equivalent. Procedures requiring access to the iliac fossa (iliac vessels, deep inguinal ring, testicular vessels or lower ureter) may, in a rectus sheath approach, be seriously hindered by the posterior leaf of transversalis fascia and indeed by a low lateral insertion of the arcuate line. A similar caution applies to the 10 per cent of individuals[96] in whom the posterior rectus sheath is preserved in the midline down to the pubic symphysis. In the former case, a direct puncture technique will allow the surgeon to develop the space laterally: sharp or blunt dissection, adhering strictly to the juxtaperitoneal plane, lateralizing the loose connective tissue and fat, reaches the psoas major belly without embarrassment to branches of the lumbar plexus. In the latter only direct puncture can avoid accessing an inappropriately superficial (and haemorrhagic) plane.

Flank approach

The muscles of the flank are loosely bundled, permitting shearing in thoracolumbar rotation. The peritoneum is loosely adherent, especially posteriorly, and well-separated from the muscle by loose fatty fascia. Initial access to this plane is easily achieved in the mid-axillary line, if incision of the skin and aponeurotic layer is followed with blunt dissection of the muscle by haemostat or finger. The latter, or the overinflated balloon of a standard Foley catheter, easily creates a space into which a cannula can be passed without a trocar and retained with a skin suture.

However, the distance between costal margin and iliac crest is short and the patient must be carefully positioned on the operating table to permit maximum lateral extension. Access to organs situated at this level (ureter, sympathetic chain, aorta) is easy, but the costal margin dictates a steeply cephalad angle to the sagittal plane in approaching the organs of the upper retroperitoneum (kidney, adrenal, liver, duodenum, pancreas, access to lesser sac). This angle, combined with the distance from the puncture site, has to be weighed against the access conferred by the alternative posterior approach (see below).

Posterior approach

The approach – by which a 2 cm incision below the tip of the twelfth rib is carried through skin muscle and fascia of Gerota, first described by Gaur[33] as a means of retroperitoneoscopy – has a long heritage from nephroscopy[8] and is no more than an adaptation of the Royal Road to the kidney in open surgery. Balloon compression of the loose connective tissue within the cone of Gerota's fascia provides a working space, a landmark contribution to minimally invasive access to kidney and upper ureter. The technique has been employed as an approach to the adrenal, with the great advantage that bilateral surgery can be undertaken without repositioning.[60] This is to be set against a relatively unfavourable approach to the vascular axis of the adrenal, virtually in line with the optical axis of a forward-viewing telescope. In principle the posterior approach offers access to the back of the right lobe of the liver, but this approach will be essentially blind and may require advanced technical support (see below, page 296). The intervening renal (and adrenal) pedicles render the posterior approach less attractive as access to the great vessels or digestive tract.

Developing a working space

Surgical access to the appropriate extraperitoneal plane needs to permit development of an adequate working space – both for the insertion of auxiliary trocars and to permit instruments inserted through them to operate on the target organ.

This enlargement can be achieved either by insufflation and formal blunt or sharp dissection under visual control ('pneumodissection') or by expanding a balloon in a chosen access space ('balloon dissection'), thereby splitting the fascial layers along a plane of least mechanical resistance. The former may seem anatomically taxing and time consuming and the latter swift and seductively simple, but whichever is preferred, the techniques differ in fundamental principle as follows.

Hypogastrium

Despite its anatomical contradiction a rectus sheath approach may, with careful and controlled dissection, be expanded into the juxtaperitoneal plane lateral to the epigastric vessels and bladder. Formal dissection seeks this plane by perforating the medial, sparse posterior leaf of transversalis fascia dorsal and medial to the epigastric vessels by blunt pledget dissection, sweeping its tough lateral extension anteriorly. Alternatively the scissors may be used to create a similar window and snip the fibrous strands between posterior transversalis fascia and preperitoneal fascia in a plane which, correctly entered, is virtually bloodless. This correct lateral plane is not reliably that of least resistance. Balloon dissection, with or without vision, may rather split the anterior from the posterior fascia transversalis across a vascular plane, denuding the epigastric vessels (or injuring them), so that the intervening fatty areolar tissue and the posterior leaf are left overlying the retroperitoneal organs of the iliac fossa. This layer will remain to be transected, sparing its neurovascular contents, before these organs can be reached. It is my personal counsel, therefore, that balloon dissection be used only to create a space between the left and right epigastric pedicle, into which initial working trocars can be inserted.

If these principles are respected, a wide pre-peritoneal space is easy to develop, permitting trocar placement that subtends an optimal angle between operating instruments. Only in the superior and lateral recess of this space may the posterior rectus sheath become an obstacle in rectus sheath approaches. By either access detachment of the peritoneum from the abdominal wall at this point must be scrupulous: a double fold of peritoneum left adherent to the muscle may be inadvertently perforated on insertion of an iliac cannula. Note that neurovascular elements of the abdominal wall are at risk from a cutting trocar: the muscle is loose here and a conical trocar may be safer. Insertion of both operating trocars anteriorly near the midline[3] avoids some of these difficulties, but may result in poor instrument angles.

Flank

Initial access to the extraperitoneal plane can be extended posteriorly close to muscle or anteriorly at least to the lateral border of the rectus sheath, where the peritoneum is quite firmly adherent. The juxtaperitoneal plane can then be traced posteriorly on the ventral aspect of the extraperitoneal fat, which may be the preferred route to ureter, great vessels and sympathetic chain. The access space is also easily extended into the iliac fossa, permitting the ureter to be followed into the pelvis. Balloon dissection can be employed directly or the telescope itself used to extend the space, permitting insertion of auxiliary cannulae and pneumodissection. One diameter of the working space can thus be developed from the lateral margin of the intrinsic muscles of the spine to the lateral border of the rectus sheath to form the base of a conical working space. The arc across which additional cannulae can be distributed in the transverse plane determines the usefulness of this approach to the upper abdominal retroperitoneum. The telescope may be transferred to the most convenient cannula.

Cephalad, however, a fascial sheet diverts dissection by either method to a plane lateral or dorsal to the kidney, thereby hindering access to the great vessels, digestive organs and adrenals. The paraconal fascia, known to radiologists in the era of pneumoretroperitoneography and recently re-emphasized by Himpens,[10] largely awaits rediscovery by retroperitoneoscopic surgeons. This tough layer represents a lateral fusion of the anterior and posterior leaves of Gerota's fascia, sweeping anterolaterally as a concave sheet, inserting into the preperitoneal fascia of the paracolic gutter. Fresh cadaver studies have confirmed this configuration, which can be seen during pneumodissection and which equally results in a real obstacle to uninformed balloon access to the cephalad retroperitoneum.

A distal working space must first be established, by pneumo- or balloon dissection, from which the caudal border of the paraconal fascia can be approached. Depending on the intended target, dissection may then proceed dorsolateral to it (to reach the sympathetic chain or spine), within the cone of Gerota's fascia (kidney, adrenal, vena cava, aorta, renal vessels, upper ureter) or by division of the paraconal fascia to access an anterior pararenal compartment (duodenum, mesenteric vessels, pancreas, splenic vessels). Although the cone of Gerota's fascia is open below, instrument access to organs within it may require that its anterior leaf or its lateral extension as paraconal fascia, be divided to widen the angle of access.

Posterior approach

The posterior approach of Gaur leads straight through the posterior pararenal compartment into the perinephric space. Initial balloon access could be restricted to the former compartment, permitting access to the bare area of the liver cranial to the upper pole of the kidney: the posterior recess of the pleura will be at risk from more medially placed cannulae. The initial access space created in either compartment will be shallow, but sufficiently wide to admit additional cannulae with a minimum of additional space creation. The space will once again be inherently restricted unless the fascial cone is incised, this time posterolaterally, to permit working cannulae out toward the mid-axillary line. As already emphasized, this approach is convenient for bilateral surgery but imposes limitations if the telescope axis is in line with the vascular axis of the organ being operated on (for example the adrenal).

Balloon or guided pneumodissection?

Given the difficulties of negotiating balloon dissectors into the correct plane relative to these major fasciae, formal pneumodissection may seem a preferable technique that offers to display the fasciae individually amid a gas-filled space. However, the space will not be found filled only by gas, fascial sheets and organs. In well-nourished subjects, particularly, the dense fascial planes and associated organs (especially those within the cone) are encased also in loose fatty areolar tissue, the compression and sweeping away of which is the seduction of balloon dissection. More time consuming but potentially less traumatic, pneumodissection challenges the surgeon not only to a greatly enhanced knowledge of the retroperitoneal fasciae but furthermore to direct the telescope toward an initially unseen target like a blindfold archer. Integration of imaging and information technology into image-based passive surgical guidance systems has been achieved in ENT,[97,98] orthopaedic[99] and neurological surgery.[100,101] The level of sophistication of a system that would guide the front lens of a rigid telescope into a target volume of, say, 20 mm diameter is by comparison to these applications very low.

Significant reductions in endoscopic operating time in the high retroperitoneum may depend on future developments of this nature. Meanwhile, a variety of balloon dissection techniques are available.

In its simplest form, balloon dissection requires nothing more than introduction of a Foley catheter with a 30 ml balloon, which is easily inflated with saline to a volume of 100 ml. Cheap and simple, such a balloon cannot be steered in any sense and has a limited size and compliance.

Gaur's original device was made of glove rubber, inflated with an ordinary sphygmomanometer bulb.[33] Introduced directly into the fascial cone of Gerota, its larger size and air inflation, coupled to the tough constraint of the fascia, results in acceptably wide and directed dissection.

A simple reusable device has recently been introduced, by which saline-inflated balloon dissection can be undertaken under visual control. A condom-like sac or a finger stall is attached to an outer sheath with fluid inlet and outlet ports and a fluid lock enables the telescope to be inserted into the inflated balloon without loss of volume.[9,102] The device is still being evaluated, but has obvious economic and technical attractions.

Two disposable balloon dissectors are commercially available. One is inflated with an air bulb and accepts a standard laparoscope to permit visual control of the dissection process.[103] Since no method is provided to steer the balloon, should it be seen to dissect the wrong plane, this feature may be of limited value. A separate cannula is introduced after removal of the balloon dissector. The Spacemaker (GSI Inc., Cupertino, California, USA)[93] is a relatively inelastic balloon, pre-shaped from polyurethane foil, inflated with saline and attached to a guide rod. The latter can be left *in situ* after balloon removal to guide a pre-loaded cannula into the dissected space, a convenient and time-saving feature. Initial evaluation[104] suggests this device can be a useful dissection aid, but neither a shaped balloon nor visual control prevent the balloon from seeking the wrong plane in lateral dissection of the hypogastric pre-peritoneum.

Morbidity from balloon rupture has not been reported, but saline inflation may offer significant safety advantages over air.

Summary

Initial access and development of the working space may be achieved either by pneumodissection or by balloon dissection. The choice may rest in individual preference, but both require more detailed knowledge of the retroperitoneal fasciae. The future role of pneumodissection may be enhanced by image-based guidance support.

Instrumental access ─────────────

The above considerations of surgical anatomy and access should clarify both the potential advantages of retroperitoneal endoscopic surgery and the constraints of anatomy on the technical feasibility of operation: in the hypogastrium, groin and pelvic inlet a working space can be developed to permit nearly ideal instrument angles. This is not so easily the case in the upper abdomen, approached via the flank or from behind. The distance between access points at the costal margin and targets high in the retroperitoneum may dictate a relatively acute angle between operating instruments. The disposition of the costal margin, the retroperitoneal fasciae, the solid organs and the pleura may direct the entire operating space toward the target organ at an unfavourable angle.

The instrumental remedies to these difficulties concern telescopes, video equipment and operating instruments.

Telescopes

A 0° rigid Hopkins telescope offers optimal brightness and sharpness, but may be unable, in retroperitoneoscopy, to view the target organ from the desired angle. Forward oblique telescopes (30° or 45°) offer an obvious solution but impose technical limitations of brightness and sharpness. Performance should be evaluated critically prior to purchase. Furthermore the forward oblique optic introduces an additional degree of freedom, that of axial rotation, to be mastered by the camera operator and understood by the surgeon in order to maintain anatomical orientation. Use of such a telescope inherently destroys the natural straight-ahead eye–camera–screen axis, further taxing the operator.

A dirigible telescope might in principle solve some of these difficulties. Fibre-optics systems have not generally provided adequate sharpness, but 'chip-on-a-stick' technology, which places the camera chip on the intracoporeal end of a rigid illumination tube has been adapted (Baxter–V. Mueller) to provide a dirigible telescope with motorized pitch and yaw of the chip within the body cavity. At first sight attractive, the usefulness of this device is limited by the weight of the motor unit and the heat generated in it. The definition and brightness of the image are acceptable, but the only link by which camera operator and surgeon could know the orientation of the video image – the position and orientation of the telescope objective – is now completely broken, adding to the difficulties found with rigid forward oblique telescopes.

A very high quality forward oblique telescope, of the smallest angle that permits the desired view, remains a good compromise solution.

Video equipment

Low lighting levels further compromise the optical performance of telescopes. The serous lining of the peritoneum or thorax reflect ambient light in a way which does not occur in the interstitial planes. Analogue cameras operating under poor lighting conditions require high video gain with consequent deterioration of signal to noise ratio and loss of definition. Gain control based on average brightness of the whole field may cast the very feature the surgeon most needs to see into shadow or into 'white-out'.

In consequence, retroperitoneal endoscopic surgery can only be safely conducted using a camera with digital image processing (preferably of three-chip design) in conjunction with a high power light source appropriately interfaced to the video processor.

Operating instruments

Anatomy constrains even more than in intracavity surgery the angle by which conventional straight instruments can approach the tissues. A variety of mechanisms have been developed to overcome this constraint, as follows.

Bead chain instruments

Steel beads threaded onto a steel cable lock into a rigid instrument shaft of predetermined shape when the cable is tightened.

Initial examples were limited to retractors, but scissors and graspers are now available, based on the same pattern and with excellent ergonomic hand grips, providing accomplished instruments (Endoflex, Surgical Innovations Ltd, Leeds UK). The instrument jaws can approach the tissue from whatever angle is pre-set in the manufacture of the instrument, but rigidity is impaired if the instrument is only partially tightened into this shape.

Shape-memory alloy instruments

Super-elasticity technology has been employed (Autosuture UK Ltd) to provide angled instruments that can be used in a similar way and which are undoubtedly convenient to use. Designed to be disposable, they are expensive and of limited rigidity.

Curved instruments

Rigid curved instruments designed for thoracoscopy[105] can be introduced through flexible cannulae (Keymed Olympus Ltd). The latter have either no valve or only a simple gland mechanism, but with the patient in the prone or lateral position, gas leak from the extraperitoneal space is not a serious issue: the weight of the viscera flopping away from the posterior abdominal wall tends to hold the space open despite low gas pressure.

Angulating instruments

A range of rigid instruments (Microfrance SA, 03160 Bourbon L'Archambault, France) with a single pivot joint interposed between the end mechanism and the shaft and operated by an additional lever near the handgrip has been available for some time. Simple to use and extremely robust, these instruments were designed for intra-cavity use, require a certain amount of space to manoeuvre and are 10 mm in diameter.

Summary

Appropriate instrumentation can mitigate the technical difficulties imposed by the anatomy of retroperitoneal access. The optimal combination will depend on individual preference and on the procedures to be undertaken. Bead-chain instruments, digital three-chip cameras and very high quality telescopes are probably indispensable for advanced retroperitoneal operating.

Anatomical perspective ───────────

Much anatomy has already been presented. It remains to place three related issues in sharp focus: the compartments of the abdomen, the perception of interfascial planes as spaces and the configuration of the retroperitoneal fasciae themselves.

The abdominal cavity comprises three separate compartments – the pelvic cavity, the upper abdomen (surrounded by chest wall) and the general, lower abdomen. In transperitoneal laparoscopic surgery, however, the abdominal cavity is regarded as a continuum from the diaphragm to the pelvic floor. No attention is paid to the fourth compartment, the retroperitoneum, on which this chapter has focused. The reader must judge – as will history – whether that disregard is warranted or whether it results solely from the mental habits of open surgery and of diagnostic laparoscopy.

The opening up of this forgotten surgical compartment as an endosurgical arena – the recognition that fascial planes can be converted to working spaces without compromise to the principle of minimal invasion – is the wider achievement of Dulucq,[1] and reaches beyond the practical concept of totally extra-peritoneal hernia surgery. This approach is, however, predicated on knowledge of the fascial planes on the deep aspect of the abdominal wall in a detail that has not been of relevance to open surgery. In relation to hernia repair these difficulties have been largely solved,[69,95] but that solution stands only at the beginning of a wider understanding concerning the whole set of extraperitoneal planes, explored by Himpens[10] and alluded to in previous paragraphs.

Our present picture then, from the work of Read,[95] Dulucq and Himpens, is as follows. Hypogastric access can be made to a pre-peritoneal compartment, chiefly above, before and beside the bladder and bounded by a bilaminar fascia transversalis anteriorly, by pre-peritoneal fascia posteriorly and by perivesical fascia inferiorly and posteriorly. Behind and lateral to the upper abdominal cavity lies a retroperitoneum, subdivided by Gerota's fascia into an anterior pararenal, perinephric and posterior pararenal space. Anterolaterally the anterior and posterior pararenal compartment are separated by the paraconal fascia, a fusion of anterior and posterior fascia of Gerota, sweeping anterolaterally, concave medially, to fuse with paracolic peritoneum.

At the intermediate level, between the lower pole of the kidney and the true pelvic brim, the situation is less clear. The extraperitoneal space is filled with loose fatty tissue and it is not easily demonstrated how the fascial confines of the upper abdominal and pelvic extraperitoneal compartments relate to one another. Does the fascia of Gerota, for example, correspond embryologically to perivesical fascia, or does the ureter penetrate a fascial plane? Is the stabilizing structure of the transversalis fascia reflected in that of the paraconal, or are the two separated completely by the extraperitoneal fat of the flank?

Clearly further research is needed and its outcome will be of practical consequence in retroperitoneal endoscopic surgery. Delineated by pneumodissection, the fascial planes may be recognized and serve both as guide and obstacle, the surgeon electing which side of each sheet to operate. Compressed unwittingly by balloons, the fasciae may act as unrecognized barriers to the point of frustrating the aim of minimal invasion. Hence the importance of the direction in which Himpens has pointed.

Conclusion

Surgery to extraperitoneal structures is appropriately conducted by a wholly extraperitoneal approach, a principle which has been demonstrated in a variety of procedures to the genito-urinary tract, endocrine, vascular, lymphoreticular and autonomic nervous systems and to the body wall. There is scope for development in digestive surgery. Extraperitoneal endoscopic surgery is in an early state of development and procedures demonstrated as possible today may either stand the test of time or become obsolete as treatment modalities. Numerous challenges of technique and technical support remain.

If pneumodissection has been presented as less invasive in this context than balloon dissection, a word of caution should be added. In the peritoneum we orientate by finding known organs within a known space. In the retroperitoneum there is no space and no orientation save that created by dissection. Our understanding of the fascial framework must be completed, but a future perspective on endoscopic surgery of the retroperitoneum may show that least invasive navigation around this framework required the support of image-based guidance technology.

Postscript

This chapter was originally written at the end of 1994. In the interim further developments have occurred in several areas, with, for example, growing interest in the totally retroperitoneal approach to the urinary tract and the adrenals.[116]

Laparoscopic anterior lumbar spinal interbody fusion is now a reality, both in animal models[109,110] and in clinical studies from several countries.[106–109,111–114] Laparoscopic anterior lumbar discectomy alone was recognized to be vitiated, like the conventional posterior approach, by the problem of disc space narrowing and instability, with the additional disadvantage of potentially incomplete excision of protruded material. Most clinical studies have therefore procured fusion by insertion of an interbody prosthesis,[106,111–113] usually a titanium cage,[111] although carbon fibre devices have also been used.[108] It remains unclear whether insertion of a prosthesis is superior to simple compression loading of autologous bone material.[108,114]

It should be stressed that all these studies have employed a transperitoneal approach and have only addressed the L5–S1 level, occasionally the L4–L5.[109,112] Radiological studies[107] have emphasized the narrow zone of access by this route, dictated by the anatomy of the great vessels. Bladder injuries have also occurred.[108] Even at the L4–L5 level a lateral approach is enforced by the aorta and vena cava.[112] These difficulties, combined with the hazard of posterior displacement of an end-plate fracture segment[113] suggest that, at least in the higher lumbar levels, a lateral extraperitoneal endoscopic approach may offer significant advantages.

Finally it has recently been demonstrated[115] that access to the extraperitoneal spaces in the groin can also be obtained via the femoral canal. This approach has at least the theoretical advantage of carrying dissection into the correct plane, deep to the posterior leaf of fascia transversalis. Time will show whether that advantage is offset by a risk of femoral vein injury and whether the usual advantages of minimal invasion can be maintained.

References

1. Dulucq J-L. Traitement des hernies del'aine par mise en place d'un patch prothetique sous-peritoneal en retro-peritoneoscopie. *Cahiers de Chirurgie* 1991; **79**: 15–16.

2. Begin G-F. Laparoscopic extraperitoneal treatment of inguinal hernias in adults. A series of 200 cases. *End Surg* 1993; **1**: 204–206.

3. McKernan JB. Laparoscopic extraperitoneal repair of inguinofemoral herniation *End Surg* 1993; **1**: 198–203.

4. Bartel M. Die Retroperitoneoskopie. Eine endoskopische Methode zur Inspektion und bioptischen Untersuchung des retroperitonealen Raumes. *Zentralbl Chir* 1969; **94**: 377.

5. Wittmoser R. Die Retroperitoneoskopie als neue Methode der lumbalen Sympathikotomie. *Fortschr Endoskopie* 1973; **4**: 219–223.

6. Sommerkamp H. Lumboskopie: ein neues diagnostisch-therapeutisches Prinzip der Urologie. *Acta Urol* 1975; **5**: 183.

7. Kaplan LR, Johnston GR, Hardy RM. Retroperitoneoscopy in dogs. *Gastrointest Endosc* 1979; **25**: 13.

8. Wickham JEA. The surgical treatment of renal lithiasis. In: Wickham JEA (ed.) *Urinary Calculus Disease* Churchill Livingstone, New York, 1979, pages 145–198.

9. Rassweiler JJ, Henkel TO, Stock C, Frede T, Alken P. Retroperitoneoscopic surgery – technique, indications and first experience. *Min Invas Ther* 1994; **3**(4): 179–195.

10. Himpens J, Van Alphen P, Cadière GB, Verroken R. Balloon dissection in extended retroperitoneoscopy. *Surg Lap Endosc* 1995; **5**(3): 193–196.

11. Franklin ME, Pharand D, Rosenthal D. Laparoscopic common bile duct exploration. *Surg Lap Endosc* 1994; **4**(2): 119–124.

12. Evoy DA, Regan MC, Attwood SEA, Stephens RB. The role of ERCP and laparoscopic cholecystectomy in gallstone-related pancreatitis. *Min Invas Ther* 1994; **3**(3): 149–152.
13. Watkin DS, Haworth JM, Leaper DJ, Thompson MH. Assessment of the common bile duct before cholecystectomy using ultrasound and biochemical measurements: validation based on follow-up. *Ann R Coll Surg Eng* 1994; **76**(5): 317–319.
14. Fabiani MD, Kathkouda N, Iovine L, Mouiel J. Laparoscopic fenestration of biliary cysts. *Surg Lap Endosc* 1991; **1**(3): 162–165.
15. Cappuccino H, Campanile F, Knecht J. Laparoscopy-guided drainage of hepatic abscess. *Surg Lap Endosc* 1994; **4**(3): 234–237.
16. Yanaga K, Kitano S, Hashizumi M, Ohta M, Matsumata T, Sugimachi K. Laparoscopic drainage of pyogenic liver abscess. *Br J Surg* 1994; **81**(7): 1022.
17. Mompean JAL, Paricio PP, Campos RR, Ayllon JG. Laparoscopic treatment of a liver hydatid cyst. *Br J Surg* 1993; **80**: 907–908.
18. Zamora A, Mucio M. Partial hepatectomy by laparoscopy: experimental phase. *Min Invas Ther* 1992; **1**(6): 389–391.
19. Croce E, Azzola M, Russo R, Golia M, Angelini S, Olmi S. Laparoscopic liver tumour resection with the argon beam. *End Surg* 1994; **2**(3/4): 186–188.
20. Catona A, Gossenberg M, LaManna A, Mussini G. Laparoscopic gastric banding: preliminary series. *Obesity Surgery* 1993; **3**: 207–209.
21. Amaral JF, Meltzer RC. Laparoscopic surgery for morbid obesity. *Min Invas Ther* 1994; **3**(supp 1): 61.
22. Cadière G-B, Bruyns J, Himpens J, Favretti F. Laparoscopic gastroplasty for morbid obesity. *Br J Surg* 1994: **81**(10): 1524.
23. Morino M, Toppino M, Garrone C, Morino F. Laparoscopic adjustable silicone gastric banding for the treatment of morbid obesity. *Br J Surg* 1994; **81**(8): 1169–1170.
24. Anderson PE, Pilkington TRE, Gazet J-C. Reversal of jejunoileal bypass in patients with morbid obesity. *Br J Surg* 1994; **81**(7): 105–1017.
25. McFarland RJ, Gazet J-C, Pilkington TRE, Grundy A. Gastric partition – experience at St George's Hospital, London. *Clin Nutr* 1986; suppl: 47–50.
26. Gigot JF, Healy ML, Ferrant A, Michaux JL, Njinou B, Kestens PJ. Laparoscopic splenectomy for idiopathic thrombocytopenic purpura. *Br J Surg* 1994; **81**(8): 1171–1172.
27. Sardi A. Laparoscopic splenectomy for patients with idiopathic thrombocytopenic purpura. *Surg Lap Endosc* 1994; **4**(4): 316–319.
28. Dexter SPL, Martin IG, Leindler L, Fowler R, McMahon MJ. Laparoscopic enucleation of a solitary pancreatic insulinoma. *Surg Endosc* 1994; **8**(8): 977.
29. Weber Sanchez A, Serrano Berry F, Cueto Garcia J, Rodriguez Weber G. Laparoscopic treatment of pancreatic serous cystadenoma. *Surg Lap Endosc* 1994; **4**(4): 304–307.
30. Hunt N, Stacey A, Darzi A. Retroperitoneoscopy and retroperitoneal mobilisation of the colon; A new approach in colo-rectal surgery. *Min Invas Ther* 1994; **3**(supp 1): 66.
31. Regan MC, Boyle B, Stephens RB. Laparoscopic repair of colonic perforation occurring during colonoscopy. *Br J Surg* 1994; **81**(7): 1073.
32. Gaur DD. Retroperitoneoscopy; the balloon technique. *Ann R Coll Surg Eng* 1994; **76**(4): 259–263.
33. Gaur DD. Laparoscopic operative retroperitoneoscopy: use of a new device. *J Urol* 1992; **148**: 1137.
34. Gaur DD, Agarwal DK, Purohit KC. Retroperitoneal laparoscopic nephrectomy: initial case report. *J Urol* 1993; **149**: 103.
35. Dauleh MI, Townell NH. Laparoscopic nephrectomy and nephroureterectomy. Argument for morselation or retrieval of intact specimens. *Min Invas Ther* 1994; **3**(1): 51–53.
36. Eden CG, Carter PG, Haigh AC,

Sherwood RA, Green DW, Coptcoat MJ. The metabolic response to laparoscopic and open nephrectomy. *Min Invas Ther* 1994; **3**(1): 34–50.

37. Gaur DD, Agarwal DK, Purohit KC. Retroperitoneal laparoscopic Gil-Vernet pyelolithotomy: an initial report. *Min Invas Ther* 1994; **3**(1): 55–58.

38. Lipsky H, Wuernschimmel E. Laparoscopic lithotomy for ureteral stones. *Min Invas Ther* 1993; **2**(1): 19–22.

39. Gaur DD, Purohit KC, Agarwal DK, Darshane AS. Laparoscopic ureterolithotomy for impacted lower ureteral calculi: initial case report. *Min Invas Ther* 1993; **2**(5): 267–269.

40. Notley RG. Anatomy and physiology of the ureter. In: Blandy J. (ed.) *Urology.* Blackwell Scientific Publications, Oxford, 1976, pages 568–598.

41. Walshe A. Ureterostomy in situ. *Br J Urol* 1967; **39**: 744–748.

42. Mandressi A, Buizza, C, Antonelli D, Belloni M, Chisena S, Zaroli A, Bernasconi S. Retro-extraperitoneal laparoscopic approach to excise retroperitoneal organs: kidney and adrenal gland. *Min Invas Ther* 1993; **2**(5): 213–220.

43. Sewell RW, Waddell RL. Complications of laparoscopic inguinal hernia repair. In: Arregui ME, Nagan RF (eds) *Inguinal Hernia, Advances or Controversies.* Radcliffe, Oxford, 1994, pages 488–493.

44. Mauermayer W. *Transurethral Surgery.* Springer, Berlin, 1981, pages 74–82.

45. Chapple CR, Osborne JL. Laparoscopic colposuspension – a new procedure. *Min Invas Ther* 1993; **2**(2): 59–62.

46. Nezhat C, Nezhat F, Nezhat CR, Rottenberg H. Laparoscopic retropubic cystourethropexy. *J Am Ass Gyn Lap* 1994; **1**(4): 339–349.

47. Ou C-S, Presthus J, Beadle E. Laparoscopic bladder neck suspension using hernia mesh and surgical staples. *J Laparoendosc Surg* 1993; **3**(6): 563–566.

48. Darzi A, Carey P, Menzies-Gow N, Monson JRT. Laparoscopic varicocoelectomy. *Surg Lap Endosc* 1994; **4**(3): 210–212.

49. Pisani E, Austoni E, Zanetti G. Clinical laparoscopic surgery: renal cyst excision, varicocoelectomy, pelvic lymph node dissection. *Min Invas Ther* 1992; **1**: 115.

50. Coptcoat MJ, Joyce AD. Laparoscopic varicocoelectomy. In: Coptcoat MJ, Joyce AD (eds) *Laparoscopy in Urology.* Blackwell Scientific Publications, Oxford, 1993, pages 67–77.

51. Gracey L. Endocrine surgery. In: Kirk RM (ed.) *General Surgical Operations.* Churchill Livingstone, Edinburgh, 1978, pages 366–372.

52. Schlinkert RT, Whitaker M. Laparoscopic left adrenalectomy offers advantages to standard resection techniques in selected patients. *Min Invas Ther* 1993; **2**(3): 119–121.

53. Matsuda T, Terachi T, Yoshida O. Laparoscopic adrenalectomy: the surgical technique and initial results of 13 cases. *Min Invas Ther* 1993; **2**(3): 123–127.

54. Gagner M, Lacroix A, Bolte E. Laparoscopic adrenalectomy in Cushing's syndrome and phaeochromocytoma. *New Engl J Med* 1992; **327**: 1033.

55. Lepsien G, Luedtke FE, Neufang T. Laparoscopic resection of Phaeochromocytoma. *Min Invas Ther* 1993; **2** (suppl 1): 52.

56. Lepsien G, Neufang T, Luedtke FE. Laparoscopic resection of phaeochromocytoma. *Surg Endosc* 1994; **8**(8): 906–909.

57. Edye MB, Pertsemlidis D. Laparoscopic lateral transperitoneal adrenalectomy. *Surg Endosc* 1994; **8**(8): 1013.

58. Brunt LM, Molmenti EP, Kerbl K, Soper NJ, Stone M, Clayman RV. Retroperitoneal endoscopic adrenalectomy: an experimental study. *Min Invas Ther* 1992; **1** (suppl 1): 41.

59. Taylor RS. Laparoscopic extraperitoneal adrenalectomy. Personal Communication, 1993.

60. Mercan S, Seven R, Ozarmagan S, Bozbora A, Budak D. Videoscopic retroperitoneal adrenalectomy. *Surg Endosc* 1994; **8**(8): 990.

61. Terachi T, Kawakita M, Kakehi Y, Terai A, Ogawa O, Matsuda T, Mikami O,

Yoshida O. Laparoscopic adrenalectomy: results of 31 cases. *Min Invas Ther* 1994; **3** (suppl 1): 11.

62. Sardi A, McKinnon WMP. Laparoscopic adrenalectomy in patients with primary aldosteronism. *Surg Lap Endosc* 1994; **4**(2): 86–91.

63. Stuart RC, Wyman A, Lau J, Chan A, Chung SCS. Laparoscopic adrenalectomy: transperitoneal approach. *Surg Endosc* 1994; **8**(8): 991.

64. Amaral JF, Uddo JF, Hoenig DM, Stein BS. Direct retroperitoneoscopic adrenalectomy using balloon dissection. *Min Invas Ther* 1994; **3** (suppl 1): 12.

65. Heintz, A Junginger Th. Retroperitoneal Endoscopic Adrenalectomy. *Min Invas Ther* 1994; **3** (suppl 1): 12.

66. Janetschek G, Reissigl A, Peschel R, Bartsch G. Laparoscopic retroperitoneal lymphadenectomy for testicular tumour: Animal studies and first clinical experience. *Min Invas Ther* 1992; **1** (suppl 1): 68.

67. Dulucq J-L, Himpens J. Iliac and obturator nodal sampling under retroperitoneoscopy. *Min Invas Ther* 1992; **1** (suppl 1): 111.

68. Hald T, Rasmussen F. Extraperitoneal pelvioscopy: a new aid in staging of lower urinary tract tumours. A preliminary report. *J Urol* 1979; **124**: 248–254.

69. Mudan SS, Thomas PRS, Read RC, Dulucq J-L, Fiennes AGTW. The extraperitoneal laparoscopic approach for groin hernias: Role of the fascia transversalis. *Clin Anat*, in press.

70. Jorgensen JO, Lalak NJ, North L, Hanel K, Hunt DR, Morris DL. Venous stasis during laparoscopic cholecystectomy. *Surg Lap Endosc* 1994; **4**(2): 128–133.

71. McMahon AJ, Baxter JN, Murray W, Imrie CW, Kenny G, O'Dwyer PJ. Helium pneumoperitoneum for laparoscopic cholecystectomy: ventilatory and blood gas changes. *Br J Surg* 1994; **81**(7): 1033–1036.

72. Bagley JS, Krukowski ZH. Case report. Laparoscopic splenectomy for dermoid cyst. *Min Invas Ther* 1994; **3**(1): 29–31.

73. Caroll BJ, Phillips EH, Semel CJ, Fallas M, Morgenstern L. Laparoscopic Splenectomy. *Surg Endosc* 1992; **6**: 183–185.

74. Cuschieri A, Shimi S, Banting S, Vander Velpen G. Technical aspects of laparoscopic splenectomy: hilar segmental devascularisation and instrumentation. *J R Coll Surg Edin* 1992; **37**: 414–416.

75. Kusminsky RE, Tiley EH, Lucente FC, Boland JP. Laparoscopic staging laparotomy with intra-abdominal manipulation. *Surg Lap Endosc* 1994; **4**(2): 103–105.

76. Hagemeister FB, Fuller LM, Martin RG. *Hodgkin's Disease and Non-Hodgkin's Lymphomas in Adults and Children.* Raven Press, New York, 1988, pages 170–185.

77. Taylor MA, Kaplan HS, Nelsen TS. Stageing laparotomy with splenectomy for Hodgkin's Disease: The Stanford experience. *World J Surg* 1985; **9**: 449–460.

78. Dion Y-M, Katkhouda N, Rouleau C, Aucoin A. Laparoscopy-assisted aorto-bifemoral bypass. *Surg Lap Endosc* 1993; **3**(5): 425–429.

79. Dulucq J-L. Totally extraperitoneal iliofemoral bypass. Video presentation in 'Emerging Procedures'. *2nd Int Congress EAES*, Madrid, Sept 15–17th, 1994.

80. Sayers RD, Thompson MM, Nasim A, Bell, PRF. Endovascular repair of abdominal aortic aneurysm: limitations of the single proximal stent technique. *Br J Surg* 1994; **81**(8): 1107–1110.

81. Dulucq J-L, Himpens J. Retroperitoneoscopically guided lumbar sympathectomy. *Min Invas Ther* 1992; **1** (suppl 1): 116.

82. Helms B, Schwanitz P, Czametzki H-D, Retroperitoneoscopic and thoracoscopic sympathectomy for periphery vessel diseases. *Min Invas Ther* 1994; **3** (suppl 1): 11.

83. Baker DM, Lamerton AJ. Operative lumbar sympathectomy for severe lower limb ischaemia: still a valuable treatment option. *Ann R Coll Surg Eng* 1994; **76**(1): 50–53.

84. Janetschek G, Flora G, Biedermann H,

Bartsch G. Lumbar sympathectomy by means of retroperitoneoscopy. *Min Invas Ther* 1993; **2**(5): 271–273.

85. Attwood EAS, Kelly IP, Hederman W, Fitzpatrick JM. Repair of Spigelian hernia by laparoscopy. *Min Invas Ther* 1992; **1** (suppl 1): 63.

86. Estour E. Eventrations et coelioscopie. *Journal de Coelio-chirurgie* 1994; **10**: 42–46.

87. Aebi M, Webb JK. The spine: thoracolumbar spine. In: Mueller ME, Allgoewer M, Schneider R, Willenegger H (eds) *Manual of Internal Fixation*. Springer, Berlin, 1991, pages 657–682.

88. Aichholzer M, Muehlbauer MK, Ferguson JG, Losert UM. The pig as a model for laparoscopic and thoracoscopic approaches to the spine. *Min Invas Ther* 1994; **3** (suppl 1): 52.

89. Marsh GDJ, New CH, Marshman D, Taylor TKF. Thoracoscopic anterior disc release in scoliosis: A sheep model. *Min Invas Ther* 1994; **3** (suppl 1): 55.

90. Muehlbauer MK, Ferguson JG, Losert UM. Experimental laparoscopic and thoracoscopic spinal interbody fusion with carbon fiber cage, iliac bone graft, plates and screws: A pilot study in the pig. *Min Invas Ther* 1994; **3** (suppl 1): 84.

91. Retzius AA. Some remarks on the proper design of the semilunar lines of Douglas. *Edinburgh Med J* 1858; **3**: 685.

92. Bogros AJ. *Essai sur l'anatomie chirurgicale de la region iliaque et description d'un nouveau procede pour faire la ligature des arteres epigastrique et iliaque externe*. (Thesis) Didot le Jeune, Paris, 1823.

93. Kieturakis MJ. Advances in extraperitoneal dissection and hernia repair. In: Arregui, ME, Nagan RF (eds) *Inguinal Hernia, Advances or Controversies*. Radcliffe, Oxford, 1994, pages 465–473.

94. Berthou JC. Personal communication, 1994.

95. Read RC, Cooper's posterior lamina of transversalis fascia. *Surg Gyn Obst* 1992; **174**: 426.

96. McVay CB, Anson BJ. Composition of the rectus sheath. *Anat Rec* 1940; **77**: 213.

97. Nitsche N, Margot H, Lamm C, Tummler HP, Schulz HJ, Kosak J. A new sonar stereometric system for intraoperative orientation – first experiences in endonasal sinus surgery. *Min Invas Ther* 1992; **1** (suppl 1): 50.

98. Adams L, Krybus W, Meyer-Ebrecht D, Rueger R, Gilsbach JM, Moesges R, Schloendorff G. Computer-assisted surgery. *IEEE Computer Graphics and Applications* 1990; **10**(3): 43–51.

99. Matsen FA, Garbini JL, Sidles JA. Robotic assistance in orthopaedic surgery. *Clin Orthop* 1993; **296**: 178–186.

100. Nabavi A, Blomer U, Klinge H, Mehdorn HM. Neuronavigation – 'Frameless Stereotaxy' using a mechanical arm. *Min Invas Ther* 1994; **3** (suppl 1): 28.

101. Zamorano LJ, Nolte L, Kadi AM, Jiang Z. Interactive intraoperative localization using an infrared-based system. *Neurological Research* 1993; **15**: 290–298.

102. Rossweiler J. Retroperitoneoscopic surgery. *Min Invas Ther* 1994; **3** (suppl 1): 11.

103. McKernan JB. Laparoscopic extraperitoneal prosthetic inguinal herniorrhaphy. In: Arregui ME, Nagan RF (eds) *Inguinal Hernia, Advances or Controversies*. Radcliffe, Oxford, 1994, pages 263–271.

104. Fiennes AGTW. The Kieturakis balloon dissector – an aid to the extraperitoneal approach for laparoscopic repair of groin hernias? *End Surg* 1994; **2**(3/4): 221–225.

105. Cuschieri A, Shimi S, Banting S, Van Velpen G, Dunkley P. Coaxial Curved Instrumentation for Minimal Access Surgery. *End Surg* 1993; **1**(5/6): 303–305.

106. Scholz-Jäger A, Kemen M, Willburger RE, Steffen R, Zumtobel V. Die videolaparoskopische transperitoneale Freilegung der lumbalen Wirbelsäule zur ventralen Fusion. *Langenbecks Archiv*

für Chirurgie 1996; **113**(suppl): 956–959.

107. Norotte G, Aimard P, Champey JC, Panel N. Abords du disque L5–S1 par coelioscopie transperitoneale. Interêt d'une étude tonodensitometrique préalable. *Revue de Chirurgie Orthopédique et Reparatrice de l'Appareil Moteur* 1996; **82**(7): 615–619.

108. Olsen D, McCord D, Law M. Laparoscopic discectomy with anterior interbody fusion of L5–S1. *Surg Endosc* 1996; **10**(12): 1158–1163.

109. Regan JJ, McAfee PC, Guyer RD, Aronoff RJ. Laparoscopic fusion of the lumbar spine in a multicenter series of the first 34 consecutive patients. *Surg Lap Endosc* 1996; **6**(6): 459–468.

110. Hildebrandt U, Pistorius G, Olinger A, Menger MD. First experience with laparoscopic spine fusion in an experimental model in the pig. *Surg Endosc* 1996; **10**(2): 143–146.

111. Mahvi DM, Zdeblick TA. A prospective study of laparoscopic spinal fusion. Technique and operative complications. *Ann Surg* 1996; **224**(1): 85–90.

112. Olinger A, Hildebrandt U, Pistorius G, Lindemann W, Menger MD. Laparoskopische 2-Etagenfusion der lumbalen Wirbelsäule mit Bagby-and-Kulisch (BAK)-Implantaten. *Chirurg* 1996; **67**(4): 346–350.

113. Zucherman JF, Zdeblick TA, Bailey SA, Mahvi D, Hsu KY, Kohrs D. Instrumented laparoscopic spinal fusion. Preliminary Results. *Spine* 1995; **20**(18): 2029–2034.

114. Matthews HH, Evans MT, Molligan HJ, Long BH. Laparoscopic discectomy with anterior lumbar interbody fusion. A preliminary review. *Spine* 1995; **20**(16): 1797–1802.

115. Read RC, de la Torre RA, Scott JS. Balloon dissection of the space of Bogros via the femoral canal for the total extraperitoneal laparoscopic herniorrhaphy. *Surg Endosc* 1997; **11**(6): 687–692.

116. Rassweiler JJ, Henkel TO, Stock C, Greschner M, Becker P, Preminger GM, Schulman CC, Frede T, Alken P. Retroperitoneal laparoscopic nephrectomy and other procedures in the retroperitoneum using a balloon dissection technique. *Eur Urol* 1994; **25**: 229–236.

SECTION IV

Other considerations

16

Medico-legal aspects of laparoscopy

J.H. Scurr

Introduction

Laparoscopy is not new, but in the last five years there have been significant advances in instrumentation, extending the role of the laparoscope from pure diagnosis to treatment. Prior to 1989 the laparoscope was widely used by gynae-cologists, and only occasionally used by general surgeons, principally for diag-nosis. The dangers and complications of laparoscopy, when applied to gynaecology, have been recognized and are subject to review.

The introduction of laparoscopic surgery is akin to the industrial revolution with rapid widespread acceptance by both patients and doctors. Laparoscopic techniques require different skills, different hand–eye co-ordination control and are totally different from the normal surgical procedures carried out. The demand for laparoscopic procedures, driven partly by patients and partly by economic factors, has resulted in the widespread introduction of these procedures without first establishing proper training programmes, without accreditation and without any controlled trials to assess the efficacy of the procedures when compared with conventional surgery. Many of these issues are now being addressed: training programmes are being established, there is discussion about accreditation and who should or should not perform laparoscopic procedures, which procedures can be performed and which procedures should remain experimental, and more recently, studies to evaluate laparoscopy with conventional surgery have been undertaken.

The benefits of laparoscopy and laparoscopic procedures must be considered against the disadvantages. Many surgeons remain on a learning curve, the procedures can take longer, and even where considerable experience has been obtained in, for example, removing the gallbladder, the incidence of complications is greater. A patient who experiences a complication or whose discharge is delayed, may seek legal advice. A defence can be entered against any allegation of negligence if a reasonable and reputable body of medical opinion supports the action taken by the surgeon. When performing new laparoscopic procedures it is important not to stray too far from standard practice without having first warned the patient and preferably obtained the agreement and support of a colleague. The introduction of new drugs requires clinical studies and ethical committee approval. The introduction of new surgical techniques have not required prior ethical committee approval. This is, however, an area which may change.

Consent

It is important that a patient is informed about the procedure and truly understands what the procedure involves, the potential benefits and the potential risks. Common complications should be explained to the patient and rare complications only need to be explained if they are likely to have a serious consequence. It is important that patients realize that it is a new procedure, that damage to other structures can occur and may require conventional surgery to correct for this. Patients need to know the benefits as well as the disadvantages of these procedures. All patients undergoing a laparoscopic procedure must be warned that if the procedure fails it will be converted to an open and standard operation. Patients should also be advised that complications can arise following a laparoscopic procedure which may not be immediately recognized, but which may in themselves require further treatment.

If a new procedure is being undertaken then the patient should be consented as though this were an experimental procedure. Where this truly is a new procedure then the support of a colleague who has considered the procedure and who agrees with it will assist if there are subsequent problems.

Pre-operative preparation

It should be remembered that patients undergoing laparoscopic procedures are at the same risk of developing chest complications, deep vein thrombosis, wound infections, incisional hernias, cardiac and renal problems as any other patient. DVT prophylaxis should be employed. The evidence for this is partly anecdotal, although a number of studies are currently being carried out. Prophylactic antibiotics, if indicated, should also be employed and post-operative physiotherapy for chest complications given if needed. The increased length of operation and early hospital discharge may mean that complications such as deep vein thrombosis occur once the patient has left hospital. An awareness of this problem and adequate documentation stating that the risk was considered and adequate prophylaxis given is essential.

Complications of laparoscopy

Complications may result from the Verres needle, insertion of the trocar and cannula, or the insertion of small cannulae used to manipulate structures within the abdominal cavity. When inserting the Verres needle it is important not to damage intra-abdominal structures and to make sure that the needle is in the peritoneal space before insufflating air. There have been a number of fatalities where air has been injected into large vessels. Sudden death can occur when air is injected into the inferior vena cava or a large vein, particularly in the presence of a patent foramen ovale. During the introduction of gas into the peritoneal cavity the patient should be fully monitored.

When inserting the trocar into the anterior abdominal wall it is important to avoid previous scars and to aim the point away from major retroperitoneal structures.

Damage to the bowel, if recognized, is an acceptable complication of laparoscopy. Damage to retroperitoneal structures including the aorta, inferior vena cava, iliac vessels, ureter and kidneys have all been reported, and are unacceptable complications, given a proper technique.

Damage caused by the trocar, if recognized and treated appropriately, is usually defensible except when it involves structures on the posterior abdominal wall. These structures are fixed, their position known, and therefore steps must be taken to avoid them. It is the failure to recognize the damage and inappropriate post-operative treatment, often culminating in a severe peritonitis, that is difficult to defend. In this situation the nursing records and the temperature, pulse and respiration charts may clearly display a problem which remains apparently unrecognized by the treating doctor. These records can be used to show that there was a problem, and yet despite this, inappropriate action or no action at all was taken.

A high index of suspicion regarding perforation of the bowel is a safe policy, and if in doubt repeat laparoscopy or a laparotomy is a wise precaution. The 'It can't happen to me' syndrome is extremely dangerous. A patient presenting with signs of peritonism following a laparoscopy can be safely explored. Failure to explore a patient with signs of peritonism may result in an extensive procedure being necessary at a later date and inevitably leads to litigation.

Laparoscopic cholecystectomy ———

This is now the commonest method of removing the gallbladder. Injuries to the common bile duct are four times greater than when performing a conventional cholecystectomy. Damage to the bowel and surrounding structures also occurs. When performing a laparoscopic cholecystectomy it is important to record the operative details. It is difficult to justify an 'easy' laparoscopic cholecystectomy when the operation time is recorded as five hours. The presence of dense adhesions, a thick-walled gallbladder and uncertain anatomy should lead the surgeon to revert to an open procedure. To record these difficulties and yet persist with a laparoscopic procedure, which then results in complications, is again difficult to defend.

It is important that every surgeon performing this procedure takes care to avoid the known complications, which include failure to identify accurately the anatomy and failure to secure the cystic duct and cystic artery, resulting in a severe bile leak, or bleeding. Despite careful and meticulous surgical techniques, complications will arise. It is important to have adequate follow-up and to review any patients who are not recovering at the expected rate. A complication may result in litigation, but failure to recognize a complication, and certainly failure to do anything about it will definitely result in litigation, which will probably be successful.

The development of biliary peritonitis following a laparoscopic procedure may arise simply because of a leak from a cystic duct or an unrecognized biliary radical draining directly into the gallbladder. If there is a significant collection and this cannot be dealt with percutaneously then early surgery is indicated. If there is any doubt about the integrity of the bile ducts early investigation should be carried out and reconstructive surgery, if indicated, performed by somebody experienced in these techniques.

Inguinal hernias

The laparoscopic repair of inguinal hernias has received considerable publicity and many patients now arrive requesting this procedure. There are relatively few surgeons carrying out this procedure on a routine basis, and the long-term results are unknown. The procedure itself is simple enough, and using a prosthetic mesh a repair can be effected from behind the inguinal ligament. As with any new method of repairing a hernia, a long period of follow-up is required before one can say whether the technique is as good or better than existing methods. When obtaining consent from a patient for laparoscopic repair of an inguinal hernia it is important that the patient realizes that it is a new procedure and that the outcome cannot be guaranteed. The patient should understand that as with any laparoscopic procedure there are complications and these complications include the complications of laparoscopy in addition to the complications of repairing an inguinal hernia. Damage to cord structures should not occur, but as the procedure involves dissecting an indirect sac at the internal ring the testicular artery and veins are in close proximity and can be compromised. As with any laparoscopic procedure there is a learning curve, and it is important that surgeons carrying out these procedures at an early stage in their training should have the support of an experienced colleague. While I have seen many medical negligence claims resulting from laparoscopic cholecystectomy procedures I have yet to see a claim from a laparoscopic procedure following the repair of an inguinal hernia. This may reflect only the relatively small number of cases being done.

Laparoscopic colectomy

It is now possible to perform many procedures, both laparoscopically and laparoscopically-assisted. Colonic mobilization using a laparoscope is a relatively straightforward procedure. If the colon is delivered through a small incision a segment can be resected and anastomosis performed outside the abdomen before returning it to the abdominal cavity. The advantages of this procedure are that it limits the surgical incision, but the disadvantages include the increased time taken to perform the operation. To date there are relatively few surgeons performing general abdominal procedures apart from laparoscopic cholecystectomy, but it is probable that more and more colonic procedures will be performed using these techniques.

It is important to remember that the same problems arise following laparoscopic colectomy as do following a normal colectomy. Adequate pre-operative preparation, appropriate consent and good post-operative follow-up are essential to avoid medical litigation.

Other surgical procedures

Other laparoscopic procedures currently being carried out include removal of the spleen or kidney and repair of a hiatus hernia. The problems and complications associated with these procedures include those that might be encountered using a conventional procedure, but in addition include those arising from the laparoscope itself. Again patients should be advised that these procedures are not routine, they are in a stage of development and may lead to a standard surgical procedure.

Appendicectomy

Laparoscopic treatment of acute appendicitis is not without its problems. Removal of a normal appendix via the laparoscope is a relatively simple procedure. The removal of a severely inflamed and stuck appendix can be extremely difficult. To remove the appendix it is necessary to insert at least three trocars and probably four. The incisions necessary are in combination often as great as a simple skin crease incision in the right iliac fossa. Given that the laparoscopic procedure may be unsuccessful, serious consideration should be given to removing the appendix by a standard method and not a laparoscopic procedure, when it is known that the appendix is probably inflamed.

Removal of the appendix itself, even under difficult circumstances, can probably be justified. If complications arise it is important that these complications are recognized early and appropriate treatment given.

Incisional hernia – a complication of laparoscopy

There have been a number of cases where small incisional hernias have developed, particularly around the peri-umbilical region. This has led some surgeons to close the fascia formally, either using staples or sutures. An incisional hernia is a recognized complication of any surgical procedure and the development of an incisional hernia does not necessarily imply negligence. The development of a prolonged ileus with abdominal distension may predispose to a loop of bowel becoming stuck in either the laparoscopic or port incision. This diagnosis should be considered in a patient whose ileus/obstruction is not resolving.

Again, it is failure to recognize an incisional hernia and failure to offer the patient appropriate treatment which leads to litigation.

Damage to retroperitoneal structures

Damage to retroperitoneal structures, particularly the aorta and the inferior vena cava, are usually indefensible.

If a significant injury to these vessels occurs the patient usually collapses extremely rapidly and an urgent laparotomy is required. There have been a number of operative deaths directly attributable to injuries to the inferior vena cava and aorta. It is best to avoid the retroperitoneal structures by using a technique introducing the trocar away from these structures. Once the laparo-scope is inserted all other trocars can be inserted under direct vision. It must be remembered that the field of vision through the laparoscope is relatively small and the trocar with an instrument can stray outside the area of direct vision. Damage at a remote site can occur without the operator necessarily being aware of it. Under these circumstances it is important to note excess bleeding or bowel contents if there is any doubt then a laparotomy should be performed.

Summary

Laparoscopic procedures are in their infancy. There are undoubtedly benefits to this technology and it is important that we avoid complications and medical litigation during the early learning period. Most medico-legal claims can be avoided by better communication, a greater understanding of the procedure, the complications of the procedure and what may be involved to sort out any predictable and indeed unpredictable complications. Good pre-operative assess-ment, sensible selection of patients, the use of any necessary prophylactic mea-sures, and good post-operative monitoring will both reduce the incidence of complications and allow for early detection of those complications that require intervention.

If in doubt it is much safer to intervene at an early stage, even if this proves to be unnecessary. When problems do arise they are probably better sorted out by specialist surgeons in specialist centres. This will avoid repeated surgical proce-dures and an escalation of the damages. The majority of medical negligence claims start as a result of poor communication, a lack of understanding on behalf of the patient, and surgical arrogance.

Afterword

The contributors to this book have, in describing laparoscopic surgery, high-lighted many kinds of general problem that all modern medical practitioners face. The problems themselves are not new, but they present with greater urgency in an age when the general public's interest in all matters medical is rivalled only by its interest in crime and the law.

The more difficult the manipulations involved in a method of treatment, the more important become the methods of training, the more stringent must be the assessment of trainees if the public weal is to be protected. The fact that the only animal available for surgical training in this country is the human poses a particularly difficult problem. The facts that the laparoscopic approach is still relatively new and unfamiliar, is clearly powerful, and in certain areas carries obvious advantages, add up to a strong incentive to use this technique without careful evaluation of its role in comparison with other, more prosaic, methods. One must remain aware that there is even a possibility that a laparoscopic procedure might be advised in circumstances where no procedure is justified.

Then there are the problems of weighing dangers and inadequacies against temporary symptoms: does an earlier return to work (even supposing that this thesis has been proved) compensate for a definitely larger incidence of bile duct injuries? In the absence of prolonged follow-up results of laparoscopic hernia repair, should the operation be offered to patients outside a controlled trial? There can be no firm answers to these questions, although answers may present themselves as experience increases. The answers will come more quickly if surgeons keep careful records and are prepared to publish all their results.

Despite these doubts and difficulties, there is no doubt that laparoscopic surgery is here to stay: in some fields, such as simple cholecystectomy, it would seem that already the laparoscopic is the operation of choice. Some of the areas described in this book may turn out to be unsuitable for the technique, but it is almost inevitable that some areas not mentioned at present will become fruitful in the future. The initial phase of exciting and rapid progress may have reached its zenith, but in our crystal ball, the progress in the future, even if not quite as exciting, will continue to be rapid.

Two things are certain: a book on laparoscopic surgery in five years' time will be completely different from the present one; and a large number of patients will have benefited from the technique.

Michael Hobsley   Tom Treasure   John Northover

Index

Note: page numbers in *italics* refer to figures and tables

see also apprenticeship
audit 75
    innovative treatment 67

balloon dissectors 296
Barrett's oesophagus 156, 157
Bassini repair 259
bead chain instruments 298, 299
beneficial outcome 64
Bernstein test of mucosal sensitivity 156
bile
    bacterial contamination 127
    leak 312
bile duct
    imaging 125
    laparoscopic exploration 130–5
    see also common bile duct
bile duct injury 12
    laparoscopic cholecystectomy 120, 121
    peroperative cholangiography 129
Billroth II reconstruction 168
binocular disparity 30
bipolar diathermy 103, 107
bipolar electrosurgical dessication
        (ESD) 100
bladder 288
blood vessels, major abdominal 290
body form, plastic 49
bowel damage 311
breast cancer treatment 65
buildings costs 84
Burch colposuspension, totally
        extraperitoneal laparoscopic 288

capital investment 84
Cardiac Surgical Register 77–8
cave of Retzius 288
cavernous sinus surgery 64
Certificate of Completion of Specialist
        Training (CCST) 45, 47, 71
certification 58
cervical carcinoma 109
charges 83
cholangiography, peroperative 118, 119,
        129, 132
cholangitis 133
cholecystectomy, laparoscopic 6, 115
    abdominal wall metastases 116
    adverse incidents 37
    and bile duct exploration 131
    common bile duct exploration 126
    complications 120–1

contraindications 115–16
conversion risk 119
cost comparison with open
        cholecystectomy 85–7
difficulties 119
haemorrhage 116, 120
indications 115–16
introduction in UK 43–4
medico-legal aspects 311–12
operation 117–19
partial 119
peroperative cholangiography 118, 119
plus ERCP 131
pneumoperitoneum 117, 118
pre-operative preparation 117
return to normal activity 88
thromboembolic disease risk 116, 117
training
    guidelines 511
    in UK 44
cholecystectomy, open
    comparison with laparoscopic
        cholecystectomy 121
    costs 85–7
    senior trainees 94
cholecystitis, acute 116
cholecystoscopy, laparoscopic *215*, 216
choledochoduodenostomy 135
choledocholithiasis 131–2
    elderly unfit patient 133
    expected 131–2
    recurrent 127–8
    unexpected 132–3
choledocholithotomy, open 126, *127*
choledochoscopy
    operative 126
    transcystic duct 129
choledochotomy, laparoscopic 129–30
ciliary muscle 30
clinical competence predictors 33–4
CO_2 embolism, fatal 120
co-operation, selection of surgical
        trainees 33
cognitive factors 22–3
colectomy
    laparoscopic-assisted total abdominal
        with Brooke ileostomy/total
        proctocolectomy 226–8
    preliminary total 225
colectomy, laparoscopic 56–7, 226–8
    malignancy 57
    medico-legal aspects 312–13